OXFORD MEDICAL PUBLICATIONS

IATROGENIC DISEASES

IATROGENIC DISEASES

P. F. D'ARCY

B.Pharm., Ph.D., F.P.S., F.R.I.C.

Professor of Pharmacy,
The Queen's University of Belfast,
Formerly Professor of Pharmacology and Dean,
Faculty of Pharmacy, University of Khartoum

and

J. P. GRIFFIN

B.Sc., Ph.D., M.B. B.S.

Senior Medical Officer, Medicines Division, Department of Health and Social Security,
and Honorary Clinical Assistant, Institute of Diseases of the Chest,
Brompton Hospital, London

LONDON
OXFORD UNIVERSITY PRESS
NEW YORK   TORONTO

Oxford University Press, Ely House, London W.I

GLASGOW   NEW YORK   TORONTO   MELBOURNE   WELLINGTON
CAPE TOWN   SALISBURY   IBADAN   NAIROBI   DAR ES SALAAM   LUSAKA   ADDIS ABABA
BOMBAY   CALCUTTA   MADRAS   KARACHI   LAHORE   DACCA
KUALA LUMPUR   SINGAPORE   HONG KONG   TOKYO

Clothbound edition ISBN 0 19 264150 6
Paperbound edition ISBN 0 19 264157 3

Printed in Great Britain at the Pitman Press, Bath

PREFACE

The use of any therapeutic agent is inevitably attended by a small risk that the patient may react adversely to the prescribed agent. Adverse reactions can be caused by several different factors. In correlating the data for this book, it has been apparent that two factors are the major contribution to the manifestation of iatrogenic disease. These are the abnormal patient reaction to a drug, and the development of unexpected toxicity when several drugs are given in combination.

Predictable toxicity is the manifestation of secondary pharmacological actions; this is a hazard that can be well elucidated in the battery of tests to which the drug is subjected during its development stage. In such instances, assuming that the drug has a worthwhile place in therapy, the ratio of dosage of drug to produce the major effect, to dosage to produce a secondary (toxic) effect is the real factor which should be considered and not the 'built in' potentiality to the side-effect itself. Nevertheless, certain groups of patients exist who may be at risk from these predictable manifestations of toxicity. These patients are at peculiar risk because of a genetically determined defect of metabolism, or because their metabolism has been impaired by concomitant hepatic disease, or because their excretory function has been reduced by either liver or renal malfunction. In these instances, the drug or its metabolites may rapidly build up to toxic levels in the body, even at normal accepted therapeutic doses.

Intolerance is a lowered threshold to the normal pharmacological action of drugs. Individuals may vary widely from the well established norm in their reaction to drugs. The very old and the very young are liable to be more sensitive to drugs possibly because the metabolic and excretory mechanisms essential for the disposal of the drug are less efficient than in the adult. In addition, the reactions of the old or the young may also differ qualitatively from those of the adult.

Adverse reactions may follow the use of a drug, and these reactions may be unexpected, in that they are completely unrelated to the known toxicity of the drug. These reactions include hypersensitivity to the agent, in which the patient develops antibodies to the drug. The antigenic factor is usually a combination of drug with body protein. Skin rashes and eruptions are the most common symptoms of this type of allergic reaction, although haemolytic anaemia is not infrequent.

Idiosyncrasy involves a qualitatively abnormal response on the part of the patient to the drug; an example of this is drug-induced porphyria, in which a qualitatively abnormal response of porphyrin metabolism is induced by barbiturates in susceptible subjects. Similarly, mepacrine-induced haemolytic anaemia in glucose-6-phosphate dehydrogenase deficient subjects is an idiosyncratic reaction.

The role of polypharmacy in iatrogenic disease is not insignificant, since toxicities not shown by either drug singly may develop when used in combination. This ill-begotten offspring of medicine and pharmacy has been nurtured through the ages and William Withering wrote in 1785 that 'the ingenuity of man has ever been fond of exerting itself to varied forms and combinations of medicines'. This is equally true today and one objective of this book is to emphasize that the risk of untoward reaction bears a direct relation to the number of drugs prescribed at any one time.

The practice of treating trivial complaints by the simultaneous administration of a wide variety of drugs has been satirized by Moat (1969) in his article 'Life without Leeches' in the *Daily Telegraph Supplement* (255). He humorously described the treatment taken by a guest at his home:

> The other day a friend from the big world came to stay, and when I took him his breakfast I found him swallowing pills. He'd been depressed recently, which was why he took the yellow pills, antidepressants. The white pills were tranquillizers, and he took those because the yellow pills were inclined to agitate him. The mixture of white and yellow made him itch unbearably and affected his vision—hence the blue pills. He found this particular dosage of pills constipating, and for that he took a strong aperient. 'And just look at these', he said excitedly, waving at me a bottle of large multi-coloured pills. 'And what are those?' I asked. 'I don't know', he said, 'but I like to keep them till last'.
>
> I then asked him how he was feeling. He said he felt fine, except that the pills made him feel lethargic, which he personally found depressing.

Laurence, writing in the latest edition of his *Clinical Pharmacology*, expressed similar views when he said that 'habitual polypharmacy is sure to blur the outline of rational thought which should precede the use of any drug'. Unfortunately the danger of polypharmacy is somewhat concealed from the physician, since a patient, blissfully unaware of the hazards of drug interaction, may indulge in self-medication. For example, a prescribed monoamine oxidase inhibitor is taken together with a self-prescribed proprietary common cold remedy containing ephedrine, phenylephrine or other sympathomimetic amine. A life threatening hypertensive crisis may ensue.

In presenting the data in this book, it was felt that classification of drug-induced reactions into a systematic pathological approach would result in the most readable and useful presentation for the prescribing physician, for the student of medicine, for the pharmacist and the pharmacologist. We have attempted in this volume to produce an adjunct for the study of therapeutics and at the same time provide a reference book on the clinical aspects of drug toxicity.

Where we have referred to specific iatrogenic effects of drugs we have used the approved name rather than suggest that the reaction had been exhibited by any particular brand of drug. Nevertheless, to increase the usefulness of the book, we have given, in an appendix, the British, American and continental proprietary names of each drug, together with the approved name.

In conclusion, let all of us who contribute to the ultimate treatment of patients reflect on the prayer of Sir Robert Hutchinson which hangs on the wall of the Children's Ward at The London Hospital:

> From inability to let well alone:
> from too much zeal for the new
> and contempt for what is old:
> from putting knowledge before wisdom,
> science before art, and cleverness before
> common sense,
> from treating patients as cases, and from
> making the cure of the disease more
> grievous than the endurance of the same,
> Good Lord, deliver us.

Acknowledgements

We gratefully acknowledge the assistance of Mrs. Brenda Chapman and Mrs. Hazel Sainsbury for seeking out our references, Mr. A. Bailey for classifying the examples of known drug interactions and Dr. A. McQueen for contributing his chapter on 'Iatrogenic Skin Disease'.

Permission to reproduce figures and tables and to quote directly from the writings of some authorities has been generously granted, and we thank them and their publishers for this. We also thank Dr. C. Brown, Dr. P. Hansell, Dr. A. McQueen, Dr. D. J. Pollock, Dr. F. J. Prime and Professor R. E. Steiner for allowing us to reproduce photographs and photomicrographs from their case records. Reference to all these are made with acknowledgements individually in the text.

We are indebted to our respective wives for giving us the time to write this book and for their many assistances in its preparation. Finally, we would like to thank Dr. J. C. Gregory and the staff of Oxford University Press for unfailing help and courtesy during the preparation of this volume.

Pattishall   P. F. D'Arcy
Welwyn   J. P. Griffin
January 1971

CONTENTS

1

EPIDEMIOLOGICAL ASPECTS OF IATROGENIC DISEASE

INCIDENCE OF DRUG-INDUCED DISEASE

The problem of assessing the incidence of drug-induced disease is multifarious. The reported incidence of reactions is variable, reflecting the different methods of surveillance, the populations under study, and the habits of medical care. There are surprisingly few reports in the literature on the incidence of drug reactions in general, hospital or specialized practice.

Those studies that have been published in recent years are, however, most enlightening and informative. For example in the Johns Hopkins Hospital, between 1 January and 31 March 1964, 184 adverse drug reactions were seen in 122 patients out of a total of 714 patients admitted to general medical beds. Drug reactions following admission were seen in 13·6 per cent of patients and reactions present on admission were seen in 5 per cent of patients and were the major cause for their admission. There were six fatal hospital-acquired adverse reactions (Seidl *et al.*, 1966).

The same group of workers (Smith, Seidl, and Cluff, 1966) also investigated the incidence of drug-induced adverse effects in a 33-bed medical ward between 1 January and 31 December 1965. Nine hundred patients were included in the survey, and reactions were detected in 10·8 per cent of patients. Reactions were most common in patients who were seriously ill and who had received many drugs. Patients with abnormal renal function or with previous drug reactions appeared to be predisposed to drug reactions, and allergic reactions were common in patients with gastro-intestinal disease. Altogether 133 drugs were incriminated in 114 adverse drug reactions; barbiturates, meprobromate, codeine, penicillins and thiazide diuretics produced 70 per cent of the adverse reactions although they accounted for only 17 per cent of all medication.

In 1967 Ogilvie and Ruedy surveyed adverse drug reactions in 731 patients admitted to a general medical unit over a twelve-month period, and 193 patients (18 per cent) suffered undesirable consequences of drug therapy. One-quarter of the 67 deaths on the unit were due to adverse drug reactions. The majority of the reactions was caused by drugs that had been in common use for many years; indeed 60 per cent were caused by digitalis, antimicrobials, insulin and diuretics. Most of the reactions (81 per cent) were caused by the primary pharmacological action of the drug or overdosage or side-effects or cytotoxic effects; these reactions were dose related and predictable. Nineteen per cent of reactions were due to interaction of the drug with special predisposing factors that were constitutionally-induced, disease-induced, drug-induced or environmentally-induced.

Another recent study by Montgomery and Jackson (1968) reviewed 100 patients with drug-induced skin reactions. They found that these skin reactions accounted for one in every 61 dermatological patients seen in their practice. Causative drugs were classified in five main groups: (i) tranquillizers and sedatives accounted for 33 cases of drug-induced skin reaction; (ii) antibiotics caused 9 cases; (iii) diuretics were responsible for 9 cases of dermatological eruptions; (iv) topical agents caused 13 cases and (v) 22 cases were caused by a miscellaneous group of 18 drugs.

The general appearance of the cutaneous reactions seen were classified as shown in TABLE 1.1.

TABLE 1.1

REACTION TYPE

	per cent
Urticaria	28
Generalized toxic erythema	16
Contact dermatitis	10
Papulo-squamous eruptions	6
Erythema multiforme	6
Purpura	5
Eczematous dermatitis	4
Photosensitivity	3
Serum sickness	3
Other conditions	19
	100

It is difficult to reconcile the relatively high incidence of drug-induced reactions obtained in the quoted individual studies with official figures published on the incidence of adverse drug reactions. For example, the Australian Drug Evaluation Committee in their *Report on Adverse Drug Reactions* recorded a total of only 628 reactions during the period October 1965 to December 1967, which was only 3 per 100,000 of the population at risk. Furthermore, during 1968 the Committee on Safety of Drugs received a total 3,446 notifications of adverse reactions occurring in the United Kingdom, during which period approximately 306,000,000 prescriptions were issued.

It may well be that not all adverse drug reactions are reported to official bodies; indeed the Committee on

Safety of Drugs has repeatedly reminded physicians to fill in their 'yellow cards' on which statistics are dependent. In the United States there may be a further complication in collecting accurate statistics; the F.D.A. report of 1966 states that 'physicians are becoming increasingly fearful of reporting deaths or adverse reactions because of the fear of legal reprisals'.

In a recent publication of the Office of Health Economics (1969) it was stated that in 'medicine in the 1990s more rational attitudes to adverse reactions are expected to develop. A sounder epidemiological approach, with better monitoring, the development of record linkage, and the use of computers and possibly local "recording officers", will identify more precisely the risks of adverse reactions occurring with particular medicines. "False" reports of adverse reactions, which have in fact arisen from other causes, will be reduced. The risks of adverse reactions will then be able to be logically balanced against the expected benefits from the use of the medicine. In addition, these improvements in the epidemiology of adverse reactions may sometimes identify differing degrees of risk for different types of patient and effects arising from the interaction of different preparations. The underlying mechanism of adverse reactions will be better understood and this will allow more accurate prediction and will reduce hazards. Some reactions may be avoided or minimized by specific additives in the medicine.'

An attempt has been made in this present section to pin-point some of the patients at particular risk due to a number of factors many of which must by their very nature occur together in the same patient with potentially additive effects. Age, sex and disease state are particularly relevant.

AGE

Many cases of drug reaction can be attributed to predisposing factors in the patient himself. Basically, there is the problem of the same drug having diverse effects in different clinical conditions and in different individuals, for example amphetamine is widely used as an appetite-suppressant drug in the treatment of obesity, yet the same drug is also used in patients with anorexia nervosa to stimulate appetite. In both circumstances, amphetamine provides effective therapy. Amphetamine has been used to combat physical and mental fatigue on the one hand, but conversely has been used successfully to quieten behaviourally disturbed hyperactive children.

A further example is that barbiturates and phenytoin are frequently used in combination to control grand mal epilepsy. However, in children, barbiturates may increase the incidence of fits, and better control is achieved by phenytoin alone.

There are also other well defined examples of age being a factor in drug metabolism which has a direct bearing on incidence of iatrogenic disease.

The newborn have a relatively lower glomerular filtration rate and renal plasma flow than adults and are also seriously deficient in drug metabolizing enzymes for at least the first month after birth. The latter is particularly marked in their failure of glucuronation. All these deficiencies are enhanced in premature babies; thus neonates may fail to metabolize effectively vitamin K analogues, sulphonamides, chloramphenicol, barbiturates, morphine and curare. Penicillin excretion is also delayed, although this may be a useful rather than harmful defect of renal function, since effective blood levels are maintained for longer periods.

In the geriatric patient drug overdosage is particularly likely to occur if the drug remains active in the body until it is excreted by the kidneys. This is so because renal function (glomerular filtration and tubular function) diminishes with increasing age even in the absence of clinically detectable disease. A reduction of about 30 per cent in the glomerular filtration rate and tubular function has been demonstrated in otherwise normal patients over 65 years of age when compared with normal young adults. Indeed at 90 years of age the functional capacity of the 'normal' kidney may be only half what it was at 30 years (Agate, 1963). Diminished renal function may be made worse by dehydration, congestive heart failure, urinary retention or diabetic nephropathy, all of which are more frequent in the elderly patient. Under these circumstances drugs such as streptomycin, digitalis and oral hypoglycaemic agents may prove a real hazard in some elderly patients.

Chlorpropamide has a long action (half-life 40 hours) even in the presence of normal kidney function, but elderly women are particularly prone to risk of hypoglycaemic episodes with this long acting agent because of generally poor renal function and their greater liability to urinary infection. Under such circumstances therefore tolbutamide is safer since it is inactivated by the liver and therefore has a much shorter half-life (about 5 hours). Even using tolbutamide in these elderly patients it should be borne in mind that use of other drugs, particularly phenylbutazone and sulphonamides, can prolong the half-life of tolbutamide to as much as 17 hours (Berck, 1966; Davison, 1968).

In the elderly, if a night sedative proves necessary, barbiturates are best avoided altogether since they increase nocturnal restlessness and often produce sufficient hangover to make the old person inactive, inattentive and mentally confused and unsteady on his feet next day. Safer alternatives are chloral hydrate or nitrazepam or glutethimide.

However, barbiturates are still the most popular night sedative and can be taken by younger people without trouble. Liability to mental confusion increases with age and stress and in some cases the offending agent is the normal dose of barbiturate which the patient has been taking as a night sedative for years without untoward effect. Such an acute confusional episode must be treated by withdrawal of the drug; attempts to suppress the adverse response by increasing the barbiturate dosage simply makes matters infinitely worse.

The phenothiazine group of drugs have proved invaluable in geriatric practice by decreasing anxiety, hallucinations and delusions, but with these drugs too, there are special hazards. Compared with younger subjects on phenothiazines, elderly patients are more liable to suffer from phenothiazine-induced parkinsonism. Because the phenothiazines lower body temperature, they contribute to the problem of accidental hypothermia in the elderly, more especially if there is any reduction in thyroid function (Jones and Meade, 1964; Exton-Smith, 1964). Hypotension is also an important effect of phenothiazines in the elderly causing increased risk of dizziness and falls. In those geriatric patients who develop cholestatic jaundice due to phenothiazines, their rate of recovery of liver function is greatly impaired.

The toxic effects of digitalis on the heart are essentially an extension of its therapeutic effects. The age of the patient is a predisposing factor in the development of toxic manifestations of digitalis. The elderly patient whose heart is usually more severely damaged is more likely to develop serious toxic manifestations. Indeed the incidence of digitalis intoxication increases with age out of proportion to the increasing incidence of heart disease (Mathes et al., 1952; Soffer, 1961; Crouch et al., 1956; Dall, 1965).

SEX

It is well known that the agranulocytosis due to amidopyrine, phenylbutazone and chloramphenicol occurs far more frequently in females than in males; the ratio is about 3:1 for these drugs. Pancytopenia, due to chloramphenicol, is the result of bone marrow damage through an anti-metabolic effect, and again females are more susceptible than males. The possibility that females, young girls in particular, may have an inferior defence mechanism against the toxic effect of chloramphenicol must be considered [see CHAPTER 4].

There are no other clinically important sex differences in drug action except, of course, of sex hormones. 'Women are said to be more liable to become excited by morphine than are men; in this respect they resemble cats' (Laurence, 1966).

GENETIC FACTORS

Variations in drug metabolism as a result of enzyme deficiencies or abnormal enzyme systems in the patient are classic examples of the patient component in iatrogenic disease. Two examples of enzyme abnormality causing abnormal drug reactions can be cited as illustrations. Firstly, the duration of neuromuscular blocking action of succinylcholine is prolonged in two familial abnormalities of plasma pseudocholinesterase, namely the hereditary deficiency of the normal type of pseudocholinesterase, and the familial presence of an atypical form of pseudocholinesterase [see CHAPTER 15].

Secondly there is a tendency to haemolytic anaemia in patients with glucose-6-phosphate dehydrogenase deficiency when treated with antimalarial and other drugs or even with certain normal dietary constituents such as the fava bean [see CHAPTER 4].

There are great differences in the rate at which people inactivate isoniazid and it has been found that this depends on a single gene. People may be classified either as slow inactivators (autosomal homozygous recessive) or rapid inactivators (heterozygous and homozygous dominants) (Evans et al., 1960). In fixed-dose treatment regimes the proportion of slow inactivators is slightly higher than for rapid inactivators. The relevance of this difference in metabolism is that slow inactivators get more peripheral neuritis with the drug (Fox, 1962). It is not yet known whether dosage can be altered to give the best therapeutic effect to rapid inactivators with negligibly increased risk of toxicity to slow inactivators. It is of interest to note that about 5 per cent of Eskimos, 15 per cent of Chinese, 60 per cent of Asian Indians, 45 per cent of American Negroes, 45 per cent of Europeans and 55–75 per cent of Jews are slow inactivators of isoniazid (Motulsky, 1964).

BLOOD GROUPS

Jick et al. (1969) studied the incidence of blood groups in women who developed venous thrombo-embolism while taking oral contraceptives. There was a deficit of blood group O in these women. The ratio of blood groups $(A + B + AB)/O$ for women with thrombo-embolism while on the pill was 3·3 and for controls 1·2. Thus women of blood group A are nearly three times as likely to develop venous thrombo-embolism while taking oral contraceptives as women of blood group O.

DISEASE STATES

Renal Failure

The action of a drug can be prolonged or increased in the presence of renal failure; this can be illustrated by the cumulative action of phenformin and the sulphonylureas which have been described as causing profound hypoglycaemic episodes in the presence of renal failure (Bauer, 1965; Tranquada et al., 1963). Toxic manifestations of a drug are more likely to occur in the presence of diminished excretion of the drug; indeed in all the quoted cases of deafness attributed to ethacrynic acid and frusemide this toxicity has occurred in patients with reduced renal function (Pillay et al., 1969; Hanzelik and Peppercorn, 1969).

Liver Disease

It is common knowledge that morphine may precipitate coma in patients with cirrhosis and that paraldehyde causes profound sleep in some patients with liver disease. It is difficult to show that the half-life of these drugs is increased in patients with cirrhosis though recent investigations indicate that this is probably so. In other words failure to metabolize a drug due to liver failure can enhance and prolong the action of any drug metabolized by the liver.

Porphyria

Certain drugs such as barbiturates can precipitate attacks of porphyria in patients with acute intermittent porphyria; there is, however, no evidence that drugs can precipitate an attack of acute porphyria in the absence of genetic predisposition. In general, clinical experience indicates conclusively that symptoms of acute porphyria appear only in those patients who are carriers of the genetic defect in a latent state (De Matteis, 1967).

Myasthenia Gravis

A dual block of neuromuscular transmission following succinylcholine is seen in certain normal patients for no apparent reason, but this type of block is particularly prevalent in patients suffering from myasthenia gravis [see CHAPTER 15]. This dual neuromuscular block consists of a depolarizing block followed by a non-depolarizing or curare-like block.

Gout and Diabetes

Thiazide diuretics may cause diabetogenic or uricogenic effects even at normal therapeutic dosage. These unwanted effects occur in patients with a predisposition to these conditions. In addition the newer diuretics chlorthalidone and frusemide may also precipitate gout in susceptible patients and both these and the thiazide diuretics are contraindicated in severe renal and hepatic failure.

Abnormal Eyes (Shallow Anterior Chamber)

In patients with a shallow anterior chamber of the eye dilatation of the pupil with mydriatic drugs causes the iris to block the outflow of the aqueous humour, and angle closure glaucoma results. This occurrence is more likely in the elderly than in the younger patient. In addition the eyes of mongols are more sensitive to mydriatic drugs than normal patients.

Asthma

In 1917 Eppinger and Hess suggested that asthma was related to excessive cholinergic activity. Subsequent clinical studies have demonstrated that the airways of asthmatic subjects are unusually sensitive to cholinergic mediators and to histamine. Administration of acetyl-β methylcholine or histamine parenterally (Curry et al., 1950) or by inhalation (Townley et al., 1965) produced a greater impairment of ventilatory function in asthmatic patients than in controls.

Szentivanyi (1966) has suggested that the underlying abnormality in bronchial asthma is an inherited or acquired abnormality of function of β-adrenergic receptors. In human studies, support for this hypothesis has come from the observations that asthmatics have a diminished hyperglycaemic response to intravenous isoprenaline (isoproterenol) (Cookson and Reed, 1963) and adrenaline (epinephrine) (Lockley et al., 1967). Kirkpatrick and Keller (1967) found a diminished response, in the rise of plasma free fatty acids (F.F.A), to adrenaline infusion in patients with allergic asthma. In similar studies Middleton and Finke (1968) showed that patients with severe asthma failed to show an elevation of blood pyruvate, lactate and glucose after subcutaneous adrenaline whereas non-asthmatic or mild asthmatic patients responded with a significant increase. In the above cited studies most of the patients with severe asthma were receiving corticosteroids and sympathomimetic bronchodilator therapy; it is therefore impossible to decide whether the diminished response to adrenaline represented a metabolic defect in this group of patients or whether the diminished response was tachyphylaxis or tolerance induced by the previous administration of other sympathomimetics. Tolerance may well be the explanation of these results since it is known that tolerance develops to many sympathomimetic amines given in the treatment of asthma; this is true with ephedrine and with salbutamol (Choo-Kang et al., 1969). Support for tolerance to sympathomimetics being implicated is given by Paterson et al. (1968), who reported that therapeutic doses of isoprenaline administered by pressurized aerosols caused tachycardia in healthy individuals, but patients who use the aerosols continuously become relatively resistant to the cardiac stimulating effect of isoprenaline whether it be given by inhalation or by intravenous infusion. Furthermore, Atkinson and Rand (1967) showed that prolonged intravenous infusion of isoprenaline in increasing dosage resulted in the development of resistance to the cardiac stimulating effects of the drug. Resistance to intravenous isoprenaline in asthmatics is not due to increased rate of inactivation of isoprenaline since isoprenaline has a similar half-life in healthy individuals and in asthmatics; in addition normal subjects on high doses of inhaled isoprenaline also develop a relative resistance to the cardiac side-effects of this drug (Paterson et al., 1968).

Therefore, before interpreting the relative resistance of asthmatics to sympathomimetics as being a consequence of their disease state, one must exclude the possibility that their relative resistance is due to a developed tolerance to sympathomimetic bronchodilators. Nevertheless, it is highly suggestive that there is an abnormally developed receptor in asthmatics, and this can be inferred from the fact that β-blockade produces a much greater increase in airway resistance in asthmatics than in healthy people (McNeill and Ingram, 1966).

Diabetes Insipidus

The treatment of diabetes insipidus with thiazide diuretics is a classical example of how a specific disease can alter the action of a drug. In 1959 Kennedy and Crawford observed that thiazide diuretics given to patients with diabetes insipidus caused a marked reduction of urine volume, increased urine concentration, and alleviated thirst. This paradoxical phenomenon has been reviewed by Lant (1968).

Alcoholism

Kater *et al.* (1969) have compared the rate of clearance of tolbutamide, warfarin and diphenylhydantoin from the circulation in alcoholic subjects and in abstinent controls. The half-life of all three of the drugs in the blood of the alcoholics was significantly shorter than in the controls. It is possible that continued intake of alcohol induces, non-specifically, hepatic microsomal enzymes.

DRUG HYPERSENSITIVITY

Hypersensitivity is an entirely different problem in the epidemiology of drug-induced reactions since there is usually no reaction on first exposure (i.e. during the first few days of treatment) unless there has been previous exposure (and sensitization) to a similar chemical agent. Thus neomycin may cause topical skin hypersensitivity, but because of certain common chemical groupings, subsequent treatment of the patient with streptomycin or kanamycin may lead to a generalized reaction. Strangely, this cross-sensitivity principle does not necessarily extend to stereoisomers—e.g. quinidine and quinine may not cross-react.

A good example of drug hypersensitivity is the haemolytic anaemia caused by methyldopa; the possible mechanisms of auto-antibody formation in these patients have been classified by Worrledge (1969) and cover the whole spectrum of immunological probability, of which there are four basic concepts:

Hapten Theory

The drug or one of its metabolites acts as a hapten and the auto-antibodies formed react against the drug.

Alteration of the Red Cells leading to Absorption of Normal Immunoglobulin G (IgG)

A drug may alter the surface of a red cell so that normal IgG is absorbed; this postulate has been used to explain the positive direct antiglobulin test that may occur in patients receiving cephalothin and cephaloridine (Molthan *et al.*, 1967).

Altered Auto-antigens

The drug or metabolites alters auto-antigens so that a normal antibody-producing mechanism no longer recognizes them as 'self'. This might explain the Rhesus specificity of the red cell auto-antibodies. It would therefore have to be postulated that the drug or one of its metabolites becomes incorporated into the red cell at the normoblast or reticulocyte stage, thus altering the Rhesus antigens. These cells would have a normal life-span and would not reach the antibody-producing mechanism until at least 120 days had elapsed, thus explaining the delay in development of a positive antiglobulin test.

Abnormal Clone

It is postulated that the drug or metabolites acts on 'immunocytes' and in some way stimulates them to produce a clone or clones of abnormal but immunologically competent cells which fail to recognize the auto-antigens as 'self' and produces antibodies against them. As multiple antibodies are produced, more than one clone must be involved. The main difficulty in accepting this theory has been the connotation of the word 'abnormal'; the abnormality of these clones is not self perpetuating once the drug is withdrawn.

Hypersensitivity reactions can, unfortunately, develop to drugs which the patient is completely unaware of having received. Wicher *et al.* (1969) describe such a case in a 42-year-old woman who had, on a previous occasion, developed an extreme allergic sensitivity to penicillin. This patient experienced a second severe allergic reaction which was traced to the presence of 10 units/ml penicillin in milk. The patient received the penicillin unwittingly and despite the fact that she was aware of her sensitivity and avoided penicillin even to the extent of giving up her work as a nurse.

A similar example is discussed in the chapter on Drug Interaction where the para-amino group of para-phenylenediamine hair dyes may lead to cross-sensitization on subsequent treatment with sulphonamides and para-amino salicylic acid and other drugs containing the common moiety.

EPIDEMIOLOGICAL STUDY OF UNEXPECTED DEATHS IN YOUNG ASTHMATICS

An increase in mortality from asthma has been reported in Australia (Gandevia, 1967, 1968), the United States (Richards and Patrick, 1965) and Britain (Smith, 1966). The increase in mortality was particularly marked in the 5–35 year age group.

The possibility that sudden death in asthmatics was due to sympathomimetic amine therapy was suggested first by McManis (1964) who described three cases of unexpected and sudden death in young asthmatics who had initially used isoprenaline pressurized aerosols and subsequently had been given adrenaline by injection. Twenty-one further cases of sudden death were reported from Australia by Patrick and Tonge (1966); orciprenaline had been used prior to death in 16 of these cases and isoprenaline in a single case; in the remaining four cases no sympathomimetic amine had been prescribed.

In 1967 Greenberg and Pines wrote a warning letter to the *British Medical Journal* stating 'we suspect that patients with asthma may be killing themselves by the excessive use of metered or pressurized aerosols. . . . We have had four patients known to us previously as having mild or severe asthma and who have been found unexpectedly dead at home or at work. By their side has been an empty or almost empty pressurized aerosol'. Other similar reports followed rapidly (Douglas *et al.*, 1967; Pickvance, 1967; Exon, 1967) and each of these authors implicated or associated the deaths of these patients with the usage or over-usage of pressurized aerosols containing sympathomimetic amines. During the same period of time there were similar reports of association between deaths of asthmatic patients and the usage of pressurized aerosols, which appeared in the national press as reports of coroners' inquests.

In July 1967, the Committee on Safety of Drugs issued a warning to all doctors 'drawing attention to reports in the medical press which suggest a possible link between the excessive use of aerosols and a recorded rise in the death rate in asthma'.

In the United Kingdom, the first report of an increased death rate in asthmatics was reported from the Bristol area where Corner (1966) observed an increase in death from asthma among children. Smith (1966) confirmed this finding for the whole of England and Wales. Speizer, Doll and Heaf (1968) also examined the mortality figures for asthma in England and Wales from 1960 to 1965, and found that the death rate had increased annually over that period. The increase was more pronounced at ages 5–34 years than at older ages and was most pronounced at ages 10–24 years. In this last age group, the mortality increased nearly eight-fold in seven years, and in 1966 asthma accounted for 7 per cent of all deaths.

It would also seem from published reports that this increased death rate in young asthmatics is also sex related. Speizer and Doll (1968) drew attention to the fact that up until 1907 deaths in young asthmatics showed a male preponderance although since then the situation has reversed. During the sudden increase in deaths in young asthmatics in the 1960s in England and Wales this female preponderance had apparently continued.

Speizer *et al.* (1968) studied further the use of drugs by patients aged 5–34 years who subsequently died from asthma; information was obtained from the general practitioners about 177 of the 184 subjects, and necropsy data were obtained for 113 of the 124 cases in which a post-mortem examination was known to have been made. Ninety-eight per cent of these subjects for whom case histories were available were known to have been suffering from asthma, and signs of severe asthma (overdistended lungs and small bronchi plugged with mucus) were found in 91 per cent of necropsies (57 per cent of all deaths). Evidence that death might have been due to any other pathological condition was rare. Death was sudden and unexpected in 81 per cent of the subjects (137 out of 171) and 59 per cent of all deaths were referred to the coroner. In 39 per cent of cases (67 out of 171) the practitioner had not regarded these asthmatics as suffering from severe asthma in their terminal episodes. It is important to note that corticosteroids and sympathomimetic amine preparations were the only drugs used by a large proportion of the patients. Two-thirds of the patients had received corticosteroids; however, there was no suggestion that

corticosteroids had been used excessively, but 84 per cent of the patients were known to have used pressurized aerosol bronchodilators and in several instances excessive use of these devices was recorded.

Inman and Adelstein (1969) also studied the rise and fall of asthma mortality in England and Wales in relation to use of pressurized aerosols. Between 1961 and 1967, there was, at all ages, a total of more than 3,500 deaths from asthma in excess of that number which could have been expected on the basis of experience of the two years (1959 and 1960) that preceded the large scale use of pressurized aerosols. The workers stated that 'after the publication of letters in the medical press and the distribution by the Committee on Safety of Drugs of a warning to all practitioners mortality fell; there has also been a decline in the use of pressurized aerosols although this has not been as pronounced, proportionately, as the decline in mortality'.

In the course of these epidemiological studies, no mechanism has been advanced to explain sudden deaths from asthma; all post-mortem examinations of the children and young people who died suddenly, have shown only classical changes of over-inflated lungs with mucus plugging.

The situation has probably been frankly and honestly summarized by Inman and Adelstein (1969) in their final paragraph: 'Fortunately, the high mortality has now been reduced (although it is still higher than it was before the introduction of the aerosols). This in itself is likely to make it difficult or impossible in the future to evaluate all the factors that were responsible or to prove a direct link with aerosol bronchodilators. In the absence, however, of any other satisfactory explanation for the changes that have been observed, it is concluded that the increase in mortality from asthma that was observed during the years 1961 to 1966, was likely to have been due to the excessive use of pressurized aerosol bronchodilators and that the subsequent reduction in mortality resulted from a greater awareness among the medical profession and the patients themselves of the hazards of these devices if improperly used'.

It must also be recalled that sudden death from asthma did occur before the introduction of sympathomimetic aerosols (Ellis, 1908; Murphy and Case, 1930; Maxwell, 1955). Sudden death from asthma has also been reported by McLaren (1968) of a 48-year-old woman who died suddenly after inhaling an ignited powder of lobelia and stramonium which she took when her asthma attacks were severe.

Straub *et al.* (1969) showed that in eleven episodes of status asthmaticus in nine patients, there was significant haemoconcentration and diminished blood volume. The haematocrit during attacks was raised by a mean of 7 per cent. After the relief of airway obstruction the pulse rate rose and blood pressure fell and was accompanied by clinical signs of hypovolaemic collapse in four of the patients. Rapid volume replacement in these patients led to immediate circulatory improvement. A possible relation of hypovolaemia to unexplained death was suggested by these authors. It is salutatory to bear in mind that toxicity of aminophylline (Bresnick *et al.*, 1948), adrenal failure in steroid-treated patients (El-Shaboury, 1966) and overdose of pressurized aerosols

have all been incriminated on separate occasions as causing sudden unexpected death in asthmatics in whom mucus plugging was not present at necropsy. In fact, a drug-induced factor may not even be involved.

RECOMMENDED FURTHER READING

VESSEY, M. P. (1970) Epidemiological and public health aspects of oral contraceptives and thromboembolic disease, *J. clin. Path.*, **23**, Suppl. (Ass. Clin. Path.), **3**, 62–6.

REFERENCES

AGATE, J. (1963) *The Practice of Geriatrics*, London, pp. 217–22, 355–7.

ATKINSON, J. M., and RAND, M. J. (1967) Pressurized aerosols in asthma, *Brit. med. J.*, **3**, 239.

BAUER, H. G. (1965) Severe and prolonged hypoglycemic shock during sulfonylurea treatment, *Metabolism*, **14**, 220–8.

BERCK, H. (1966) Les accidents vasculaires cérébraux chez diabetiques ages traites par les sulphonylureas, *Rev. franç. Géront.*, **12**, 91.

BRESNICK, E., WOODARD, W. K., and SAGEMAN, C. B. (1948) Fatal reactions to intravenous administration of aminophylline; report of 3 cases, *J. Amer. med. Ass.*, **136**, 397–8.

CHOO-KANG, Y. F. J., SIMPSON, W. T., and GRANT, I. W. B. (1969) Controlled comparison of the bronchodilator effects of three β-adrenergic stimulant drugs administered by inhalation to patients with asthma, *Brit. med. J.*, **2**, 287–9.

COMMITTEE ON SAFETY OF DRUGS (1967) Aerosols in asthma and vaccines, *Adverse Reaction Series*, No. 5.

COMMITTEE ON SAFETY OF DRUGS (1969) *Report for Year ended December 31st, 1968.*

COOKSON, D. U., and REED, C. E. (1963) A comparison of the effects of isoproterenol in the normal and asthmatic subject. A preliminary report, *Amer. Rev. resp. Dis.*, **88**, 636–43.

CORNER, B. (1966) Paper presented to a joint meeting of the British Tuberculosis Association and West of England Thoracic Society, 1 April 1966.

CROUCH, R. B., HERRMANN, G. R., and HEJTMANCIK, M. R. (1956) Digitalis intoxication, *Tex. St. J. Med.*, **52**, 714–19.

CURRY, J. J., FUCHS, J. E., and LEARD, S. E. (1950) The effect of dihydroergocornine on the pulmonary response to methacholine and histamine in subjects with bronchial asthma, *J. clin. Invest.*, **29**, 439–43.

DALL, J. L. C. (1965) Digitalis intoxication in elderly patients, *Lancet*, **i**, 194–5.

DAVISON, W. (1968) Drug hazards in the elderly, in *Drug-Induced Diseases*, Vol. 3, eds. Meyler, L., and Peck, H. M., Excerpta Medica Foundation, Amsterdam, pp. 307–21.

DE MATTEIS, F. (1967) Disturbances of liver porphyrin metabolism caused by drugs, *Pharmacol. Rev.*, **19**, 523–59.

DOUGLAS, E. M., HILLIER, T., and JOHNSON, I. C. (1967) Pressurized aerosols in asthma, *Brit. med. J.*, **2**, 53.

ELLIS, A. G. (1908) Pathological anatomy of bronchial asthma, *Amer. J. med. Sci.*, **136**, 407–29.

EL-SHABOURY, A. H. (1966) Adrenal failure complicating status asthmaticus in steroid-treated patients, *Brit. med. J.*, **2**, 1478–81.

EPPINGER, H., and HESS, L. (1917) *Vagotonia. A Clinical Study in Vegetative Neurology*, Nervous and Mental Disease Monograph Series No. 20, 2nd ed., trans. Kraus, W. M., and Jelliffe, S. E., New York, pp. 47–8.

EXON, P. D. (1967) Pressurized aerosols in asthma, *Brit. med. J.*, **2**, 178.

EXTON-SMITH, A. N. (1964) Accidental hypothermia in the elderly, *Brit. med. J.*, **2**, 1255–8.

EVANS, D. A. P., MANLEY, K. A., and McKUSICK, V. A. (1960) Genetic control of isoniazid metabolism in man, *Brit. med. J.*, **2**, 485–91.

FOX, W. (1962) The chemotherapy and epidemiology of tuberculosis. Some findings of general applicability from the tuberculosis chemotherapy centre, Madras, *Lancet*, **ii**, 413–17, 473–8.

GANDEVIA, B. (1967) The changing pattern of mortality from asthma in Australia, *Aust. Ann. Med.*, **16**, 184.

GANDEVIA, B. (1968) The changing pattern of mortality from asthma in Australia, 2. Mortality and modern therapy, *Med. J. Aust.*, **1**, 884–91.

GREENBERG, M. J., and PINES, A. (1967) Pressurized aerosols in asthma, *Brit. med. J.*, **1**, 563.

HANZELIK, E., and PEPPERCORN, M. (1969) Deafness after ethacrynic acid, *Lancet*, **i**, 416.

INMAN, W. H. W., and ADELSTEIN, A. M. (1969) Rise and fall of asthma mortality in England and Wales in relation to use of pressurized aerosols, *Lancet*, **ii**, 279–85.

JICK, H., SLONE, D., WESTERHOLME, B., INMAN, W. H. W., VESSEY, M. P., SHAPIRO, S., LEWIS, G. P., and WORCESTER, J. (1969) Venous thromboembolic disease and ABO type, *Lancet*, **i**, 539–42.

JONES, I. H., and MEADE, T. W. (1964) Hypothermia following chlorpromazine therapy in myxoedematous patients, *Geront. clin. (Basel)*, **6**, 252–6.

KATER, R. M. H., ROGGIN, G., TOBORN, F., ZIEVE, P., and IBER, F. L. (1969) Increased rate of clearance of drugs from the circulation of alcoholics, *Amer. J. med. Sci.*, **258**, 35–9.

KENNEDY, G. C., and CRAWFORD, J. D. (1959) Treatment of diabetes insipidus with hydrochlorothiazide, *Lancet*, **i**, 866–7.

KIRKPATRICK, C. H., and KELLER, C. (1967) Impaired responsiveness to epinephrine in asthma, *Amer. Rev. resp. Dis.*, **96**, 692–9.

LANT, A. F. (1968) The antidiuretic effect of diuretics in diabetes insipidus, *J. roy. Coll. Phycns Lond.*, **2**, 298–309.

LAURENCE, D. R. (1966) *Clinical Pharmacology*, 2nd ed., London, p. 632.

LOCKLEY, S. D., GLENNON, J. A., and REED, C. E. (1967) Comparison of some metabolic responses in normal and asthmatic subjects to epinephrine and glucagon, *J. Allergy*, **40**, 349–54.

MATHES, S., GOLD, H., MARSH, R., GREINER, T., PALUMBO, F., MESSELOFF, C., and PEARLMUTTER, M. (1952) Comparison of the tolerance of adults and children to digitoxin, *J. Amer. med. Ass.*, **150**, 191–4.

MAXWELL, J. (1955) Unexpected death in asthma, *Dis. Chest*, **27**, 208–12.

McLaren, G. (1968) Sudden death in asthma, *Brit. med. J.*, **4**, 456.

McManis, A. G. (1964) Adrenaline and isoprenaline: A warning, *Med. J. Aust.*, **2**, 668.

McNeill, R. S., and Ingram, C. G. (1966) Effect of propranolol on ventilatory function, *Amer. J. Cardiol.*, **18**, 473.

Middleton, E. and Finke, S. R. (1968) Metabolic response to epinephrine in bronchial asthma, *J. Allergy*, **42**, 288–99.

Molthan, L., Reidberg, M. M., and Eichman, M. F. (1967) Positive direct Coombs test due to cephalothin, *New Engl. J. Med.*, **277**, 123–5.

Montgomery, D. C., and Jackson, R. (1968) One hundred consecutive patients with drug reactions, *Canad. med. Ass. J.*, **99**, 712–14.

Motulsky, A. G. (1964) in *Progress in Medical Genetics*, New York.

Murphy, J. A., and Case, E. A. (1930) Sudden death from bronchial asthma, *J. Allergy*, **1**, 434–7.

Ogilvie, R. I., and Ruedy, J. (1967) Adverse drug reactions during hospitalization, *Canad. med. Ass. J.*, **97**, 1450–7.

Paterson, J W., Conolly, M. E., Davies, D. S., and Dollery, C T. (1968) Isoprenaline resistance and the use of pressurized aerosols in asthma, *Lancet*, **ii**, 426–9.

Patrick, R. R., and Tonge, J. I. (1966) Asthma and aerosol sprays, *Med. J. Aust.*, **2**, 668.

Pickvance, W. (1967) Pressurized aerosols in asthma, *Brit. med. J.*, **1**, 756.

Pillay, V. K. G., Schwartz, F. D., Aimi, K., and Kark, R. M. (1969) Transient and permanent deafness following treatment with ethacrynic acid in renal failure, *Lancet*, **i**, 77–9.

Richards, W., and Patrick, J. R. (1965) Deaths from asthma in children, *Amer. J. Dis. Child.*, **110**, 4–23.

Seidl, L. G., Thornton, G. F., Smith, J. W., and Cluff, L. E. (1966) Studies on the epidemiology of adverse drug reactions, III. Reactions in patients on a General Medical Service, *Bull. Johns Hopk. Hosp.*, **119**, 299–315.

Smith, J. M. (1966) Death from asthma, *Lancet*, **i**, 1042.

Smith, J. W., Seidl, L. G., and Cluff, L. E. (1966) Studies on the epidemiology of adverse drug reactions, *Ann. intern. Med.*, **65**, 629–40.

Soffer, A. (1961) The changing picture of digitalis intoxication, *Arch. intern. Med.*, **107**, 681–8.

Speizer, F. E., and Doll, R. (1968) A century of asthma deaths in young people, *Brit. med. J.*, **3**, 245–6.

Speizer, F. E., Doll, R., and Heaf, P. (1968) Observations on recent increase in mortality from asthma, *Brit. med. J.*, **1**, 335–9.

Speizer, F. E., Doll, R., Heaf, P., and Strang, L. B. (1968) Investigation into use of drugs preceding death from asthma, *Brit. med. J.*, **1**, 339–43.

Straub, P. W., Bühlmann, A. A., and Rossier, P. H. (1969) Hypovolaemia in status asthmaticus, *Lancet*, **ii**, 923–6.

Szentivanyi, A. (1966) The biochemical pharmacology of adrenergic action as related to the pathogenesis of bronchial asthma, *Ann. Allergy*, **42**, 203–32.

Townley, R. G., Dennis, M., and Itkin, I. H. (1965) Comparative action of acetyl-beta-methylcholine, histamine and pollen antigens in subjects with hayfever and patients with bronchial asthma, *J. Allergy*, **36**, 121–37.

Tranquada, R. E., Bernstein, S., and Martin, H. E. (1963) Irreversible lactic acidosis associated with phenformin therapy. Report of three cases, *J. Amer. med. Ass.*, **184**, 37–42.

Wicher, K., Reisman, R. E., and Arbesman, C. E. (1969) Allergic reaction to penicillin present in milk, *J. Amer. med. Ass.*, **208**, 143–5.

Worrledge, S. M. (1969) Autoantibody formation associated with methyl-dopa therapy, *Brit. J. Haemat.*, **16**, 5–8.

2

DRUG INTERACTION

Today there is much concern about drug interaction because patients so often receive more than one drug at a time. Many doctors have been unaware of the risks to which their patients are exposed when being treated with multiple drugs. Occasionally these risks are predictable on the basis of known pharmacology, but too often they have emerged only after the exposure of many patients.

With the present awareness of this problem, it is becoming increasingly apparent that it is in the realms of psychopharmacology and cardiovascular pharmacology that drug interaction may be of the greatest inconvenience and danger to the patient. In 1965 a symposium on 'Clinical Effects of Interaction between Drugs' was held at the Royal Society of Medicine in London and most of the possible mechanisms of drug interaction were reviewed and considered in detail. Perhaps the one salient feature that could be concluded from these discussions was that with greater understanding of underlying mechanisms, many of the untoward interactions being reported might be foreseen and avoided (Symposium, 1965).

The majority of drug interactions may be explained in terms of antagonism or synergism, the latter term including both summation and potentiation. It is now also clear that apart from simple drug interaction there can also be a related problem of interaction between an administered drug and a known or unknown component of normal diet. It would, however, be grossly misleading to think that all drug interactions are of potential hazard to the patient. This is obviously not so; synergistic actions of drugs can be of considerable benefit to the patient, provided that the potential side-effects of each component are not also exaggerated by their combination. A recent example of this is the combination of trimethoprim and sulphamethoxazole (*Bactrim, Septrin*) which attacks folic acid metabolism at different sites in the bacterium.

There are a number of ways in which drugs are known to interact and probably at least twice that number are as yet undiscovered. These have been reviewed by Macgregor (1965). The presence of one drug may accelerate or retard the metabolism of a second drug; concomitant administration of a second drug may replace the first drug during transport by displacing it from a particular plasma or tissue protein. The first drug, by causing an electrolyte imbalance, may increase the toxicity of the second drug and physiological antagonism or competitive antagonism at the receptor site, or at some other site in the same biological system, can greatly modify drug action. Modification of absorption or excretion mechanisms by one drug can drastically change the metabolism of another administered at the same time.

Much of the detailed knowledge of drug interaction has been gained by animal experimentation and, although such observations are of undisputed importance, it should not be overlooked that the speed and pathway of drug metabolism in man may be quite different from that which has been determined in many species of laboratory animal. Indeed Brodie (1962) and later Modell (1964) have emphasized that trial in man is the only valid way of establishing drug interaction in man, and that such studies should be performed ideally during the early stages of drug development. The problems and practical aspects of such a course of action are only too obvious, and it is relevant at this stage to examine, if only in brief detail, some of the evidence of drug interaction that has been revealed.

ACCELERATION OR SLOWING OF DRUG METABOLISM

Animal experiments have shown that many of the interactions between drugs are due to drug-metabolizing enzymes, particularly in the liver, being affected by the previous administration of other drugs (Burns and Conney, 1965). In their simplest form such studies have shown that pre-treatment with a drug may increase the activity of the enzyme system responsible for metabolizing that drug; for example, pre-treatment of rats with phenylbutazone will enhance the ability of the liver to metabolize phenylbutazone and pre-treatment with imipramine will likewise enhance the ability of liver microsomes to metabolize imipramine. The major interest in this type of study, however, arises when one drug cross-stimulates or inhibits the metabolism of another drug; for example, pre-treatment with nikethamide results in enhanced pentobarbitone-metabolizing activity in the liver (Brazda and Baucum, 1961) and prior pentobarbitone administration augments zoxazolamine hydroxylase activity (Conney *et al.*, 1961).

It has been suggested that such augmenting actions are due to the stimulation of the synthesis of enzyme protein by polycyclic hydrocarbons and drugs, since several groups of workers have shown that this induction of increased microsomal enzyme activity is completely prevented by the amino acid antagonist, ethionine, which prevents the incorporation of methionine and glycine into liver protein (cited by Macgregor, 1965).

Stimulation of drug-metabolizing enzymes may

explain the altered therapeutic responses observed in some patients when they receive several drugs at the same time. Indeed Dollery (1965) has well summarized this position by his statement, 'Every time a physician adds to the number of drugs a patient is taking he may devise a novel combination that has special risk'. It is obvious therefore that new drug combinations require separate investigation, with full animal toxicity and efficacy studies and then clinical evaluation; these studies to be carried out just as thoroughly as the primary trial of a single new drug.

Drug combinations are, however, only one facet of the whole potential problem. Substances present in the environment, such as insecticides, have been shown in animals to stimulate drug-metabolizing enzymes in the liver. So far the significance of such exposure to man is not known but the widespread use of such household insecticide sprays, although non-toxic in themselves, might well present a potential hazard to the patient on a therapeutic regimen with specific drugs.

Keeri-Szanto and Pomeroy (1971) have shown that the rate of pentazocine metabolism is greater in city dwellers than in patients from a rural community. Similarly, smokers metabolize the drug more rapidly than non-smokers.

Drugs which stimulate drug metabolism also enhance the hydroxylation of testosterone, oestradiol, progesterone and cortisol by enzymes in liver microsomes and obviously further research is required to establish the physiological importance of this interaction of drugs in the metabolism of steroids.

Stimulation of drug-metabolizing enzymes also occurs where barbiturates are used at the same time as anticoagulants. Rats treated with pentobarbitone showed a marked increase in the liver microsomal enzyme activity responsible for the metabolism of dicoumarol (Cucinell et al., 1965), and prior barbiturate administration accelerates the breakdown of coumarin anticoagulant drugs in man (Dayton et al., 1961). This latter finding can explain earlier reports that barbiturates decreased the anticoagulant activity of the coumarins (Avellaneda, 1955).

The danger of such barbiturate-anticoagulant combination is that the barbiturate, in stimulating the anticoagulant metabolism, induces a rise in prothrombin level. Therefore the dose of the anticoagulant has to be increased to reduce the prothrombin level. If the barbiturate is suddenly withdrawn, without adjusting the anticoagulant dosage, the anticoagulant activity is then far too great, the prothrombin level will fall rapidly and dangerously and bleeding may result.

The slowing or inhibition of the metabolism of one drug by another drug is an effect already well documented in animal studies and there are many examples where drugs can inhibit the metabolic detoxification of other drugs and thus cause an increase in both their duration and intensity of pharmacological action (Gillette, 1963). Burns and Conney (1965) reviewing this aspect of drug interaction listed the following

compounds as examples of inhibitors of drug metabolism. SKF-525A (β-diethylaminoethyldiphenylpropyl acetate), iproniazid, pheniprazine, nialamide, triparanol, chloramphenicol, p-aminosalicylic acid and the two narcotics pethidine (meperidine) and morphine. SKF-525A is an interesting compound and is worthy of further mention in this context since, apart from showing a wide spectrum of drug metabolism inhibition, it also shows a curious biphasic effect of inhibition or stimulation of drug metabolism. SKF-525A decreases the rate of phenylbutazone metabolism in dogs (Burns et al., 1955) and inhibits the metabolism of phenacetin (acetophenetidin) in rats (Burns et al., 1963). In acute doses SKF-525A markedly inhibits the metabolism of hexobarbital and thus prolongs its hypnotic action; however, when given for a long time to rats, the compound accelerates the metabolism of the barbiturate whose hypnotic effect is drastically reduced.

Other examples of compounds which can inhibit or stimulate drug metabolism by enzymes in liver microsomes, depending whether they are administered acutely or chronically, are chlorcyclizine, phenylbutazone and glutethimide (Burns and Conney, 1965).

Although the ability of drugs to inhibit the metabolism of other drugs has been well documented in experimental animals, this effect has been studied only recently in man. Oxyphenbutazone potentiates the anticoagulant action of warfarin sodium (Fox, 1964), and in related studies in man Weiner et al. (1965) reported that the plasma levels of bishydroxycoumarin and the anticoagulant response to the drug were prolonged after treatment with oxyphenbutazone. The same group also showed that the anabolic steroid, methandienone, slowed the metabolism of oxyphenbutazone in man by inhibiting glucuronyl transferase, an enzyme required for the conjugation of oxyphenbutazone with glucuronic acid. The importance of these effects in man remains to be established.

Monoamine oxidase inhibitors (MAOI's) are a specific example of compounds that owe their therapeutic usage to their blockage of the synthesis of certain sympathomimetic amines. Such MAOI's in clinical use have an irreversible action on monoamine oxidase and their effect persists until the enzyme has been resynthesized. The biochemical effects of the MAOI's involve several substrates of MAO including dopamine, tyramine, serotonin and, to a lesser extent, noradrenaline and adrenaline. MAO probably regulates the metabolism of catecholamines and serotonin in tissues, while catechol-o-methyltransferase is responsible for the metabolism of circulating noradrenaline and adrenaline (Kopin and Axelrod, 1963).

It should be emphasized that the varied actions of MAOI's cannot be explained simply in terms of MAO inhibition. Other enzyme systems are also affected, for example those concerned with the detoxification of drugs in the liver. Unfortunately, however, the MAOI's still account for a wide range of interactions with other drugs as has been well shown by both animal and human studies (Sjöqvist, 1965). van Rossum (1963) showed that mice pre-treated with pargyline and then given methyldopa responded with a central excitation resembling amphetamine overdosage. Paykel (1966) reported the results of such combined treatment in a patient; the use of pargyline treatment for hypertension was inadequate and methyldopa was added to aid control. This combination of therapies resulted in vivid hallucinations and the removal of the patient to hospital.

Cooper and Keddie (1964) reported that mebanazine was responsible for hypoglycaemic attacks in a diabetic patient stabilized on insulin zinc suspension. Further investigation in animals and in man (Cooper and Ashcroft, 1966) showed that MAOI's potentiated the hypoglycaemic effect of insulin and the sulphonylureas. It was suggested that the interaction was due to interference with the release of adrenaline thus preventing its compensatory hyperglycaemic effect.

The general use of MAOI's and anti-parkinsonism drugs such as benzhexol or ethopropazine seems to be generally condemned. Interaction results in tremor with profuse sweating; the mechanisms involved are not known.

These are but a few examples of MAOI's interacting with other drugs; the literature has become voluminous on this topic and indeed MAOI's probably account for the widest and most numerous of interactions reported with drug combinations. Sjöqvist (1965) has reviewed this problem.

Unfortunately the problem does not only apply to MAOI's and other drug combinations; it may also occur with combinations of MAOI's and specific foods. Several reports appeared prior to 1963 in British literature relating attacks of forceful heartbeat, severe headache and hypertension to treatment with tranylcypromine sulphate. Indeed these formed the subject of a Report of the Council on Drugs in the *Journal of the American Medical Association* (1963). This syndrome had also occurred, if only in part, with other MAOI's including phenelzine sulphate, nialamide and iproniazid (Blackwell, 1963; Davies, 1963). In severe cases the episodes progressed to nausea, vomiting, stiff neck and even death from intracranial haemorrhage (McClure, 1962). Commonly the onset was noted after a meal, particularly after ingestion of cheese or, in one case, a yeast product (Blackwell, 1963). Asatoor *et al.* (1963) proposed that cheese toxicity in patients receiving tranylcypromine sulphate was attributable to the effects of the ingested amine normally degraded by MAO; they suggested that tyramine was the causative agent. Horwitz *et al.* (1964) reviewed the literature on MAOI's, tyramine and cheese and also demonstrated marked potentiation of the pressor effects of tyramine in patients receiving MAOI's; a pressor response in pargyline-treated patients could be provoked by as little as 6 mg of tyramine given by mouth.

Examination of various foods and drinks for tyramine content has revealed that certain cheeses are rich in tyramine and 20 grams of New York cheddar was sufficient to provoke a pressor response in two MAOI-treated patients. Chianti contained sufficient tyramine in 400 ml to provoke a pressor response and smaller amounts of tyramine were found in certain beers. Fortunately, however, with the latter beverage precise calculations revealed that intoxication would be reached before the quantity of imbibed tyramine reached dangerous levels. A severe reaction to tyramine in schmaltz pickled herrings was reported by Nuessle *et al.* (1965) in a patient treated with tranylcypromine and trifluoperazine. Chemical investigation showed the high level of 3·03 mg/gram of tyramine in the herring. Other food stuffs notably fruits and caffeine-containing drinks may cause bizarre effects in patients on MAOI therapy due to their dopamine, tyramine or serotonin content. Indeed, in view of the large number of foods which are likely to cause interaction, MAOI therapy, even in the presence of a normal diet, must still be regarded as potentially complicated and dangerous. Sjöqvist (1965) has reviewed some of these complications.

DISPLACEMENT OF ONE DRUG BY ANOTHER FROM CARRIER OR RECEPTOR SITES

Brodie (1965), in a very comprehensive review, has explained how one drug may affect the action of another by altering its concentration at receptor sites. It may act directly by displacing the other drug from its specific site of action or it may act indirectly by displacing the second drug from proteins in plasma or tissues. In the former direct situation the biological activity of the first drug is diminished and in the other its activity is enhanced since it makes more unbound drug available at the receptor sites. The term 'drug receptors' is used somewhat empirically since little is known of their nature. However, a number of drug receptors are known to be enzymes and it is now suspected that receptors, even in the field of general pharmacology, are either enzyme processes or are closely integrated with such processes.

There are many simple pharmacological examples of a drug acting by displacing another drug from a receptor site; this is competitive inhibition. Atropine has no intrinsic activity but displaces acetylcholine from receptors at parasympathetic nerve endings; antihistamines are competitive antagonists of histamine at receptor sites and anticholinesterases compete with cholinesterases for an acetylcholine substrate. Guanethidine competes with noradrenaline at sympathetic nerve endings and it in turn can be displaced by amphetamine-like drugs. It is, however, when the first drug acts indirectly by displacing the second drug from protein binding that danger may arise with drug combinations.

Almost all drugs are reversibly bound to proteins in plasma and tissues. The bound drug, often a high proportion of the total, acts as a reservoir and prevents wild fluctuations between ineffective levels of the biologically unbound faction on one hand, and toxic levels on the other. Thus when the limited carrying capacity of the plasma proteins is filled, any unbound surplus is usually soon metabolized or excreted, so that the plasma level becomes re-stabilized.

Many acidic drugs, phenylbutazone, sulphonamides, coumarin anticoagulants and salicylates are highly bound to one or two sites on albumin molecules and are capable of displacing more loosely bound drugs. Thus sulphonamides administered to patients on tolbutamide may result in hypoglycaemia due to a massive release of unbound tolbutamide; bleeding may result when phenylbutazone is given to patients on coumarin anti-coagulants. Anti-rheumatic drugs of the non-steroidal type may displace cortisol from specific protein sites of attachment and this may explain their mechanism of action. Likewise sulphonylurea drugs may act by displacing insulin from protein in the pancreas, plasma or elsewhere. Brodie (1965) has speculated on the possibility and usefulness of developing 'silent antago-nists' for various classes of drug—that is to develop an agent that would have no intrinsic action but would act indirectly simply by replacing bound drugs from receptor sites. Benzquinamide, a compound which has little or no sedative action of its own, prevents the action of reserpine. Presumably it blocks the access of reserpine to its receptors (Sulser et al., 1964); a further example 3-hydroxyphenyltriethylammonium, a com-pound related to edrophonium chloride, is reported to be a potent anti-curare drug although intrinsically it evokes little excitatory action of its own on skeletal muscle (Randall, 1950).

EFFECT OF URINARY pH ON DRUG EXCRETION

The elimination of many drugs is markedly dependent on urinary pH and thus the excretion of a drug may be accelerated or retarded by concomitant administration of a compound that alters urinary pH. Drugs which are weak bases, examples are amphetamine, pethidine, mepacrine, chloroquine, mecamylamine, imipramine, amitriptyline and procaine, are excreted more rapidly in urine of low pH and more slowly at high pH. Con-versely weak acids such as phenobarbitone, salicylic acid, nitrofurantoin, nalidixic acid and some sulphon-amides are excreted more rapidly at high urinary pH and more slowly at low pH.

About 30–40 per cent of a dose of amphetamine is excreted in the urine as unchanged drug over 48 hours under normal conditions of fluctuating urinary pH. However, if the urine is rendered acidic (about pH 5) for the same period the proportion of unchanged drug excreted increases to 60–70 per cent. If the urine is rendered alkaline (about pH 8) this percentage falls to below 10 per cent (Beckett and Rowland, 1964, 1965). Thus concurrent self-medication with sodium bicarbon-ate during amphetamine treatment could raise urinary

pH and so delay the normal excretion of the drug and the patient would experience a more prolonged pharma-cological effect. Conversely administration of ammon-ium chloride would, by producing an acid urine, enhance the excretion of the drug and reduce its dura-tion of action.

Exercise tends to produce acidaemia and acid urine and special diets may also effect urinary pH; these factors can have profound effects also on drug action when the drug's metabolism is affected by changes in urinary pH. The influence of urinary pH does not seem to be well documented as far as drug interactions are concerned although urinary pH has already become a factor of importance in the treatment of drug poisoning and in the diagnosis of addiction to drugs. Elimination of potentially toxic drugs, for example salicylates and barbiturates may be accelerated by appropriate adjust-ment of urinary pH. Recognition and identification of addictive drugs, especially pethidine and amphetamine, are facilitated by the acidification of urine, and a general procedure for the analysis in urine of basic drugs and their metabolites, some of which may be misused as stimulants in sport, has been developed by Beckett and his colleagues (Beckett and Tucker, 1966; Beckett et al., 1967).

Many drugs, other than diuretics, have a direct effect on the kidney mechanism and this also can lead indirectly to interaction between drugs. Probenecid is one such drug; it has a selective action on the renal tubules and prevents the reabsorption of uric acid, hence its use in the treatment of gout. It delays the excretion of penicillin, sodium aminosalicylate and phenolsulphonphthalein and also raises the plasma level of sulphonamides.

The oral diuretic agents which easily cause hypo-kalaemia will promote digitalis intoxication; this is unfortunate since digitalis and its glycosides have retained a unique position in the treatment of cardiac disease and yet must still be regarded as one of the group of drugs most likely to cause side-effects. A low potassium concentration in the plasma complicates the use of digitalis even further and this digitalis-diuretic combination unfortunately remains one of the better known examples of drug interaction.

Adverse pharmacological effects or allergic reactions produced by drugs and drug interactions are deter-mined not only by differences among drugs but also by differences among individuals. Some of the personal or clinical variables and factors influencing drug effects are known, but for the most part it has been difficult to predict which patients are most likely to suffer adverse reactions after administration of a drug or drugs. Smith et al. (1966) have studied the epidemiology of adverse drug reactions in 900 hospitalized medical patients over one year, and have examined the personal variable or clinical factors which may be responsible for predispo-sition to the untoward effects of drugs. Reactions were most common in patients with serious illness who received many drugs. Patients with abnormal renal function, infection or previous drug reactions, were predisposed to drug reactions and perhaps unexpectedly, patients with gastro-intestinal disease seemed predisposed to allergic episodes.

Many groups, for example Seidl *et al.* (1966), Hoddinott *et al.* (1967), Ogilvie and Ruedy (1967) and Hurwitz and Wade (1969), have found that patients with reactions had a greater total number of drugs than patients free from side-effects. Although this is indicative of drug-interaction, the finding may be partially explained by another drug being required because of, or after, the reaction had occurred; in its simplest form this could be the administration of an antihistaminic drug after a rash had occurred as a side-effect of another drug.

Age and concurrent disease appear also to promote drug interaction. Old people are particularly liable to experience the digoxin-thiazide diuretic interaction that has previously been described; the slower metabolism of digoxin in the elderly is certainly a predisposing factor in the marked potentiation of the drug's action in these patients. Similarly concurrent liver or renal disease limiting the metabolism and excretion of drugs may easily result in undesirable interaction.

Cross reactions occur between certain drugs and frequently there is a skin and/or mucosal reaction. An eruption from exposure to one drug can result in an eruption when the skin is exposed to a chemically related compound. One such example is the para-amino group which is contained in sulphonamides, para-aminosalicylic acid, procaine, benzocaine and gentian violet. Also a person who develops an allergic contact dermatitis with a paraphenylenediamine hair dye may develop a widespread eczema with procaine local anaesthesia or with sulphonamide therapy (Verbov, 1968).

Cross allergy occurs among all penicillin derivatives, which all share the 6-aminopenicillanic acid nucleus, although they may differ appreciably in their side chain. There is also cross allergy between the penicillin and cephalosporin derivatives, e.g. cephaloridine, although they have nuclei of differing chemical structure; for the cephalosporin derivatives this is 7-aminocephalosporanic acid (Thoburn *et al.*, 1966).

The influence of previous therapy on placebo responsiveness has been studied by Batterman and Lower (1968) and surely the findings of these investigators must cast some shadow on the performance of many clinical trials where the placebo-treated patient serves as his own control to a prior or later treatment with the active agent. Second trial medications may reflect the persistence of first-drug effects and subjective beneficial responses may persist for days or weeks after the effective drug has been discontinued. The results, therefore, attained by the administration of any subsequent drug during a specific time after initial responsiveness may be statistically invalid and the conclusions drawn erroneous in any comparative cross-over study. Batterman and Lower (1968) surveyed 173 patients who

received placebo therapy for 230 trials; responsiveness was obviously dependent upon the effectiveness of previous therapy. Since the interaction of drug trials was found to be highly significant, the authors concluded that the classical cross-over evaluation of drugs required modification especially relative to trials testing analgesic and anti-rheumatic agents.

Perhaps this conclusion is a fitting stage to end this particular discussion; drugs can interact and in many instances this is to the disadvantage of the patient; it would also seem that placebos can affect drug action.

The following table [TABLE 2·1] illustrates some of the more common examples of established interaction between drugs.

TABLE 2.1
EXAMPLES OF KNOWN DRUG INTERACTIONS

DRUG	IN COMBINATION WITH	EFFECT
Antibiotics Streptomycin Neomycin	Succinylcholine (7, 12) Tubocurarine (8, 12)	Potentiation of neuromuscular block
	Hypotensives (13, 14, 15) Thiazide diuretics	Potentiation of hypotensive effect
Griseofulvin	Barbiturates (8, 16)	Increased griseofulvin inactivation
Tetracyclines Chloramphenicol	Penicillin (1, 2, 9, 10, 11)	Mutual antagonism
Streptomycin	Tetracyclines (1, 3, 4) Chloramphenicol (1, 3, 4)	Bacteriostatic effect of these two antibiotics reduces bactericidal effect of streptomycin
Sulphonamides	Methotrexate (12)	Increased toxicity
	Tolbutamide (12) Chlorpropamide (12) Insulin	Increased hypoglycaemic effect
	PAS Phenylbutazone Cobalt salts Resorcinol	Hypothyroidism, pituitary and thyroid hyperplasia
	Coumarol anticoagulants (5, 12) Salicylates (5, 12) Phenylbutazone (5, 12)	Displacement of long-acting sulphonamides bound to plasma albumin
Nitrofurantoin	Nalidixic acid (6)	Inhibition of nalidixic acid

1. GARROD, L. P., and WATERWORTH, P. M. (1962) *J. clin. Path.*, **15**, 328.

2. LEPPER, M. H., and DOWLING, H. F. (1951) *Arch. intern. Med.*, **88**, 489.
3. CHABBERT, Y. (1953) *Ann. Inst. Pasteur*, **84**, 545.
4. CHABBERT, Y. A., and PATTE, J. C. (1960) *Appl. Microbiol.*, **8**, 193.
5. DRUG AND THERAPEUTICS BULLETIN (1966) **4**, 13.
6. STILLE, W., and OSTNER, K. H. (1966) *Klin. Wschr.*, **44**, 155.
7. FOLDES, F. F., *et al.* (1963) *J. Amer. med. Ass.*, **183**, 672.
8. HUSSAR, D. A. (1967) *Amer. J. Pharm.*, **139**, 215.
9. JAWETZ, E., *et al.* (1950) *Science*, **111**, 254.
10. JAWETZ, E., and GUNNISON, J. B. (1952) *Chemotherapia (Basel)*, **2**, 243.
11. MANTEN, A., and TERRA, J. I. (1964) *Chemotherapia (Basel)*, **8**, 21.
12. MCIVER, A. K. (1967) *Pharm. J.*, **199**, 205.
13. DOLLERY, C. T. (1965) *Proc. roy. Soc. Med.*, **58**, 983.
14. SMITH, W. M., *et al.* (1964) *Ann. intern. Med.*, **61**, 829.
15. DRUG AND THERAPEUTICS BULLETIN (1967) **5**, 89.
16. BUSFIELD, D., *et al.* (1963) *Lancet*, **ii**, 1042.

6. ANTLITZ, A. M., *et al.* (1968) *Curr. Ther. Res.*, **10**, 70.
7. EISEN, M. J. (1964) *J. Amer. med. Ass.*, **189**, 64.
8. HOBBS, C. B., *et al.* (1965) *Postgrad. med. J.*, **41**, 563.
9. IKEDA, M., *et al.* (1966) *Fed. Proc.*, **25**, 417.
10. MACDONALD, M. G., and ROBINSON, D. S. (1965) *Pharmacologist*, **7**, 146.
11. PYÖRÄLÄ, K., *et al.* (1965) *Ann. Med. exp. Fenn.*, **43**, 95.
12. SOLOMON, H. M., and SCHROGIE, J. J. (1967) *Clin. Pharmacol. Ther.*, **8**, 797.
13. UDALL, J. A. (1966) *Curr. ther. Res.*, **8**, 627.
14. DENICOLA, P., *et al.* (1964) *Thrombos. Diathes. haemorrh. (Stuttg.)*, Suppl. **12**, 125.
15. FUMAROLA, D., *et al.* (1964) *Haematologica*, **49**, 1248.
16. ROGERS, L. A., and FOUTS, J. R. (1964) *J. Pharmacol. exp. Ther.*, **146**, 286.
17. FOX, S. L. (1964) *J. Amer. med. Ass.*, **188**, 320.
18. WEINER, M., *et al.* (1965) *Fed. Proc.*, **24**, 153.
19. DRESDALE, F. C., and HAYES, J. C. (1967) *J. Med. Soc. N.J.*, **64**, 609.
20. KOCH-WESER, J. (1968) *Ann. intern. Med.*, **68**, 511.
21. HOFFBRAND, B. I., and KININMONTH, D. A. (1967) *Brit. med. J.*, **2**, 838.
22. BRODIE, B. B. (1965) *Proc. roy. Soc. Med.*, **58**, 946.
23. WILLIAMS, J. T., and MORAVEC, D. F. (1966) *Hosp. Mgmt.*, **1**, 28.
24. HOUGIE, C. (1958) *Proc. Soc. exp. Biol. (N.Y.)*, **98**, 130.
25. PERKINS, H. A., *et al.* (1961) *J. clin. invest.*, **40**, 1421.
26. GOLDMAN, R., and HOHF, R. P. (1962) *Arch. Surg.*, **85**, 497.

DRUG	IN COMBINATION WITH	EFFECT
Anticoagulants Coumarol derivatives	MAOI's (14, 15) *d*-Thyroxine (12) Clofibrate (12) Anabolic steroids (11, 19) Oxyphenbutazone (8, 17, 18) Phenylbutazone (1, 7) Indomethacin (21, 22)	Potentiation of anticoagulant effect with risk of severe haemorrhage
	Barbiturates (3, 4, 6, 9, 10, 16) Glutethimide (1, 2, 3) Chloral hydrate (4) Griseofulvin (2, 5) Quinidine (20)	Antagonism of anticoagulant effect; sudden withdrawal of one of these agents from patients being anticoagulated may result in severe drop in prothrombin
	Phenytoin (Diphenylhydantoin)	Inhibition of metabolism of coumarol anticoagulants and increase of half-life from 9–36 hours
Phenindione	Vitamin K (13)	Reversal of anticoagulant effect
Heparin	Penicillin (23) Protamine (24, 25, 26) Hexadimethrine (25, 26)	Antagonism of heparin

DRUG	IN COMBINATION WITH	EFFECT
Antidiabetics Chlorpropamide Tolbutamide	Sulphaphenazole (6, 12) Phenylbutazone (3, 6, 12)	Half-life of the sulphonylureas increased from 4–17 hours
	Salicylates (7, 8)	Unbound sulphonylurea increased by competition for plasma binding
	Alcohol (9)	Hypoglycaemic action increased by competition for liver inactivating system
	Thiazide diuretics MAOI's (2) Coumarol anticoagulants (4, 13) Propranolol (10, 11)	Hypoglycaemic action of sulphonylureas potentiated
Insulin	ACTH Glucocorticoids	Hypoglycaemic effect antagonized
	Thyroxine	Insulin requirements increased
	Propranolol (10, 11, 12) Sulphonamides MAOI's (1, 2)	Hypoglycaemic effect potentiated
	Beta adrenergic blockers (5)	Hypoglycaemic effect potentiated

1. AGGELER, P. M., *et al.* (1967) *New Engl. J. Med.*, **276**, 496.
2. CATALANO, P. M., and CULLEN, S. I. (1967) *Clin. Res.*, **14**, 266.
3. CORN, M. (1966) *Thrombos. Diathes. haemorrh. (Stuttg.)*, **16**, 606.
4. CUCINELL, S. A., *et al.* (1966) *J. Amer. med. Ass.*, **197**, 366.
5. CULLEN, S. I., and CATALANO, P. M. (1967) *J. Amer. med. Ass.*, **199**, 582.

1. COOPER, A. J., and ASHCROFT, G. (1966) *Lancet*, **i**, 407.
2. COOPER, A. J., and KEDDIE, K. M. G. (1964) *Lancet*, **i**, 1133.
3. FIELD, J. B., *et al.* (1967) *New Engl. J. Med.*, **277**, 889.
4. SISE, H. S. (1967) *Ann. intern. Med.*, **67**, 460.
5. BYERS, S. O., and FRIEDMAN, M. (1966) *Proc. Soc. exp. Biol. (N.Y.)*, **122**, 114.
6. CHRISTENSEN, L. K., *et al.* (1963) *Lancet*, **ii**, 1298.
7. STOWERS, J. M., *et al.* (1959) *Ann. N.Y. Acad. Sci.*, **74**, 689.
8. WISHINSKY, H., *et al.* (1962) *Diabetes*, **11**, Suppl., 18.
9. KRISTENSEN, M., and HANSEN, J. M. (1967) *Diabetes*, **16**, 211.
10. KOTLER, M. N., *et al.* (1966) *Lancet*, **ii**, 1389.
11. LANCET (1967) Leading article, *Lancet*, **i**, 939.
12. HUSSAR, D. A. (1967) *Amer. J. Pharm.*, **139**, 215.
13. MCIVER, A. K. (1967) *Pharm. J.*, **199**, 205.

DRUG	IN COMBINATION WITH	EFFECT
Anti-inflammatory agents Salicylates	Sulphonamides (8)	Toxicity and ulcerogenic action increased
	Warfarin (8)	Anticoagulant effect increased
	Tolbutamide (9, 10) Chlorpropamide (9, 10)	Hypoglycaemic action potentiated
	Probenecid (5, 12, 13)	Uricosuric action antagonized
	Sulphinpyrazone (11)	Salicylate excretion reduced
	Methotrexate (8, 13)	Toxicity of methotrexate increased
	Phenylbutazone (2, 5)	Urate retention increased
Phenylbutazone Oxyphenbutazone	Chlorpropamide (3, 4, 5) Tolbutamide (3, 4, 5, 13)	Hypoglycaemic effect potentiated
	Warfarin (6, 7) MAOI's (13)	Anticoagulant effect potentiated
	Cortisol (1)	Metabolism of cortisol increased

1. KUNTZMAN, R. (1966) *Pharmacologist*, **8**, 195.
2. OYER, J. H., *et al.* (1966) *Amer. J. med. Sci.*, **251**, 1.
3. FIELD, J. B., *et al.* (1967) *New Engl. J. Med.*, **277**, 889.
4. CHRISTENSEN, L. K., *et al.* (1963) *Lancet*, **ii**, 1298.
5. HUSSAR, D. A. (1967) *Amer. J. Pharm.*, **139**, 215.
6. AGGELER, P. M., *et al.* (1967) *New Engl. J. Med.*, **276**, 496.
7. EISEN, M. J. (1964) *J. Amer. med. Ass.*, **189**, 64.
8. MCIVER, A. K., (1967) *Pharm. J.*, **199**, 205.
9. STOWERS, J. M., *et al.* (1959) *Ann. N.Y. Acad. Sci.*, **74**, 689.
10. WISHINSKY, H., *et al.* (1962) *Diabetes*, **11**, Suppl., 18.
11. YU, T. F., *et al.* (1962) *Fed. Proc.*, **21**, 175.
12. PASCAL, L. R., *et al.* (1955) *J. Lab. clin. Med.*, **45**, 771.
13. DRUG AND THERAPEUTICS BULLETIN (1967), **5**, 89.

DRUG	IN COMBINATION WITH	EFFECT
Barbiturates	Alcohol (8, 9)	Increased intoxication; respiratory depression
	Warfarin (references given in section on anticoagulants)	Increased liver metabolism of warfarin; antagonism of anticoagulant effect
	Griseofulvin (7)	Increased rate of inactivation of griseofulvin by liver
	Thyroxine	Phenobarbitone metabolism inhibited
	Cortisol (6)	Hydroxylation of cortisol stimulated
	Zoxazolamine (4)	Metabolism enhanced, muscle relaxant effect almost abolished
	Phenytoin (Diphenylhydantoin) (5)	Metabolism stimulated by phenobarbitone
	Phenylbutazone (1) Aminopyrine (1)	Increased hypnosis
	Anticholinesterases (2)	Increased muscle depolarization
Thiopental	Cyclopropane (3)	Potentiation of cyclopropane induced cardiac arrhythmias
Phenobarbitone	Hexobarbitone (4)	Metabolism of hexobarbitone enhanced

1. ECKHARDT, E. T. (1958), *Proc. Soc. exp. Biol. (N.Y.)*, **98**, 423.
2. WEISS, L. R., and ORZEL, R. A. (1967) *Toxicol. appl. Pharmacol.*, **10**, 334.
3. MACANNEL, K. L., and DRESEL, P. E. (1964) *Canad. J. Physiol. Pharmacol.*, **42**, 627.
4. CONNEY, A. H., *et al.* (1960) *J. Pharmacol. exp. Ther.*, **130**, 1.
5. CUCINELL, S. A., *et al.* (1963) *J. Pharmacol. exp. Ther.*, **141**, 157.
6. BURSTEIN, S., and BHARNANI, B. R. (1967) *Endocrinology*, **80**, 351.
7. BUSFIELD, D., *et al.* (1963) *Lancet*, **ii**, 1042.
8. CAMPS, F. E. (1953) *Pharm. J.*, **170**, 278.
9. NICKOLLS, L. C. (1953) *Pharm. J.*, **170**, 209.

DRUG	IN COMBINATION WITH	EFFECT
Diuretics Thiazides	MAOI's (6)	Hypotension
	Aminophylline	Potentiation of diuretic effect
	Hypotensives (3, 4, 5)	Potentiation of hypotensive effect
	Corticosteroids (5)	Increased risk of hyperglycaemia
	Digitalis (1, 2)	Potentiation of hypokalaemic effect
	Tubocurarine (1) Gallamine (1)	Persistent curarization due to K+ depletion
	Spironolactone	Reduction of K+ loss
Organomercurials	Ammonium chloride Sulphonamides Acetazolamide	Potentiation of diuretic effect

1. McIver, A. K. (1967) *Pharm. J.*, **199**, 205.
2. Hussar, D. A. (1967) *Amer. J. Pharm.*, **139**, 215.
3. Dollery, C. T. (1965) *Proc. roy. Soc. Med.*, **58**, 983.
4. Smith, W. M., *et al.* (1964) *Ann. intern. Med.*, **61**, 829.
5. Drug and Therapeutics Bulletin (1967), **5**, 89.
6. Goldberg, L. I. (1964) *J. Amer. med. Ass.*, **190**, 456.

DRUG	IN COMBINATION WITH	EFFECT
Muscle relaxants Succinylcholine	MAOI's (9) Anticholinesterases (1, 4)	Potentiation of muscle depolarization
	Procaine (3, 8) Lignocaine (3, 8)	Increased duration of neuromuscular block
	Promazine hydrochloride (2) Lignocaine (3, 8)	Prolonged apnoea
Succinylcholine Tubocurarine Gallamine	Streptomycin (7, 8) Neomycin (7, 8) Kanamycin (7, 8)	Prolonged paralysis of respiratory muscles
Tubocurarine Gallamine	Thiazide diuretics	Persistent curarization due to K+ depletion
	Quinidine (5, 8)	Recurarization even after recovery from neuromuscular blockade

1. Drug and Therapeutics Bulletin (1964) **2**, 18.
2. Regan, A. G., and Aldrete, J. A. (1967) *Anesth. Analg. Curr. Res.*, **46**, 315.
3. Usubiaga, J. E., *et al.* (1967) *Anesth. Analg. Curr. Res.*, **46**, 39.
4. Himes, J. A., *et al.* (1967) *J. Amer. vet. med. Ass.*, **151**, 54.
5. Way, W. L., *et al.* (1967) *J. Amer. med. Ass.*, **200**, 153.
6. Foldes, F. F., *et al.* (1963) *J. Amer. med. Ass.*, **183**, 672.
7. Hussar, D. A. (1967) *Amer. J. Pharm.*, **139**, 215.
8. McIver, A. K. (1967) *Pharm. J.*, **199**, 205.

DRUG	IN COMBINATION WITH	EFFECT
Tranquillizers Phenothiazines	Barbiturates (2, 9) Narcotics (9) Alcohol (8, 9) Sodium bromide (1)	Potentiation of central depressant action
	Insulin	Hypoglycaemic effect promoted
	Hypotensive agents (6, 7)	Hypotensive action potentiated
Thioridazine	Amitriptyline (3)	Severe toxic reaction to combined therapy; catatonia, coma and extrapyramidal reactions
Chlorpromazine	LSD (2, 4) Psilocybin	Reduction of hallucinogenic effects
Reserpine group	Barbiturates (2) MAOI's, Phenothiazines (6, 7, 9) Digitalis (7)	Potentiation of central depressant effect; bradycardia, hyperthermia
	Imipramine (5)	Reversal or inhibition of reserpine syndrome
	Alpha and beta adrenergic blockers (4)	Modification of reserpine-induced hyperthermia

1. Norden, L. G., and Plaa, G. L. (1963) *Toxicol. appl. Pharmacol.*, **5**, 437.
2. Child, K. J., *et al.* (1961) *Biochem. Pharmacol.*, **5**, 87.
3. Witton, K. (1965) *Amer. J. Psychiat.*, **121**, 812.
4. Jori, A., *et al.* (1967) *Arch. int. Pharmacodyn.*, **165**, 384.
5. Shepherd, M. (1965) *Proc. roy. Soc. Med.*, **58**, 964.
6. Dollery, C. T. (1965) *Proc. roy. Soc. Med.*, **58**, 983.
7. McIver, A. K. (1967) *Pharm. J.*, **199**, 205.
8. Drug and Therapeutics Bulletin (1967) **5**, 89.
9. Hussar, D. A. (1967) *Amer. J. Pharm.*, **139**, 215.

DRUG	IN COMBINATION WITH	EFFECT
Antidepressants Monoamine oxidase inhibitors *Fatal episode reported	*Sympathomimetic amines* Dopamine (1) Noradrenaline (1) Broad beans (Dopa) (6) *Amphetamine (2) *Methylamphetamine (3) Dextroamphetamine (25) Metaraminol (25) Phenylephrine (25) *Ephedrine (4) Methylphenidate (5)	Adrenergic effects potentiated, hypertension, hypertensive crisis, severe headache, cardiac arrhythmias, circulatory insufficiency, central excitation if compounds pass blood-brain barrier
	Tyramine containing foods *Cheese (7, 8, 9, 10, 11, 12, 14, 15) Yeast products (16) Pickled herring (13)	Hypertensive crisis
	*Imipramine (17, 18, 19, 20) Amitriptyline (21)	Excitation, tremor, hyperpyrexia, sweating, delirium, clonic and tonic convulsions, rigidity, coma
	Barbiturates (22, 23) Chloral hydrate (24) Anaesthetics (25)	Enhanced CNS depression
	Insulin (26) Tolbutamide Chlorpropamide	Hypoglycaemia potentiated
	Cocaine (27)	Hyperexcitation, hyperpnoea and hyperpyrexia
	Phenothiazines (22, 25)	Hypertension, increased extrapyramidal reactions
	Narcotics (28, 29, 30, 31, 32, 33) *Pethidine	Excitation, rigidity, coma, hypo- or hypertension, respiratory distress, hyperpyrexia, shock, prolonged narcotic effect if not fatal
	Antiparkinsonian agents (25, 34)	Potentiation
	Thiazide diuretics (25)	Hypotension
	Methyldopa (35, 36)	Hypertension and central excitation

DRUG	IN COMBINATION WITH	EFFECT
Sympathomimetic amines	MAOI's (12)	May produce fatal hypertensive crisis
	Hypotensives Hexamethonium (1) Pentolinium (1) Mecamylamine (1) Pempidine (1)	Potentiation of pressor effects of noradrenaline and indirect-amines producing hypertension
	Methyldopa (1) Reserpine (1) Bethanidine (1, 2) Guanethidine (1, 2) Bretylium (1, 2)	Depletion of endogenous noradrenaline thereby reducing pressor effect of indirect-sympathomimetic amines. Pressor effect of exogenous noradrenaline potentiated

1. HORWITZ, D., et al. (1960) J. Lab. clin. Med., 55, 747.
2. ZECK, P. (1961) Med. J. Aust., 2, 607.
3. DALLY, P. J. (1962) Lancet, i, 1235.
4. LOW-BEER, G. A., and TIDMARSH, D. (1963) Brit. med. J., 2, 683.
5. SHERMAN, M., et al. (1964) Amer. J. Psychiat., 120, 1019.
6. HODGE, J. V., et al. (1964) Lancet, i, 1108.
7. BLACKWELL, B. (1963) Lancet, ii, 414, 819.
8. DAVIES, E. B. (1963) Lancet, ii, 691.
9. WOMACK, A. M. (1963) Lancet, ii, 463.
10. CUTHILL, J. M., et al. (1964) Lancet, i, 1076.
11. HORWITZ, D., et al. (1964) J. Amer. med. Ass., 188, 1108.
12. LEONARD, J. W., et al. (1964) Lancet, i, 883.
13. NUESSLE, W. F., et al. (1965) J. Amer. med. Ass., 192, 726.
14. STRONG, F. M. (1962) Amer. J. clin. Nutr., 11, 500.
15. BLACKWELL, B., et al. (1964) Lancet, i, 722.
16. BLACKWELL, B., and MARLEY, E. (1964) Lancet, i, 530.
17. SINGH, H. (1960) Amer. J. Psychiat., 117, 360.
18. AYD, F. J. (1961) J. Neuropsychiat., 2 (Suppl. 1), 119.
19. KANE, F. J., and FREEMAN, D. (1963) Amer. J. Psychiat., 120, 79.
20. BRACHFELD, J., et al. (1963) J. Amer. med. Ass., 186, 1172.
21. JARECKI, H. G. (1963) Amer. J. Psychiat., 120, 189.
22. KLINE, N. S. (1963) Bull. Wld Hlth Org., 21, 397.
23. DOMINO, E. F., et al. (1962) Amer. J. Psychiat., 118, 941.
24. HOWARTH, E. (1961) J. ment. Sci., 107, 100.
25. GOLDBERG, L. I. (1964) J. Amer. med. Ass., 190, 456.
26. COOPER, A. J., and KEDDIE, K. M. G. (1964) Lancet, i, 1133.
27. CLEMENT, A. J., and BENAZON, D. (1962) Lancet, ii, 197.
28. SHEE, J. C. (1960) Brit. med. J., 2, 507.
29. PALMER, H. (1960) Brit. med. J., 2, 944.
30. COCKS, D. P., and PASSMORE-ROWE, A. (1962) Brit. med. J., 2, 1545.
31. TAYLOR, D. C. (1962) Lancet, ii, 401.
32. BRADLEY, J. J., and FRANCIS, J. G. (1963) Lancet, i, 386.
33. VIGRAN, I. M. (1964) J. Amer. med. Ass., 187, 953.
34. SHAW, D. M. (1964) Practitioner, 192, 23.
35. ROSSUM, J. M. VAN (1963) Lancet, i, 950.
36. NATARAJAN, S. (1964) Lancet, i, 1330.

DRUG	IN COMBINATION WITH	EFFECT
Phenylephrine	Debrisoquine (17)	Hypertensive response to phenylephrine due to MAOI action of debrisoquine or sensitization of adrenergic receptors to phenylephrine. Reversal by phenylephrine of adrenergic-neurone blockade induced by debrisoquine in sympathetically innervated preparation
Sympathomimetic amines (contd.)	Propranolol (16)	Blocks beta effects
	Phentolamine (3) Phenoxybenzamine (3) Dibenamine (4)	Block alpha effects; blockade is increased in presence of noradrenaline or other alpha blocker
	Ergot alkaloids (5)	Block or reverse alpha effects but produce pronounced hypertension due to vasoconstrictor action
	Chlorpromazine (6)	Blocks or reverses a variety of actions of adrenaline; antagonizes adrenaline-induced hypertension by depressing the vasopressor carotid sinus reflex
	Atropine (7)	Prolongs beta effects
	Antihistamines (11) Chlorpheniramine (11) Desipramine (11) Tripelennamine (11)	Potentiation of cardiovascular actions of noradrenaline and potentiation of noradrenaline toxicity

DRUG	IN COMBINATION WITH	EFFECT
Digitalis glycosides	Thiazides and other oral diuretics (12, 13)	Hypokalaemia due to inhibition of ion transport Low K^+ increases ATP-ase inactivation by digitalis glycosides
	Ca^{++} (8)	High concentration of calcium inhibitory to positive inotropic action of digitalis and potentiates its toxic effects. Causes a dangerous increase in ATP-ase inhibition
	Reserpine (12)	Undue bradycardia
	Procainamide (10)	Suppresses ventricular extrasystoles and tachycardia caused by digitalis intoxication but can precipitate ventricular asystole or fibrillation
	Aminophylline (9)	Potentiates digitalis
Reserpine	Phenothiazines (1, 12)	Potentiation of central depressant effects; hypotension by noradrenaline depletion
	Digitalis (12)	Undue bradycardia
Hypotensives	Sympathomimetic amines (1, 2, 12)	Antagonize each other
	MAOI's (12)	Potentiate each other
	Anaesthetics (1, 12) Barbiturates (1)	Potentiate hypotension
Guanethidine	Imipramine (14) Sympathomimetic amines (1, 14) Amitriptyline (15)	Hypotensive effect antagonized

1. Dollery, C. T. (1965) *Proc. roy. Soc. Med.*, **58**, 983.
2. Boura, A. L. A., and Green, A. F. (1963) *Brit. J. Pharmacol.*, **20**, 36.
3. Nickerson, M., and Gump, W. S. (1949) *J. Pharmacol. exp. Ther.*, **97**, 25.
4. Furchgott, R. F. (1954) *J. Pharmacol. exp. Ther.*, **111**, 265.
5. Goodman, L. S., and Gilman, A. (1965) *Pharmacological Basis of Therapeutics*, 3rd ed., New York, p. 555.
6. Ibid, p. 169.
7. Ibid, p. 540.
8. Ibid, p. 679.
9. Ibid, p. 363.
10. Ibid, p. 712.
11. Jori, A. (1966) *J. Pharm. Pharmacol.*, **18**, 824.
12. McIver, A. K. (1967) *Pharm. J.*, **199**, 205.
13. Hussar, D. A. (1967) *Amer. J. Pharm.*, **139**, 215.
14. Drug and Therapeutics Bulletin (1967), **5**, 89.
15. Meyer, J. F., *et al.* (1970) *J. Amer. med. Ass.*, **213**, 1487.
16. Shanks, R. G. (1970) *Irish J. med. Sci.*, **3**, 247.
17. Aminu, J., *et al.* (1970) *Lancet*, **ii**, 935.

RECOMMENDED FURTHER READING

BURKE, C. W. (1970) The effect of oral contraceptives on cortisol metabolism, *J. clin. Path.*, **23**, Suppl. (Ass. Clin. Path.), **3**, 11–18.

KEERI-SZANTO, M., and POMEROY, J. R. (1971) Atmospheric pollution and pentazocine metabolism, *Lancet*, **i**, 947–9.

MEYLER, L., and PECK, H. M., eds. (1962, 1965, 1968) *Drug-Induced Diseases*, Vols. 1, 2, and 3, Excerpta Medica Foundation, Amsterdam.

MEYLER, L., *et al.*, eds. (1957, 1958, 1960, 1963, 1966, 1968) *Side Effects of Drugs*, Vols. I, II, III, IV, V, and VI, Excerpta Medica Foundation, Amsterdam.

SOUTHGATE, J., COLLINS, G. G. S., PRYSE-DAVIES, J., and SANDLER, M. (1970) Effect of contraceptive steroids on monoamine oxidase activity, *J. clin. Path.*, **23**, Suppl. (Ass. Clin. Path.), **3**, 43–8.

REFERENCES

ASATOOR, A. M., LEVI, A. J., and MILNE, M. D. (1963) Tranylcypromine and cheese, *Lancet*, **ii**, 733–4.

AVELLANEDA, M. (1955) Interferencia de los barbitúricos en la acción del tromexan, *Medicina (B. Aires)*, **15**, 109–15.

BATTERMAN, R. C., and LOWER, W. R. (1968) Placebo responsiveness—influence of previous therapy, *Curr. ther. Res.*, **10**, 136–43.

BECKETT, A. H., and ROWLAND, M. (1964) Rhythmic urinary excretion of amphetamine in man, *Nature (Lond.)*, **204**, 1203–4.

BECKETT, A. H., and ROWLAND, M. (1965) Urinary excretion kinetics of amphetamine in man, *J. Pharm. Pharmacol.*, **17**, 628–39.

BECKETT, A. H. and TUCKER, G. T. (1966) A method for the evaluation of some oral prolonged-release forms of dex-amphetamine in man, using urinary excretion data, *J. Pharm. Pharmacol.*, **18**, Suppl., 725–55.

BECKETT, A. H., TUCKER, G. T., and MOFFAT, A. C. (1967) Routine detection and identification in urine of stimulants and other drugs, some of which may be used to modify performance in sport, *J. Pharm. Pharmacol.*, **19**, 273–94.

BLACKWELL, B. (1963) Hypertensive crisis due to monoamine-oxidase inhibitors, *Lancet*, **ii**, 849–51.

BRAZDA, F. G., and BAUCUM, R. W. (1961) The effect of Nikethamide on the metabolism of pentobarbital by liver microsomes of the rat, *J. Pharmacol. exp. Ther.*, **132**, 295–8.

BRODIE, B. B. (1962) Difficulties in extrapolating data on metabolism of drugs from animal to man, *Clin. Pharmacol. Ther.*, **3**, 374–80.

BRODIE, B. B. (1965) Displacement of one drug by another from carrier or receptor sites, *Proc. roy. Soc. Med.*, **58**, 946–55.

BURNS, J. J., and CONNEY, A. H. (1965) Enzyme stimulation and inhibition in the metabolism of drugs, *Proc. roy. Soc. Med.*, **58**, 955–60.

BURNS, J. J., CONNEY, A. H., COLVILLE, K. I., and SANSUR, M. (1963) Relationship of phenacetin metabolism to its analgesic-antipyretic activity in rats, *Pharmacologist*, **5**, 250.

BURNS, J. J., ROSE, R. K., GOODWIN, S., REICHENTHAL, J., HORNING, E. C., and BRODIE, B. B. (1955) The metabolic fate of phenylbutazone (Butazolidin) in man, *J. Pharmacol. exp. Ther.*, **113**, 481–9.

CONNEY, A. H., MICHAELSON, I. A., and BURNS, J. J. (1961) Stimulatory effect of chlorcyclizine on barbiturate metabolism, *J. Pharmacol. exp. Ther.*, **132**, 202–6.

COOPER, A. J., and ASHCROFT, G. (1966) Potentiation of insulin hypoglycaemia by MAOI antidepressant drugs, *Lancet*, **i**, 407–9.

COOPER, A. J., and KEDDIE, K. M. G. (1964) Hypotensive collapse and hypoglycaemia after mebanazine—a monoamine oxidase inhibitor, *Lancet*, **i**, 1133–5.

COUNCIL ON DRUGS (1963) Paradoxical hypertension from tranylcypromine sulfate, A Report of the Council on Drugs, *J. Amer. med. Ass.*, **186**, 854.

CUCINELL, S. A., CONNEY, A. H., SANSUR, M., and BURNS, J. J. (1965) Drug interactions in man, I. Lowering effect of phenobarbital on plasma levels of bishydroxycoumarin (Dicoumarol) and diphenylhydantoin (Dilantin), *Clin. Pharmacol. Ther.*, **6**, 420–9.

DAVIES, E. B. (1963) Tranylcypromine and cheese, *Lancet*, **ii**, 691–2.

DAYTON, P. G., TARCAN, Y., CHENKIN, T., and WEINER, M. (1961) The influence of barbiturates on coumarin plasma levels and prothrombin response, *J. clin. Invest.*, **40**, 1797–1802.

DOLLERY, C. T. (1965) Physiological and pharmacological interactions of antihypertensive drugs, *Proc. roy. Soc. Med.*, **58**, 983–90.

FOX, S. L. (1964) Potentiation of anticoagulants caused by pyrazole compounds, *J. Amer. med. Ass.*, **188**, 320–1.

GILLETTE, J. R. (1963) Metabolism of drugs and other foreign compounds by enzymatic mechanisms, *Fortschr. Arzneimittelforsch.*, **6**, 11–73.

HODDINOTT, B. C., GOWDEY, C. W., COULTER, W. K., and PARKER, J. M. (1967) Drug reactions and errors in administration on a medical ward, *Canad. med. Ass. J.*, **97**, 1001–6.

HORWITZ, D., LOVENBERG, W., ENGELMAN, K., and SJOERDS-MA, A. (1964) Monoamine oxidase inhibitors, Tyramine, and cheese, *J. Amer. med. Ass.*, **188**, 1108–10.

HURWITZ, N., and WADE, O. L. (1969) Intensive hospital monitoring of adverse reactions to drugs, *Brit. med. J.*, **1**, 531–6.

KOPIN, I. J., and AXELROD, J. (1963) The role of monoamine oxidase in the release and metabolism of norepinephrine, *Ann. N.Y. Acad. Sci.*, **107**, 848–55.

MACGREGOR, A. G. (1965) Review of points at which drugs can interact, *Proc. roy. Soc. Med.*, **58**, 943–6.

McCLURE, J. L. (1962) Reactions associated with tranyl-cypromine, *Lancet*, **i**, 1351.

MODELL, W. (1964) The extraordinary side-effects of drugs, *Clin. Pharmacol. Ther.*, **5**, 265–72.

NUESSLE, W. F., NORMAN, F. C., and MILLER, H. E. (1965) Pickled herring and tranylcypromine reaction, *J. Amer. med. Ass.*, **192**, 726–7.

OGILVIE, R. I., and RUEDY, J. (1967) Adverse drug reactions during hospitalization, *Canad. med. Ass. J.*, **97**, 1450–7.

PAYKEL, E. F. (1966) Hallucinosis on combined methyldopa and pargyline, *Brit. med. J.*, **1**, 803.

RANDALL, L. O. (1950) Anticurare action of phenolic quaternary ammonium salts, *J. Pharmacol. exp. Ther.*, **100**, 83–93.

Rossum, J. M. van (1963) Potential danger of mono-amineoxidase inhibitors and α methyldopa, *Lancet*, **i**, 950–1.

Seidl, L. G., Thornton, G. F., Smith, J. W., and Cluff, L. E. (1966) Studies on the epidemiology of adverse drug reactions, 111. Reactions in patients on a general medical service, *Bull. Johns. Hopk. Hosp.*, **119**, 299–315.

Sjöqvist, F. (1965) Psychotropic drugs, 2. Interaction between monoamine oxidase (MAO) inhibitors and other substances, *Proc. roy. Soc. Med.*, **58**, 967–78.

Smith, J. W., Seidl, L. G., and Cluff, L. E. (1966) Studies on the epidemiology of adverse drug reactions, V. Clinical factors influencing susceptibility, *Ann. intern. Med.*, **65**, 629–40.

Sulser, F., Bickel, M. H., and Brodie, B. B. (1964) The action of desmethylimipramine in counteracting sedation and cholinergic effects of reserpine-like drugs, *J. Pharmacol. exp. Ther.*, **144**, 321–30.

Symposium of the Royal Society of Medicine (1965) Clinical effects of interaction between drugs, *Proc. roy. Soc. Med.*, **58**, 943–98.

Thoburn, R., Johnson, J. E., and Cluff, L. E. (1966) Studies on the epidemiology of adverse drug reactions, IV. The relationship of cephalothin and penicillin allergy, *J. Amer. med. Ass.*, **198**, 345–8.

Verbov, J. L. (1968) Drug eruptions, *Brit. J. clin. Pract.*, **22**, 229–32.

Weiner, M., Siddiqui, A. A., Bostanci, M., and Dayton, P. G. (1965) Drug interactions: The effect of combined administration on the half-life of coumarin and pyrazolone drugs in man, *Fed. Proc.*, **24**, 153.

3

SKIN DISEASE

A. McQUEEN

Department of Dermatology University of Glasgow

Dermatologists have recognized the adverse effects of drugs on the skin for generations, and in the hey-day of Latin terminology they bestowed the diagnosis of 'dermatitis medicamentosa' or 'toxicoderma' on the unfortunate sufferers. The literature of dermatology at the turn of the century abounded with the detailed description of curious skin manifestations resulting from the use of the alkaloids and galenicals available at that time, and it is indeed a tribute to the powers of observation and correlation of these older practitioners that there was so clear an awareness of the possible range of medicament-induced rashes.

The skin in disease has a very limited range of reaction although manifestations of these reactions vary considerably. This is also the case with drug-induced skin diseases and today the recognition of a specific drug-induced skin disorder must still largely rely upon the simple clinical observation of patients under treatment. Studies in experimental animals are of limited value since it is difficult if not impossible to produce recognizable drug-induced skin changes in animals that simulate the multifarious lesions seen in man.

Iatrogenic dermatological reactions vary very considerably in site, extent and severity. In the Stevens-Johnson syndrome, for example, the condition is at first indistinguishable from erythema multiforme but rapidly progresses to a state where the skin is covered with lesions varying from vesicular to haemorrhagic, and the patient's life is in real danger. On the other hand, an injection of insulin may produce a mild urticaria which can easily be controlled by the use of antihistamines.

Any untoward drug reaction on the skin may mimic a classical skin disorder and dermatologists are very well aware of this. Likewise the General Practitioner knows that cutaneous eruptions are the most common indication of untoward reaction by the body to drugs. Furthermore, the same drug may produce different types of skin lesions in different people and these lesions may be modified by genetic or environmental factors as well as by current health status. Thus, a certain dose of belladonna will produce a scarlatiniform type of rash on the neck and upper trunk in some infants, whereas others will tolerate as much as twice that dose before erythema appears.

In general, cutaneous manifestations of drug toxicity abate when dosage is reduced or when the drug is withdrawn, although in some cases, for example 'arsenical dermatitis', there is a considerable delay before the skin resumes its normal appearance, and indeed if squamous carcinoma has resulted from the long-term use of arsenicals then the neoplastic process is intractable.

Skin lesions may be produced by topical or systemic administration of drugs and indeed the causative agent may not be recognized strictly as being a drug. 'Enema rash' is an example of this and was once common when soap and water enemas were routinely administered to patients being prepared for abdominal surgery. Today cases may be encountered in the domiciliary treatment of old people.

It is not always easy to define the pathogenesis of the skin reaction since precise knowledge of the specific mechanisms underlying the hypersensitivity reaction is far from complete. At best the mechanisms involved can be classified in a somewhat broad fashion (D'Arcy, 1965, 1966a) as toxicity, idiosyncrasy, allergy and photosensitivity.

The toxic mechanisms are dependent on the pharmacological properties of the drug, and the severity of the reaction is related to the dose; all persons are potentially susceptible, provided the dose is high enough. Idiosyncrasy is an inborn predisposition to respond to a specific stimulus in a qualitatively abnormal way independent of antigen-antibody reaction. Allergy is a true antigen-antibody reaction where the drug, if not already a protein, may combine with protein in the body to form an antigenic combination. The mechanism involved in photosensitivity may be similar since it has been suggested that the causative drugs, whose site of attack is the malpighian layer of the epidermis, are metabolized or conjugated with a protein in such a way as to form a photosensitizing substance with an absorption spectrum different from that of the administered drug.

An attempt has been made in this chapter to present the clinically more important and common examples of iatrogenic skin disease. For convenience and easy reference these have been classified in simple alphabetical order.

ACNEIFORM RASHES

The lesions of acne are well recognized and are typically seen between puberty and the age of about 25 when they tend to clear up spontaneously. The most striking abnormality is the presence of the comedo or blackhead accompanied by a varying degree of inflammatory changes in the subjacent pilo-sebaceous follicle which produces the swelling, followed by pitting of the skin surface as scarring takes place. The truly interesting feature of pure acne vulgaris is that it is only seen in the skin above the nipple line. A variety of drugs produce similar pustulo-nodular, swollen, rather umbilicated lesions which can, however, be differentiated from true acne by their absence of comedo formation, their atypical distribution, their abrupt onset, and often by their presence in older age groups.

The following drugs have all been implicated in the production of acneiform lesions which tend to regress on withdrawal or even adjustment of dosage: glucocorticoids, ACTH (Sullivan and Zeligman, 1956), androgens (Kennedy, 1965), bromides and iodides, isoniazid (Hesse, 1966), prothionamide, ethionamide (Lees, 1963), cyanocobalamin (Fellner and Baer, 1965) and the oxazolidine group of anticonvulsants, for example troxidone.

BULLOUS ERUPTIONS

A number of drugs may produce transient erythematous blistering eruptions; these bullae vary considerably in their extent, size, disposition, contents and degree of tension. Characteristic large bullae are found in about 6·5 per cent of cases of acute barbiturate poisoning [see PLATE 2A] and Beveridge and Lawson (1965) and Gröschel et al. (1970) have suggested that any unconscious patient displaying such bullae should be routinely screened for barbiturates. Bullae associated with barbiturates can occur during early or late stages of treatment and they have a tendency to heal with residual pigmentation. In this respect, it is well to recall that many intravenous anaesthetics are barbiturate derivatives and serious reactions can occur if they are used in sensitive patients.

Erythema multiforme can develop during the course of long-term sedation with chloral hydrate; bromides are more frequently implicated and with these the bullae may progress to involve the mucous membranes. Bullous lesions have been reported after the use of acetazolamide, the thiazide diuretics, sulphonamides and the phenazone-like antipyretic-analgesics. Salicylates are notoriously liable to lead to a number of severe skin reactions and these include bullous urticaria, bullous erythema multiforme and dermatitis-herpetiformis-like eruptions. Several cases of photosensitization and phototoxicity have been reported with the urinary antiseptic nalidixic acid; the lesions began as erythematous areas and progressed to frank bullous eruptions (Burry and Crosby, 1966; Mathew, 1966).

ERYTHEMA NODOSUM

These erythematous lesions are nodular and tender and generally occur on the shins of the legs, but occasionally elsewhere, varying in size from about 1–4 cm in diameter. They tend to resolve slowly over a few weeks undergoing a variety of colour changes as they do so, from red to bluish-green to blue and purple and eventually to a mottled brown which takes some time to disappear.

The basis of the lesion is probably a state of hypersensitivity affecting the vessels in the subcutaneous fat.

Drugs can produce identical skin changes and it is important to consider this probability in the differential diagnosis. Sporadic reports in the literature have held an assortment of drugs responsible, including sulphonamides, the sulphonylurea group of oral hypoglycaemics, penicillin, salicylates and thiouracil. Sudden withdrawal of corticosteroids has also been implicated (Browne, 1965) as also the use of oral contraceptives (Holcomb, 1965).

EXFOLIATIVE DERMATITIS

This is a generalized inflammatory skin disease; it is occasionally fulminating in onset and is characterized by redness, dryness and peeling of dry hyperkeratotic scales. Often there is considerable itching and irritation and secondary infection due to scratching is common. The nails and hair may also be affected with loss or damage to both.

The condition in its ripest form renders the patient very ill indeed (Abrahams et al., 1963) and the outcome may even be fatal (Rostenberg and Fagelson, 1965).

Over the past few years a number of reports have entered the literature of patients developing fatal exfoliative dermatitis consequent upon the use of many disparate drugs, so that the appearance of the disorder during any therapeutic regime must be regarded as an emergency. It should also be mentioned that other acute drug eruptions can develop into the picture of generalized exfoliative dermatitis. As with so many of the skin reactions to drugs, the number of drugs reported in association with this condition is large, but the most important of these include the antibiotics, especially the penicillins, arsenicals, barbiturates, chloroquine (Granirer, 1958), anticonvulsants, sulphonamides, griseofulvin (Goldblatt, 1961), mercurial diuretics, gold salts, immunological agents, thiouracil, phenothiazines and salicylates.

FIXED DRUG ERUPTIONS

A fixed drug eruption is a reaction in the skin to a drug which has reached it by way of the circulation. A localized skin lesion is produced rather suddenly and this usually subsides quickly when the drug is stopped, and reappears in an identical manner at the same site when drug treatment is renewed. It is often a diagnostic puzzle, since patients may be taking medicines of which the physician is unaware, and which may indeed seem harmless to both doctor and patient. The appearance of recurrent lesions with long intervals between may easily escape the attention of both parties and the significance of their relationship with drug therapy may be missed.

In appearance the lesion is that of a slightly raised reddish patch or cluster of macules which may feel hot or itchy or may evoke no subjective sensation at all. After each occurrence and disappearance, a little more reactive melanin is deposited in the upper dermis and basal layer of the epidermis, so that eventually there is a definite, though very slightly indurated area of pigmentation left.

Weiss and Kile (1935) described an unusual phenolphthalein-induced eruption and through the years this has been recognized as the classical example of a fixed drug eruption [see PLATE 2B], so much so in fact that any such eruption stimulates inquiry concerning the possible ingestion of proprietary laxatives containing phenolphthalein.

The number of drugs reported as being responsible for this type of eruption is dauntingly high; Welsh (1961) has produced an excellent survey of the field in his book *The Fixed Eruption* and Derbes (1964) implicated 57 drugs in this eruption. Today the count is well into the 80s and of these drugs the most important from the practical point of view are the antihistamines, barbiturates, anticonvulsants, penicillin, tetracyclines, sulphonamides, the rauwolfia alkaloids and a number of non-narcotic analgesics and antipyretic combinations containing aspirin and phenacetin.

HAIR DISORDERS

HAIR LOSS

Hair loss varying from thinning and glabrous patches to a total loss, usually from the scalp but on occasion from all the normally hirsute areas of the body, has been reported in connexion with a remarkable variety of drugs, many of which are in common use today.

In some instances hair loss may begin many weeks after administration of the incriminating agent, for example the anticoagulants and occasionally the antithyroid agents (Papadopoulos and Harden, 1966), while other drugs require only a few days before effects become noticeable, sometimes in a dramatic manner.

Ethionamide (Baran, 1966), clofibrate, vitamin A (Morrice *et al.*, 1960; Rook, 1965), and the oral contraceptives (Cormia, 1962; Vallings, 1965; Merklen and Melki, 1966; Peterkin and Khan, 1969) have all been reported as causal agents in greater or less degree. Other drugs implicated have included para-aminosalicylic acid (Griffiths and Watts, 1965), chloroquine, the proprietary preparation *Felsol* used in asthma (Chapman and Main, 1967), mephenesin, the anticonvulsant troxidone (trimethadione) (Holowach and Sanden, 1960), and nicotinyl alcohol (Zöllner and Gudenzi, 1966).

The most spectacular types of drug-induced alopecia, however, are seen in thallium poisoning and during treatment with the cytostatic drugs notably cyclophosphamide, melphalan and its *dl*-isomer merphalan

(sarcolysine), triethylenethiophosphoramide, triaziquone, hydroxyurea, a specific inhibitor of DNA synthesis, procarbazine, the antimetabolites 5-fluorouracil, 6-mercaptopurine, and methotrexate, the alkaloids colchicine, vinblastine, and vincristine, and the cytostatic antibiotic meractinomycin (dactionmycin, actinomycin D). With such agents distressing total baldness may occur rapidly and would seem to be dose-related, global in distribution but, curiously enough, reversible in most cases.

Although these effects are seen mainly during the treatment of neoplastic disorders, it should be remembered that other conditions, for example psoriasis, may be treated with drugs such as cyclophosphamide and that adjustment of dosage can usually mitigate the adverse effects of this therapy.

Allied to the production of alopecia by cytostatic drugs is that due to the effects of radiation; in these cases the hair follicles are destroyed and no regrowth of hair can be expected.

HIRSUTISM

Hypertrichosis occurs frequently during the systemic administration of corticosteroids, and in a large series of patients suffering from a variety of dermatological conditions, both hair loss and hypertrichosis have been attributed to the use of oral contraceptives (Merklen and Melki, 1966). The same curiously ambivalent kind of reaction has also been seen in patients treated with androgens or anabolic steroids as part of the virilizing effect associated with these hormones.

The virilizing effects seen in babies due to the maternal administration of some hormones may include a degree of hirsutism, as can also the use of the anticonvulsant diphenylhydantoin by pregnant women. This latter agent has also been reported as causing a generalized type of hypertrichosis in children and adults; fortunately, however, this regresses, albeit slowly, on cessation of treatment.

Chlorpromazine, in addition to producing amenorrhoea, weight increase and hyperactivity of the sebaceous glands in women patients, has also been implicated in hypertrichosis.

HAIR COLOUR

In view of the number of drugs which are associated with some disorder of skin pigmentation it is remarkable that so few appear to have noticeable effects on the colour of the hair. When colour change does occur it takes the form of depigmentation, resulting in a greying or a varying degree of bleaching of the hair. Haloperidol, a tranquillizer now in use in psychiatric units and in general practice, has been reported as having this side-effect (Simpson *et al.*, 1964), while chloroquine has been reported to have caused a lightening of hair colour in blonde, brunette and red-haired patients (Saunders *et al.*, 1959).

Mephenesin carbamate, which is used in the treatment of muscle spasm in rheumatic and neurological disorders, has been associated by Spillane (1963) with a number of cases in which loss of hair colour occurred in both male and female patients who had been taking the drug over a period of several months. Of interest is the fact that with three of these female patients hair colour was restored in 3 months after the drug was withdrawn.

Triparanol, formerly used as a cholesterol biosynthesis inhibitor, has been withdrawn from the market because of its association with the formation of irreversible cataracts. Among its other side-effects was a tendency to discolour the hair as well as causing a light-brown pigmentation of the skin (Winkelmann et al., 1963).

LUPUS ERYTHEMATOSUS

There are two schools of thought about drug-induced systemic lupus erythematosus. The first believes that the syndrome is quite distinct from the conventional L.E., whereas the second suggests that L.E. is latent in some patients and may be exhibited by certain drug therapy. Whatever the nature of this disorder a number of drugs have been implicated; Sternberg and Bierman (1963) have reported that 10 per cent of patients treated with hydrallazine for long periods suffered from lupus erythematosus. Similar reports have been made by Heine and Friedman (1962) in which it was suggested that L.E. induced by hydrallazine was associated with anti-hydrallazine antibodies.

A lupus-like illness has also been precipitated by procainamide (Ladd, 1962; Kaplan et al., 1965), and lupus-like syndromes have followed treatment with propylthiouracil (Best and Duncan, 1964), and with degraded tetracycline (Sulkowski and Haserick, 1964). A comprehensive review on drug-induced systemic lupus erythematosus has recently been published by Lee and Siegel (1968).

PHOTOSENSITIVITY

Photosensitivity has been reported as accompanying therapy with certain tetracyclines, sulphonamides, sulphonylurea derivatives, phenothiazines, thiazide diuretics, griseofulvin, chlorpromazine, chlordiazepoxide, pyridines, certain tar preparations and nalidixic acid. Recent reviews on drugs implicated in photosensitivity reactions have been published by Kirshbaum and Beerman (1964), and D'Arcy (1966).

Drug-induced photosensitivity, phototoxicity and photoallergy are of particular concern in tropical countries where climatic conditions and local customs permit large areas of the body to be exposed to strong and prolonged sunlight. They are also of equal concern in more temperate climates where a lesser degree of sunlight but perhaps a greater degree of medication may be experienced.

It has been suggested that the implicated drugs, whose site of action is in the malpighian layer of the epidermis, are metabolized or conjugated with protein in such a way as to form a photosensitizing substance. Discontinuation of the offending drug is usually followed by regression of the skin lesions.

These lesions vary from an exaggeration of the normal tanning and blistering effects associated with strong sunlight to oedema, flaking, eczema, maculopapular eruptions, urticaria and an appearance strikingly similar to contact dermatitis.

Although not strictly classified as photosensitizing agents, the psoralens, for example methoxsalen (8-methoxypsoralen), are examples of drugs producing intolerance to sunlight when taken orally or applied topically in the form of a cream or paint. Various psoralen-containing compounds have been used for centuries in Egypt to induce re-pigmentation of the skin in vitiligo or leucoderma; treatment is accompanied by exposure of the depigmented skin areas to sunlight rich in ultra violet rays. Frequently the successful course of such treatment depends entirely on the degree to which the patient can discipline himself to remain in the sun (D'Arcy, 1966). Such compounds have sometimes been used as suntan accelerators, often with disastrous and painful results.

PIGMENTATION

Disorders of skin pigmentation are well recognized in certain pathological conditions such as Addison's disease, haemochromatosis, the Peutz-Jeghers syndrome, pellagra, jaundice, Addisonian anaemia, vitiligo (leucoderma), pinta and albinism. However, it is probably true nowadays that, in terms of numbers of patients affected, drugs are responsible for the greater proportion of pigmentation disorders of skin seen in medical practice. This present section therefore deals with some of the known causal agents and applies in particular to effects seen in the white skin races. The various iatrogenic 'contact' types of pigmentation disorders have not been described since their causal relationships are generally self evident, while fixed drug eruptions and the effects of photosensitivity have already been discussed in this chapter.

OLDER REMEDIES (ARSENIC, GOLD AND SILVER SALTS)

Arsenic used to be a popular remedy for a variety of conditions but it is distinctly unfashionable at the present time. However, effects on the skin have been recognized in patients many years after use of the drug, and, of course, occupational hazards are still present in relation to arsenical compounds. In addition to their well documented association with carcinoma of the skin, arsenicals can produce a diffuse melanosis which occasionally is limited to the palms of the hands and the soles of the feet together with a flaking hyperkeratosis.

Gold salts are still in use today for the treatment of rheumatoid disorders and a rare complication of such treatment is chrysiasis. This is characterized by a grey-brown colour of the skin of exposed parts of the body and is due to the deposition of gold granules mainly within cells in the upper dermis. There is also a concomitant increase in the amount of melanin present in the dermis and epidermis.

The long-term use of silver salts causes a bluish-grey, slate-coloured or almost cyanotic discoloration of the skin which is most manifest in the exposed regions. Once seen this pigmentation is not readily forgotten. Histological examination of the skin in such cases shows an increase of melanin pigment in the papillary layer of the dermis and in the basal layer of the epidermis. The silver granules tend to be scattered through the tissue of the dermis rather than within cells, and have a tendency to aggregate around the eccrine sweat glands.

ANTIMALARIALS

Antimalarial drugs although not widely used as such in the United Kingdom, are sometimes prescribed for other conditions, and on occasion may produce colour changes in the skin. The best known is the yellowish hue, generalized in distribution, seen so frequently in troops stationed in malarial countries during the Second World War due to the prophylactic use of mepacrine (quinacrine), a feature also associated with amodiaquine, on occasion, to a lesser extent. In both cases the skin coloration gradually fades after the withdrawal of the drug. However, prolonged usage of these antimalarials may lead to a greenish-grey or bluish-black discoloration of the nail beds, nose and ears. Today the 4-aminoquinolines, notably chloroquine and hydroxychloroquine have replaced the earlier antimalarials and these too may produce colour changes in the skin ranging from grey to blue to black (Tuffanelli *et al.*, 1963), particularly on the face, the pretibial skin and the nail beds.

PHENOLPHTHALEIN

Phenolphthalein, taken regularly by many people for its laxative properties has been associated with distinctly dark grey patches on the skin, distinct from the fixed eruptions notoriously encountered during the use of the drug.

SULPHONES

In recent years leprosy has entered the differential diagnosis arena in some parts of this country. Sulphones such as dapsone and solapsone are used in the treatment of this condition and may lead to the 'fifth week dermatitis' from which may develop post-inflammatory hypermelanosis in the more severely affected parts of the skin.

CORTICOSTEROIDS AND ACTH

Long-term systemic dosage of corticosteroids has been known to lead to lessening of normal skin pigmentation, while ACTH may on occasion cause the development of deepening skin pigmentation similar in appearance to that seen in Addison's disease (Rosselin *et al.*, 1966).

ORAL CONTRACEPTIVES

As oral contraceptives have grown in popularity both in Europe and the United States many reports of associated chloasma have entered the literature (Resnik, 1967). Carruthers (1966), working in Australia, found that the incidence of this distressing complication increased markedly after 5 years of medication. It is disturbing to realize that no, or at best only part regression may occur after the drug is withdrawn, and, in some instances, recourse has to be made to masking applications to soothe the intense anxiety of women so afflicted.

HYDANTOIN ANTICONVULSANTS

An interesting possible side-effect of treatment with the hydantoin series of anticonvulsants is the occurrence of a similar state of chloasma as seen with oral contraceptives, and Kuske and Krebs (1964) have recorded 13 such cases, 10 of them women.

PHENOTHIAZINES

The phenothiazines have continued their popularity in general and psychiatric medicine, and over the past few years attention has been drawn to the unusual skin colour changes which may occur, particularly in patients treated for protracted periods of time (Greiner and Berry, 1964; Satanove, 1965). These colour changes are generally confined to light-exposed skin, but the precise mechanism of their production and the true importance of the effect of light cannot yet be clearly defined.

Chlorpromazine, still the most widely used, has been held responsible for hypermelanosis, bronzing of the skin, a grey hue, and even a purplish-grey appearance similar to cyanosis. Histochemistry has shown that much of the colour is due to melanin increase, but electron microscopy (Zelickson, 1965) has also revealed dense bodies in dermal phagocytes and blood vessel walls. These are believed to be related to degradation products of chlorpromazine, but the questions relating to pathogenesis remain unanswered. Oestrogen-like effects such as intense pigmentation of the breast areolae have been noted during treatment with phenothiazines, and, incidentally, also with griseofulvin (Durand *et al.*, 1964).

NON-BARBITURATE HYPNOTICS

Carbromal sometimes produces reddish-brown patches overlying petechial haemorrhages as part of a non-thrombocytopenic purpura syndrome. These lesions are strikingly similar in appearance to dermatitis lichenoides purpurica et pigmentosa.

Glutethimide may occasionally give rise to both rashes and brownish patches on the skin after prolonged use.

METHYSERGIDE

Methysergide, a drug used in the prophylaxis of migraine, gives rise to a large number of side-effects even at normal dosage, among which is the development of dermatitis and thickened 'orange peel' reddened skin (Graham, 1964).

CYTOSTATIC AGENTS

Cytostatic agents provide a harvest crop of skin reactions, and pigmentation disturbances are well represented among these. 6-Mercaptopurine and busulphan may each lead to deepening of the normal skin colour. This effect may occur early or late in treatment or at some time afterwards. The picture is similar to that seen in Addison's disease, but for some reason the mucous membranes usually escape involvement.

Triethylenethiophosphoramide on the other hand has been associated with loss of normal skin pigmentation (Tullis, 1958).

A deepening of melanin pigment is not unusual in patients having deep X-ray therapy.

VITAMINS

Vitamins are responsible for some effects on skin colour. High doses of vitamin A (e.g. 100,000–300,000 units) can result in signs of hypervitaminosis A. Skin changes occur early in the course of intoxication and may indeed be the only noticeable changes in some patients. Dryness and scaling of the lips are early symptoms and the skin becomes dry, itchy, shows flaking hyperkeratosis, and a distinct tanning effect occurs. Such effects are more readily appreciated in children given high daily doses of the vitamin, but they are also seen in adults, and are quickly reversible as soon as the one specific measure in treating the condition is applied, namely stopping the intake of vitamin A (Oliver, 1958).

Nicotinic acid, in addition to the expected flushing effect, can also cause a browning of the skin after lengthy administration. In rare, but disturbing instances, the picture of acanthosis nigricans may develop, presenting a strenuous exercise in diagnosis to the physician (Goldsmith, 1965).

PHENACETIN AND IRON (HAEMOCHROMATOSIS)

Since this slatey-bluish-grey discoloration has a striking appearance in the skin mention is made of this condition in this present context. Phenacetin may produce a haemolytic anaemia in patients who habitually ingest the drug, and this in turn can lead to the development of haemochromatosis which may closely mimic Addison's disease in its combination of pigmentation and hypotension (Messens, 1965).

Iron itself if administered to patients with haemolytic anaemia for lengthy periods may give rise to cirrhosis and hyperpigmentation of the skin (Pletcher *et al.*, 1963). Blood transfusions have likewise been held responsible for the appearance of exogenous haemochromatosis when given in large volumes over a period of time (Oliver, 1959).

PRURITUS

Pruritus, local or generalized, is more often associated with drug therapy than is currently realized. Sometimes the precursor of overt skin lesions, the symptom may exist by itself varying hourly or daily in intensity. Allergic reactions are the probable cause of pruritus, for example neomycin-induced eczema is often characterized by diffuse redness, scaling and pruritus; with streptomycin, skin hypersensitivity is usually characterized by intense itching and sometimes the allergic reactions may progress to generalized exfoliative dermatitis (McQueen, 1965); with chloramphenicol, the clinical symptoms of local hypersensitivity are itching at the site of application of the topical preparation and development within 6 hours of a typical allergic contact dermatitis. If the patient takes an oral dose of chloramphenicol then an inflammation of that part of the skin previously exposed to the antibiotic usually appears (Manten, 1968).

FIG. 3.1. *Alteration of status of normal bowel flora by antibiotics, for example tetracyclines*
(*from D'Arcy, P. F. (1965b) J. mond. Pharm. (La Haye),* **2–3,** 79–92).

The oral administration of the tetracycline antibiotics upsets the normal balance of the micro-organisms in the intestine. This may result in a severe superinfection associated with profuse diarrhoea. The major offenders are the yeasts and fungi, especially *Candida albicans,* which proliferate unchecked when the normal saprophytes in the gut are destroyed. The balance of intestinal non-pathogens may be restored by the administration of antifungal antibiotics notably nystatin and amphotericin B. Indeed some preparations, for example *Mysteclin* contain a combination of all three of these antibiotics.

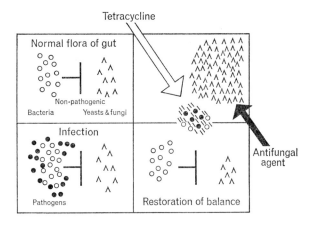

These antibiotics together with, for example, the penicillins and lincomycin are the prime offenders with regard to pruritus; the older drugs, codeine, arsenicals, bismuth, phenolphthalein and gold salts are occasionally implicated as also are the monoamine oxidase inhibitors, anticoagulants, oral contraceptives, oral hypoglycaemics, nicotinic acid, vitamin A, carbimazole, phenothiazine tranquillizers, methyprylone, imipramine, dichloralphenazone and other phenazone derivatives, and nalidixic acid.

Pruritus ani is a distressing and socially embarrassing condition which can be severe enough to deprive sufferers of sleep. Psychological factors undoubtedly play a great part in the initiation or maintenance of the itch, and when the itch cycle is established by whatever cause, it tends to be perpetuated by the emotional attitude of the patient. In bygone days, the 'toxic' or 'allergic' factor played by drugs was recognized and belladonna, morphine, and arsenic were well known as being capable of producing this symptom. Today, antibiotic-induced pruritus ani (Feinblatt and Feinblatt, 1960) is probably the most common type associated with drugs, and can often be ascribed to alteration of the status of the normal bowel flora by the antibiotic, either alone or in combined form [see Fig. 3.1].

The tetracyclines are the prime offenders in this respect and the pruritic reactions of vulva, vagina and perianal regions are usually due to an overgrowth of *Candida* species following suppression of the normal bacterial flora. Often the itch persists long after the drug has been withdrawn and may warrant further treatment which in itself may actually aggravate the situation. An example of this is the development of sensitivity to the ointment bases of topical preparations of corticosteroids, local anaesthetics, or antihistamines used to relieve the itch (Adriani, 1966).

Lincomycin, a basic sulphur-containing antibiotic useful in the treatment of Gram-positive infections, has been reported as causing pruritus ani (Kanee, 1965), proctitis, pruritus vulvae, rashes and urticaria. Some of these effects may have been due to drug allergy and others to superinfection with *Candida* or exacerbations of candidiasis (Council on Drugs, 1965).

PSORIASIS

Psoriasis is not one of the commoner iatrogenic skin diseases. However, cases have been reported following therapy with salicylates (Shelley, 1964), arsenic, gold salts, and antimalarial drugs (Kirschenbaum, 1963). An interesting report by Vickers and Sneddon, (1963) describes two patients who developed severe psoriasis following hypoparathyroidism produced by surgery, and who showed improvement after adjustment of the serum calcium in each case.

PURPURA

From the dermatological point of view purpura shows itself as petechial haemorrhages into the skin, and in the more serious cases actual ecchymoses may occur. A variety of drugs commonly prescribed in general practice may sometimes lead to any grade of this manifestation of adverse drug reaction.

A classical example of drug-induced purpura is that caused by the hypnotic apronal (apronalide, allylisopropylacetylurea). It has been suggested that platelet antibodies are formed and although apronal is relatively non-toxic in therapeutic doses, some persons show a marked idiosyncrasy to it and cases of thrombocytopenic purpura, some fatal, have been reported (Joekes and Leyden, 1938; Torrens, 1938; Miller and Rosenheim, 1938; Tatlow, 1948).

Two other urea-derivatives, the hypnotics carbromal and bromvaletone have also been associated with purpura, although with these it is of the non-thrombocytopenic type. These two hypnotics contain a bromine atom in an organic molecule, and this is thought to be the implicated radical.

The formation of platelet antibodies has been implicated in the occasional purpuric manifestations of hypersensitivity to such drugs as the amphetamines, digitoxin, phenacetin, tolbutamide, and even vitamin K. Known thrombocytopenic purpura has been attributed to hypersensitivity to chloramphenicol, and in the case report by Cahill (1962) a positive patch test was obtained to this antibiotic.

Two cases of thrombocytopenic purpura have been reported during treatment with the carbonic anhydrase inhibitor acetazolamide (Goerz *et al.*, 1964) which, formerly used as a diuretic, now finds use in reducing raised intraocular pressure. Anaphylactoid purpura may occur from the use of tetracyclines (Calnan and Lister, 1960) and purpuric eruptions are sometimes found in association with treatment by penicillin, sulphonamides, corticosteroids (Denko and Schroeder, 1957), chloroquine, colchicine (Sinaly, 1964), chloralhydrate, meprobamate, coumarin anticoagulants, and antithyroid drugs.

Of particular interest to the general practitioner is the possibility of purpuric eruptions occurring in newly-born babies as a result of medication of the mother by such drugs as quinine and thiouracil. Lastly, the possibility of purpuric eruptions of the skin arising as a result of the transfusion of stored blood should be borne in mind.

ROSACEA

There have been few reports of iatrogenic rosacea in the literature, but it has been associated with the use of oral contraceptive drugs (Ortiz, 1965), and infrequently with oral hypoglycaemic agents. Better known is the extension of an already existing rosacea by the topical application of fluorinated corticosteroids. Halogen derivatives taken internally may likewise aggravate this condition.

STEVENS-JOHNSON SYNDROME

An erythemato-bullous eruption of the erythema multiforme type, but presenting special and striking features, is seen occasionally. The onset is acute with fever which persists for 10–14 days; during this period the patient may be ill; a few cases have died. Rapid recovery follows the fall in temperature.

The cause of this condition is unknown, many cases are apparently idiopathic and it has long been associated with infections, pregnancy, food allergies, deep X-ray therapy and specific drug therapy (Rostenberg and Fagelson, 1965). The drugs especially implicated in this syndrome are sulphonamides (Bowell, 1965), barbiturates, chloramphenicol and some other antibiotics, diphenylhydantoin (Bray, 1959, Watts, 1962), chlorpropamide (Tullett, 1966), meprobamate, carbamazepine (Coombes, 1965), and thiacetazone (amithiozone).

TOXIC EPIDERMAL NECROLYSIS (LYELL'S DISEASE)

In this condition [see PLATE 2C] the skin becomes red, it loosens and is exquisitely tender presenting an appearance rather like scalded skin, although unlike scalds the skin heals without scar formation. The condition can be fatal. Causes besides drugs are known, but the drugs associated with this syndrome are hydantoins, phenylbutazone, sulphonamides, penicillin, barbiturates, antibiotics, phenolphthalein, nitrofuran derivatives, sulphones and antipyrine (Lyell, 1956; Jarkowski and Martmer, 1962; Bailey et al., 1965; Carpentier, 1965; Srivastava and Gour, 1966).

TUBEROSE LESIONS

These can be difficult to diagnose although fortunately they tend to occur as a number of lesions rather than being solitary. Bromides provide the classical type of lesion simulating tumours; the lesions are warty and mostly occur on the extremities. Their tumour-like appearance is due to a combination of papillomatosis and pseudo-epitheliomatous hyperplasia often showing some degree of secondary infection. Similar granulomatous lesions are seen occasionally as a result of iodide reaction. The gingival hyperplasia associated occasionally with phenytoin derivatives [see PLATE 2D] is too well known to warrant other than mention here.

Arsenic, while notorious for its production of arsenical keratosis, can and does on occasion proceed to actual squamous cell carcinoma, and it is of interest that in such lesions the arsenical content of the tumour can usually be demonstrated by histochemical methods.

What is fortunately a rare occurrence nowadays is the type of skin carcinoma following perhaps years after radiotherapy. Keloid formation has been seen from time to time after radiotherapy, but is perhaps more seen in this country in children as a late, rare effect of various vaccination procedures.

URTICARIA

This is one of the commonest adverse drug reactions and consists of localized patchy, or generalized single or cropping, erythematous lesions which vary from the 'heat spot' type to large wheals. In some cases the lesions are confluent and occasionally they form actual blisters or bullae. These lesions are intensely itchy and in diffuse urticaria the patient may feel that his skin is about to burst. Taken together, the picture is one of an acute hypersensitivity reaction, which, particularly in the case of injected drugs, occurs very rapidly after the administration of the offending agent.

Some cases, mild to moderate in nature, respond well to oral antihistaminics, while the more serious types, which include angioneurotic oedema, require immediate injection of adrenaline, antihistamine, or corticosteroid followed by oral therapy as necessary. The anaphylactic nature of some of these reactions is such that life is threatened, and they must therefore be treated as emergencies. In a recent paper, Montgomery and Jackson (1968) listed 100 consecutive patients with drug reactions in their dermatological practice over a period of seven months; urticaria headed that list with 28 patients, exceeding by 12 its nearest competitor.

The drugs in common use which lead to urticarial reactions are numerous and include the barbiturates, salicylates, penicillin and other antibiotics, sulphonamides, some of the tranquillizing drugs, insulin and nalidixic acid.

It should also be remembered that any vaccination procedure or desensitizing therapy for allergic disorders may bring about an allergic type of reaction, the common skin manifestation of which is a varying degree of urticaria. For this reason suitable precautions should be observed and the availability of emergency treatment checked before the injection is given.

RECOMMENDED FURTHER READING

BROWNE, S. G. (1964) Fixed eruptions in deeply pigmented subjects; clinical observations on 350 patients, Brit. med. J., 2, 1041–4.
CARROLL, O. M., BRYAN, P. A., and ROBINSON, R. J. (1968) Stevens-Johnson syndrome and long-acting sulfonamides, in Drug-Induced Diseases, Vol. 3, eds. Meyler, L., and Peck, H. M., Excerpta Medica Foundation, Amsterdam, pp. 165–9.
D'ARCY, P. F. (1966) The pharmacology of drug-cosmetics, American Perfumer and Cosmetics, 81, 45–50.
WADE, O. L. (1970) Adverse Reactions to Drugs, London.

REFERENCES

ABRAHAMS, I., McCARTHY, J. T., and SANDERS, S. L. (1963) One hundred and one cases of exfoliative dermatitis, Arch. Derm., 87, 96–101.
ADRIANI, J. (1966) Reactions to local anesthetics, J. Amer. med. Ass., 196, 405–8.
BAILEY, G., ROSENBAUM, J. M., and ANDERSON, B. (1965)

Toxic epidermal necrolysis, *J. Amer. med. Ass.*, **191**, 979–82.

BARAN, R. (1966) Les accidents cutanéo-muqueuses de l'ethionamide, *Hôpital* (*Paris*), **54**, 445.

BEST, M. M., and DUNCAN, C. H. (1964) A lupus-like syndrome following propylthiouracil administration, *J. Ky. med. Ass.*, **62**, 47–9.

BEVERIDGE, G. W., and LAWSON, A. A. (1965) Occurrence of bullous lesions in acute barbiturate intoxication, *Brit. med. J.*, **1**, 835–7.

BOWELL, G. R. (1965) Stevens-Johnson syndrome and long acting sulphonamides, *Aust. dent. J.*, **10**, 85.

BRAY, P. F. (1959) Diphenylhydantoin (dilantin) after 20 years; a review with re-emphasis by treatment of 84 patients, *Pediatrics*, **23**, 151–61.

BROWNE, S. G. (1965) Nodular panniculitis and peripheral neuropathy following sudden withdrawal of corticosteroids (poststeroid nodular panniculitis), *Int. J. Leprosy*, **33**, 893–5.

BURRY, J. N., and CROSBY, R. W. L. (1966) A case of phototoxicity to nalidixic acid, *Med. J. Aust.*, **2**, 698–700.

CAHILL, K. M. (1962) Chloramphenicol hypersensitivity: A severe haemorrhagic reaction, *Lancet*, **ii**, 277–8.

CALNAN, C. D., and LISTER, D. J. (1960) Anaphylactoid purpura from tetracycline, *Trans. St. John's Hosp. derm. Soc.* (*Lond.*), **44**, 69–72.

CARPENTIER, E. (1965) A case of Lyell's syndrome, *Arch. belges Derm.*, **21**, 363–5.

CARRUTHERS, R. (1966) Chloasma and oral contraceptives, *Med. J. Aust.*, **2**, 17–20.

CHAPMAN, R. S., and MAIN, R. A. (1967) Diffuse thinning of hair in iodine-induced hypothyroidism, *Brit. J. Derm.*, **79**, 103–5.

COOMBES, B. W. (1965) Stevens-Johnson syndrome associated with carbamazepin ('Tegretol'), *Med. J. Aust.*, **1**, 895–6.

CORMIA, F. E. (1962) Alopecia from oral contraceptives, *J. Amer. med. Ass.*, **201**, 635–7.

COUNCIL ON DRUGS (1965) A new antibiotic. Lincomycin (Lincocin), A Report of the Council on Drugs, *J. Amer. med. Ass.*, **194**, 545.

D'ARCY, P. F. (1965a) The pharmacological basis of drug treatment in dermatology, *Pharm. J.*, **194**, 637–43.

D'ARCY, P. F. (1965b) How drugs act, *J. mond. Pharm.* (*La Haye*), 2–3, 79–92.

D'ARCY, P. F. (1966) The sun and the skin, *Pharm. J.*, **196**, 477–81.

DENKO, C. W., and SCHROEDER, L. R. (1957) Ecchymotic skin lesions in patients receiving prednisone, *J. Amer. med. Ass.*, **164**, 41–3.

DERBES, V. J. (1964) The fixed eruption, *J. Amer. med. Ass.*, **190**, 765–6.

DURAND, P., BORRONE, C., SCARABICCHI, S., and RAZZI, A. (1964) Hyperpigmentation of breast areolae and external genitals with gynaecomastia following griseofulvin treatment, *Minerva med.*, **55**, 2422–5.

FEINBLATT, T. M., and FEINBLATT, H. M. (1960) Antibiotic induced rectal itch (Pruritus ani) treated with amino acid ointment, *Gastroenterology*, **38**, 247–9.

FELLNER, M. J., and BAER, R. L. (1965) Cutaneous reactions to drugs: With particular reference to penicillin sensitivity, *Med. Clin. N. Amer.*, **49**, 709–24.

GOERZ, G., IPPEN, H., and MEIERS, H. G. (1964) Sulfonamid-Uberempfindlichkeit. Gekreuzte Reaktionen zwischen anti-. bakteriellen Sulfonamiden und Diuretika, *Dtsch. med. Wschr.*, **89**, 1301–3.

GOLDBLATT, S. (1961) Severe reaction to griseofulvin. Sensitivity investigation, *Arch. Derm. Syph.* (*Chic.*), **83**, 936–7.

GOLDSMITH, G. A. (1965) Niacin: Antipellagra factor, hypocholesterolemic agent: Model of nutrition research yesterday and today, *J. Amer. med. Ass.*, **194**, 167–73.

GRAHAM, J. R. (1964) Methysergide for prevention of headache, *New Engl. J. Med.*, **270**, 67–72.

GRANIRER, L. W. (1958) Exfoliative dermatitis as a complication of chloroquine (Aralen) therapy in rheumatoid arthritis, *Arch. Derm.*, **77**, 722–4.

GREINER, A. C., and BERRY, K. (1964) Skin pigmentation and corneal and lens opacities with prolonged chlorpromazine therapy, *Canad. med. Ass. J.*, **90**, 663–5.

GRIFFITHS, H. E., and WATTS, C. (1965) Hypersensitivity to para-aminosalicylic acid; a hazard in the treatment of orthopaedic tuberculosis, *J. Bone Jt. Surg.*, **47**, 86–90.

GRÖSCHEL, D., GERSTEIN, A. R., and ROSENBAUM, J. M. (1970) Skin lesions as a diagnostic aid in barbiturate poisoning, *New Engl. J. Med.*, **283**, 409–10.

HEINE, W. I., and FRIEDMAN, H. (1962) Hydralazine lupus syndrome associated with a possible antihydralazine antibody, *J. Amer. med. Ass.*, **182**, 726–9.

HESSE, P. G. (1966) Die antituberkulöse Therapie und das akneiform Exanthem, *Derm. Wschr.*, **152**, 305–12.

HOLCOMB, F. D. (1965) Erythema nodosum associated with the use of an oral contraceptive. Report of a case, *Obstet. and Gynec.*, **25**, 156–7.

HOLOWACH, J., and SANDEN, H. V. (1960) Alopecia as a side effect of treatment of epilepsy with trimethadione: Report of two cases, *New Engl. J. Med.*, **263**, 1187.

JARKOWSKI, T. L., and MARTMER, E. E. (1962) Fatal reaction to sulphadimethoxine ('Madribon'). A case showing toxic epidermal necrolysis and leukopenia, *Amer. J. Dis. Child.*, **104**, 669–74.

JOEKES, T., and LEYDEN, M. B. (1938) Purpura haemorrhagica (Werlhof) after taking 'Sedormid', *Lancet*, **ii**, 305–6.

KANEE, B. (1965) Lincomycin in dermatological practice, *Canad. med. Ass. J.*, **93**, 220–2.

KAPLAN, J. M., WACHTEL, H. L., CZARNECKI, S. W., and SAMPSON, J. J. (1965) Lupus-like illness precipitated by procainamide hydrochloride, *J. Amer. med. Ass.*, **192**, 444–7.

KENNEDY, B. J. (1965) Systemic effects of androgenic and estrogenic hormones in advanced breast cancer, *J. Amer. Geriat. Soc.*, **13**, 230–5.

KIRSHBAUM, B. A., and BEERMAN, H. (1964) Photosensitization due to drugs: A review of some of the recent literature, *Amer. J. med. Sci.*, **248**, 445–68.

KIRSCHENBAUM, M. B. (1963) Psoriasis following administration of antimalarial drugs, *J. Amer. med. Ass.*, **185**, 1044.

KUSKE, H., and KREBS, A. (1964) Chloasma-type hyperpigmentation after treatment with hydantoin preparations, *Dermatologica* (*Basel*), **129**, 121–39.

LADD, A. T. (1962) Procainamide induced lupus erythematosus, *New Engl. J. Med.*, **267**, 1357–8.

LEE, S. L., and SIEGEL, M. (1968) Drug-induced systemic lupus erythematosus, in *Drug-Induced Diseases*, Vol. 3, eds. Meyler, L., and Peck, H. M., Excerpta Medica Foundation, Amsterdam, pp. 239–48.

LEES, A. W. (1963) Toxicity in newly diagnosed cases of pulmonary tuberculosis treated with ethionamide, *Amer. Rev. resp. Dis.*, **88**, 347–54.

LYELL, A. (1956) Toxic epidermal necrolysis: Eruption resembling scalding of skin, *Brit. J. Derm.*, **68**, 355–61.

MANTEN, A. (1968) Antibiotic drugs, in *Side Effects of Drugs*, Vol. VI, eds. Meyler, L., and Herxheimer, A., Excerpta Medica Foundation, Amsterdam, p. 287.

MATHEW, T. H. (1966) Nalidixic acid, *Med. J. Aust.*, **2**, 243–4.

McQueen, E. G. (1965) Allergic reaction to streptomycin, *N.Z. med. J.*, **64**, 663.

Merklen, F. P., and Melki, G. R. (1966) Incidences dermatologiques de contraceptifs oraux, *Bull. Acad. nat. Méd. (Paris)*, **150**, 624–32.

Messens, Y. (1965) A propos d'un cas d'intoxication chronique par la phénacétine, *Rev. méd. Liège*, **20**, 516–22.

Miller, C., and Rosenheim, M. L. (1938) Purpura after taking Sedormid, *Lancet*, **ii**, 402.

Montgomery, D. C., and Jackson, R. (1968) One hundred consecutive patients with drug reactions, *Canad. med. Ass. J.*, **99**, 712–14.

Morrice, G., Jr., Havener, W. H., and Kapetansky, F. (1960) Vitamin A intoxication as a cause of pseudotumor cerebri, *J. Amer. med. Ass.*, **173**, 1802–5.

Oliver, R. A. M. (1959) Siderosis following transfusions of blood, *J. Path. Bact.*, **77**, 171–94.

Oliver, T. K., Jr. (1958) Chronic vitamin A intoxication. Report of a case in an older child and review of the literature, *Amer. J. Dis. Child.*, **95**, 57–68.

Ortiz, Y. (1965) Anovulatorias, *Dermatologia (Méx.)*, **9**, 63.

Papadopoulos, S., and Harden, R. McG. (1966) Hair loss in patients treated with carbimazole, *Brit. med. J.*, **2**, 1502–3.

Peterkin, G. A. G., and Khan, S. A. (1969) Iatrogenic skin disease, *Practitioner*, **202**, 117–26.

Pletcher, W. D., Brody, G. L., and Meyers, M. C. (1963) Hemochromatosis following prolonged iron therapy in a patient with hereditary nonspherocytic hemolytic anemia, *Amer. J. med. Sci.*, **246**, 27–34.

Resnik, S. (1967) Melasma induced by oral contraceptive drugs, *J. Amer. med. Ass.*, **199**, 601–5.

Rook, A. (1965) Some chemical influences on hair growth and pigmentation, *Brit. J. Derm.*, **77**, 115–29.

Rosselin, G., Assan, R., Tchobroutsky, G., and Pignard, P. (1966) L'ACTH plasmatique, I. Biochimie; exploration cortico-surrénale; propriétés antigéniques, *Presse méd.*, **74**, 813–18.

Rostenberg, A., Jr., and Fagelson, H. J. (1965) Life-threatening drug eruptions, *J. Amer. med. Ass.*, **194**, 660–2.

Satanove, A. (1965) Pigmentation due to phenothiazines in high and prolonged dosage, *J. Amer. med. Ass.*, **191**, 263–8.

Saunders, T. S., Fitzpatrick, T. B., Seiji, M., Brunet, P., and Rosenbaum, E. E. (1959) Decrease in human hair color and feather pigment of fowl following chloroquine diphosphate, *J. invest. Derm.*, **33**, 87–90.

Shelley, W. B. (1964) Birch pollen and aspirin psoriasis. A study in salicylate hypersensitivity, *J. Amer. med. Ass.*, **189**, 985–8.

Simpson, G. M., Blair, J. H., and Cranswick, E. H. (1964) Cutaneous effects of a new butyrophenone drug, *Clin. Pharmacol. Ther.*, **5**, 310–21.

Sinaly, N. P. (1964) Vascular purpura due to colchicine in a patient with gout, *Ann. intern. Med.*, **60**, 470–3.

Spillane, J. D. (1963) Brunette to blonde: Depigmentation of human hair during oral treatment with mephenesin, *Brit. med. J.*, **1**, 997–1000.

Srivastava, B. N., and Gour, K. A. (1966) Cutaneous manifestations of drug toxicity, *Indian Practit.*, **19**, 465–73.

Sternberg, T. H., and Bierman, S. M. (1963) Unique syndromes involving skin induced by drugs, food additives and environmental contaminants, *Arch. Derm. Syph. (Chic.)*, **88**, 779–88.

Sulkowski, S. R., and Haserick, J. R. (1964) Simulated systemic lupus erythematosus from degraded tetracycline, *J. Amer. med. Ass.*, **189**, 152–4.

Sullivan, M., and Zeligman, I. (1956) Acneiform eruption due to corticotropin, *Arch. Derm.*, **73**, 133–41.

Tatlow, W. F. T. (1948) Acute purpura with neurological complications associated with 'Sedormid' therapy, *Brit. med. J.*, **2**, 558–9.

Torrens, J. (1938) Purpura following Sedormid, *Lancet*, **i**, 749.

Tuffanelli, D., Abraham, R. K., and Dubois, E. I. (1963) Pigmentation from antimalarial therapy. Its possible relationship to the ocular lesions, *Arch. Derm. Syph. (Chic.)*, **88**, 419–26.

Tullett, G. L. (1966) Fatal case of toxic erythema after chlorpropamide (Diabinese), *Brit. med. J.*, **1**, 148.

Tullis, J. L. (1958) Triethylenephosphoramide in the treatment of disseminated melanoma, *J. Amer. med. Ass.*, **166**, 37–41.

Vallings, R. (1965) Oral contraceptives and alopecia areata, *Brit. med. J.*, **2**, 1005.

Vickers, H. R., and Sneddon, I. B. (1963) Psoriasis and hypoparathyroidism, *Brit. J. Derm.*, **35**, 419–21.

Watts, J. C. (1962) Fatal case of erythema multiforme exudativum (Stevens-Johnson syndrome) following therapy with Dilantin, *Pediatrics*, **30**, 592–4.

Weiss, R. S., and Kile, R. L. (1935) Unusual phenolphthalein eruption. Report of a case, *Arch. Derm. Syph. (Berl.)*, **32**, 915–21.

Welsh, A. L. (1961) *The Fixed Eruption*, Springfield, Illinois.

Winkelmann, R. K., Perry, H. O., Achor, R. W., and Kirby, T. J. (1963) Cutaneous syndromes produced as side effects of triparanol therapy, *Arch. Derm. Syph. (Chic.)*, **87**, 372–7.

Zelickson, A. S. (1965) Skin pigmentation and chlorpromazine, *J. Amer. med. Ass.*, **194**, 670–2.

Zöllner, N., and Gudenzi, M. (1966) Behandlung der Hypercholesterinämie mit Beta-Pyridylkarbinol, II. Nebenwirkungen und Diskussion, *Med. Klin.*, **61**, 2036–40.

4

BLOOD DYSCRASIAS

Six types of adverse reaction to drugs may occur in the haemopoietic system. These are haemolytic anaemia, aplastic anaemia (pancytopenia), megaloblastic anaemia, granulocytopenia, followed if unrecognized by the syndrome of agranulocytosis, thrombocytopenia and erythroid hypoplasia without changes in platelets or leucocytes (Wintrobe, 1969).

DRUG-INDUCED HAEMOLYTIC ANAEMIA

It has long been known that when certain ordinarily harmless drugs are administered to some individuals an acute haemolytic anaemia results. Cases of drug-induced haemolytic anaemia fall into several categories; some have been associated with drugs that have oxidant properties, others depend on one of a number of immunological effects.

Certain antipyretics, sulphonamides, pamaquin and other antimalarials of the 8-aminoquinoline group fall into the first category. Haemolysis can be induced in many individuals if very large doses are given, but in certain instances the administration of normal doses is accompanied by accelerated red cell destruction. Susceptibility to haemolysis by ordinary doses of these drugs usually depends on a deficiency of the enzyme glucose-6-phosphate dehydrogenase (G-6-PD). Wintrobe (1967) has described the biochemical basis of the

haemolytic anaemia that ensues. Wintrobe (1969) has, however, emphasized that instances of haemolytic anaemia following administration of customary doses of these drugs are not limited to patients with G-6-PD deficiency. Haemolytic anaemia may develop on exposure to oxidant drugs in persons who, for example, inherit erythrocyte glutathione (GSH) reductase deficiency, erythrocyte GSH deficiency or the haemoglobinopathy associated with haemoglobin Zurich, also haemoglobin-H disease and possibly other unstable haemoglobins may be implicated.

A list of these haemolytic oxidant drugs is given in TABLE 4.1. In this present context discussion on the haemolytic anaemia caused by this group of drugs will be confined to the antimalarial primaquine and its association with G-6-PD deficiency.

PRIMAQUINE AND GLUCOSE-6-PHOSPHATE DEHYDROGENASE DEFICIENCY

An opportunity arose to study sensitivity to a drug-induced haemolytic anaemia in greater detail than had previously been possible when the Army Malaria Research Unit at Stateville Penitentiary, Illinois, undertook to investigate the haemolytic effect of the antimalarial drug, primaquine. Since this work presents an almost classic study to determine the precise nature of drug-induced haemolytic anaemia, it is reported in some detail in this chapter.

Primaquine is the most successful of the 8-aminoquinoline antimalarials; it was introduced into medicine about 1945 and is a very close chemical relative of pamaquin, the first successful synthetic antimalarial drug which was introduced in 1926 and is now obsolete.

In common with the other members of its series primaquine has cumulative toxic effects which have tended to prevent its widespread use. Gastro-intestinal upsets and blood dyscrasias (methaemoglobinaemia and leucopenia) are common; the most serious hazard is, however, acute haemolytic anaemia. Such haemolytic crises occur more frequently in dark-skinned and Mediterranean races. This sensitivity is linked with genetically transmitted abnormalities of the erythrocytes, the most characteristic of which is a deficiency in the enzyme glucose-6-phosphate dehydrogenase (G-6-PD). Vella and Ibrahim (1962) have recorded the incidence of G-6-PD deficiency in certain African and Middle East countries; their data tabulated in TABLE 4.2 gives a good indication of the widespread incidence of this defect, which is all the more important and

TABLE 4.1

DRUGS HAVING OXIDANT PROPERTIES ASSOCIATED WITH HAEMOLYTIC ANAEMIA
(Based on Wintrobe, 1969)

CLASS OF DRUG	MEMBERS
Antimalarials (8-amino-quinolines)	primaquine pamaquin mepacrine (quinacrine)
Sulphonamides	sulphanilamide (sulfabenz) sulphapyridine sulphasoxazole sulphamethoxypyridazine
Nitrofurans	nitrofurantoin nitrofurazone furazolidone
Sulphones	dapsone (diaminodiphenyl-sulphone) solapsone
Probenecid	
Vitamin K (water-soluble derivatives)	potassium menaphthosulphate menazodime menadiol sodium diphosphate
Acetylphenylhydrazine	formerly in use as an anti-pyretic (hydracetin, pyrodin)
Cinchona alkaloids	quinine, quinidine

TABLE 4.2

INCIDENCE OF GLUCOSE-6-PHOSPHATE
DEHYDROGENASE DEFICIENCY IN ARAB AND
AFRICAN SUBJECTS
(after Vella and Ibrahim, 1962)

COUNTRY	INCIDENCE per cent
Congo	3–30
East Africa and Tanganyika	2–28
Gambia	15
Ghana	24
Nigeria	6–17
Northern Nigeria	21
Palestine (Arab)	3·4
South Africa (Bantu)	3
Sudan (Arab)	
adults	8·1
newborn (umbilical cord)	7·3

serious since it occurs in those subjects who are living in areas where prophylaxis or treatment of malaria is an everyday occurrence.

When a daily dose of 30 mg of primaquine is given to sensitive individuals, there is no untoward reaction for about three days. Then the urine begins to darken, the haemoglobin level, red cell count and haematocrit fall, the reticulocyte count increases, Heinz bodies appear in the erythrocytes, and the patient feels ill (Beutler, 1959). In the more severe type of reaction, haemolysis is almost explosive; there is, in addition, haemoglobinaemia and immediate transfusions are necessary (Hockwald *et al.*, 1952). If, in spite of these reactions, primaquine therapy is continued, the haemo- lytic symptoms continue for about a week and then the patient slowly recovers. After about a month, during which time red cell production is speeded up to com- pensate for the haemolytic episode, the various blood parameters return to normal again. This 'self-limiting' nature of drug-induced haemolytic anaemia is charac- teristic of the disease (Dern *et al.*, 1954*a*). If therapy is stopped for a month or two and then resumed, a new haemolytic episode is observed similar in onset and in nature to the original episode. Once a self-limiting stage has been reached, an increase in the dose may induce further haemolysis for a period, until a new self-limiting phase is attained.

Clearly, the haemolysis could be caused either by factors present in the plasma which, in association with drugs, affect the erythrocyte, or by a defect in the erythrocyte itself. To resolve this point, washed red cells from both sensitive and non-sensitive individuals were 'tagged' with radioactive chromium Cr^{51} and transfused into compatible recipients (Dern *et al.*, 1954*b*). Red cells from sensitive individuals were haemolyzed in the circulations of recipients receiving primaquine irrespec- tive of whether the recipients were themselves sensitive or not. Conversely, red cells from non-sensitive donors were not haemolyzed, even when in the circulations of primaquine-treated individuals whose own red cells were being destroyed. Thus it became plain that drug- induced haemolysis was entirely a defect of the erythro- cyte itself.

By administering radioactive iron Fe^{59} for a short period, new red cells marked with this tracer were produced in susceptible individuals. A two-week course of primaquine administered to these subjects shortly afterwards, induced the expected haemolytic episode but the young labelled cells (8 to 21 days of age) were not haemolyzed. However, 55 days later these labelled cells were rapidly destroyed when primaquine was given again (Beutler *et al.*, 1954). Thus, only the older cells were lysed in a haemolytic episode, and the self-limiting phase of the disease occurred when the erythrocyte population was reduced to the younger cells.

When primaquine treatment was continued, the cells haemolyzed at about 60 days of age; however, this degree of destruction (1·7 per cent per day) was not distinguishable clinically from the normal rate (0·8 per cent per day) of red cell breakdown; a raised level of red cell production prevented anaemia. Even in the absence of drugs, the erythrocytes of sensitive subjects lyse at about 90 days of age instead of the normal 120–130 days. They are therefore undergoing a chronic haemolysis without anaemia (Brewer *et al.*, 1962).

Heinz bodies (granular inclusions) are formed in the red cells of susceptible patients when treated with haemolytic anaemia-producing drugs and this forma- tion precedes by a day or two the haemolytic episode. Indeed recognition of Heinz bodies can be used to predict haemolysis. Beutler and colleagues (1955) in *in vitro* studies showed that various substances, particularly acetylphenylhydrazine, induced the formation of many small Heinz bodies when incubated with susceptible erythrocytes. By this means a fairly reliable test was developed to detect sensitive individuals.

Other physiological and biochemical characteristics of the abnormal (i.e. susceptible) red cells have also been studied. Beutler *et al.* (1955) found that the con- centration of reduced glutathione (GSH) was only about 60 per cent of normal in sensitive red cells, and incubation of these cells for a few hours with acetyl- phenylhydrazine produced a further decrease in the GSH concentration. Similar incubation of normal red cells hardly affected the GSH concentration. This *in vitro* technique, the glutathione stability test, has been found to be a simple and useful way of screening for sensitive individuals. Flanagan *et al.* (1958), in *in vitro* studies, showed that a decreased GSH concentration occurred in erythrocytes of sensitive patients treated with pamaquin, even before the development of Heinz bodies.

Glucose-6-phosphate dehydrogenase deficiency is a further characteristic of the abnormal erythrocyte and the importance of this deficiency can only be fully understood if mention is made of the role of this enzyme in the red cell. Parr (1962) has included discussion on this deficiency in his comprehensive review on drug- induced haemolytic anaemia.

Oxidation of GSH (reduced glutathione) results in loss of the sulphydryl grouping and a linking together of pairs of glutathione molecules by a disulphide linkage to form oxidized glutathione (GSSG). There is an enzyme system present in red cells, glutathione reductase, which will reduce any GSSG which may happen to be formed, provided there is a supply of reduced nicotinamide adenine dinucleotide phosphate (reduced NADP) present. This can be represented in the following formula:

$$GSSG + \text{reduced NADP} \rightarrow 2\,GSH + NADP$$
$$\ldots \text{Reaction (1)}$$

Two dehydrogenases are known to function in erythrocytes and to produce reduced NADP, acting on the substrates glucose-6-phosphate (G-6-P) and 6-phosphogluconate (6-P-G) respectively. These reactions can be represented as follows:

$$G\text{-}6\text{-}P + NADP \rightarrow 6\text{-}P\text{-}G + \text{reduced NADP}$$
$$\ldots \text{Reaction (2)}$$

$$6\text{-}P\text{-}G + NADP \rightarrow \text{ribulose 5-phosphate} + CO_2$$
$$+ \text{reduced NADP}$$
$$\ldots \text{Reaction (3)}$$

As may be seen from the formula, 6-P-G, the product of Reaction (2), is the substrate for Reaction (3), so that the latter reaction is dependent upon the former. These two reactions (2 and 3) direct carbohydrate metabolism along the oxidative pentose phosphate pathway, which is an alternative metabolic route to the anaerobic glycolytic sequence.

In 1956, Carson and associates showed that whereas both Reaction (1), GSSG reductase, and Reaction (3), 6-P-G dehydrogenase, were about normal in erythrocytes from primaquine sensitive individuals, there was a marked deficiency in the activity of Reaction (2), G-6-P dehydrogenase, in these cells. There are several good methods for the assay of G-6-P dehydrogenase in haemolysates, for example those of Kornberg (1950), Glock and McLean (1953) and Kirkman (1959). Also, simplified procedures coupling the co-enzyme reduction with the decoloration of dyes have been evolved, for example methaemoglobin reduction by sensitive erythrocytes in the presence of methylene blue is slower than with normal cells (Brewer *et al.*, 1960; Tarlov *et al.*, 1962). With these techniques large scale surveys can be made using merely a small drop of blood from a finger prick in each subject.

Obviously age of the red cell is a factor in G-6-P dehydrogenase activity since the younger cells always contain a higher concentration of the enzyme. In sensitive individuals the older cells are practically devoid of activity (Marks and Gross, 1959).

The characteristics of red cell G-6-P dehydrogenase have been studied by a number of investigators including Carson *et al.*, 1959; Kirkman, 1959; and Marks *et al.*, 1961, in an attempt to determine whether there were any qualitative differences between the enzyme present in the red cells of normal and sensitive individuals. No such differences were evident and the enzymes from both groups were identical in a variety of physical characteristics including chromatographic behaviour, pH optima, and Michaelis constants for both substrate and co-enzyme.

The mechanism of haemolysis is still far from clear. The first detectable event before haemolysis is a drop in the erythrocyte GSH level. Then Heinz bodies are formed, granular inclusions in the erythrocyte consisting, it is thought, of denatured protein, probably altered haemoglobin. Normally this modified haemoglobin is reconverted back to its native form by reaction with GSH, which is itself oxidized to GSSG. Under normal conditions the GSSG will be then reduced again to GSH by Reaction (1), utilizing the reduced NADP produced in Reactions (2) and (3). However, in sensitive red cells there is a deficiency of G-6-P dehydrogenase and so Reaction (2) and hence Reaction (3) are blocked. No reduced NADP is forthcoming and consequently GSH cannot be regenerated in Reaction (1). When no free GSH remains in the erythrocyte, irreversible changes take place in the haemoglobin molecule leading to Heinz body formation and eventually to cell destruction.

It has been suggested that the modified haemoglobin might be methaemoglobin, which might then be converted irreversibly to sulphaemoglobin in deficient erythrocytes. There is a known enzymic reaction involving reduced NADP which converts methaemoglobin formed inside the red cell back to haemoglobin; this may be expressed as follows:

$$\text{methaemoglobin} + \text{reduced NADP}$$
$$\rightarrow \text{haemoglobin} + NADP$$

However, a lack of reduced NADP would block this reaction and methaemoglobin would accumulate. There are several arguments against this theory; for example the reaction utilizes reduced NAD (nicotinamide adenine dinucleotide) as well as reduced NADP, and it cannot be presumed that the supply of reduced NAD, from glycolysis, is also depressed in mutant erythrocytes. A further pertinent fact is that methaemoglobinaemia and sulphaemoglobinaemia occur clinically from time to time without being accompanied by gross haemolysis. The full story of the haemolysis is therefore clearly more complex than that outlined; indeed it may be quite different. Possibly, for example, both GSH depletion and G-6-P dehydrogenase deficiency are secondary to some unknown primary defect which itself leads to haemolysis.

Glucose-6-phosphate dehydrogenase deficiency has been of much interest to geneticists; it is thought to be a sex-linked trait. In the male the gene associated with G-6-P dehydrogenase deficiency is thought to be carried on the X-chromosome derived from the mother. The question immediately arises as to why females, who carry two X-chromosomes, do not have double the activity of G-6-P dehydrogenase; a possible answer is that one of the X-chromosomes in the somatic cells of women may be inactive. There is reason to believe that the inactive X-chromosome could not be derived solely from either the mother or father. The cells of women may therefore comprise a mosaic, some with active paternal X-chromosomes and some with active maternal X-chromosomes. The studies of Beutler *et al.* (1962) on heterozygous women with erythrocyte G-6-P dehydrogenase activities at intermediate levels have given some support to this hypothesis. These erythrocytes consist of a population of fully active cells together with completely inactive ones, and not a homogeneous population of cells with intermediate enzyme levels.

DRUG-INDUCED HAEMOLYTIC ANAEMIA WITH POSITIVE DIRECT COOMBS TEST

A number of drugs and chemicals have been incriminated in haemolytic processes mediated by antibodies, including penicillin, stibophen and alpha-methyldopa [TABLE 4.3].

These haemolytic anaemias are associated with a positive direct Coombs test but at least three different mechanisms are involved. These can be distinguished, in part, by means of the modification of the Coombs antiglobulin technique that recognizes the two major types of red cell coating with proteins. One is the antigamma (anti-γ) reaction that recognizes the immunoglobulin G (IgG) globulins. The second detects

TABLE 4.3

DRUGS HAVING IMMUNOLOGICAL PROPERTIES
ASSOCIATED WITH HAEMOLYTIC ANAEMIA
(based on Wintrobe, 1969)

CLASS OF DRUG	MEMBER
Hypotensive	methyldopa
Antibiotic	penicillin
Chemotherapeutic agent in schistosomiasis	stibophen (sodium antimonyl pyrocatechol disulphonate)
Cinchona alkaloids	quinine, quinidine
Analgesic/antipyretic	phenacetin (acetophenetidin) dipyrone (methampyrone)
Chemotherapeutic agent in tuberculosis	*p*-aminosalicylic acid (PAS)
Sulphonamide	sulphasalazine (salicylazo-sulphapyridine)

the presence of the complement (C′) system on the surface of the red cell. This is the anti-non-gamma or the anti-C′ reaction.

The three types of drug-induced Coombs-positive haemolytic anaemias have been termed the alpha-methyldopa type, the innocent bystander type (e.g. stibophen) and the haptene type (e.g. penicillin). FIGURE 4.1 illustrates these three different mechanisms.

FIG. 4.1. *Diagrammatic representations of types of drug-induced Coombs-reactive haemolytic anaemias (redrawn from Wintrobe, 1969).*

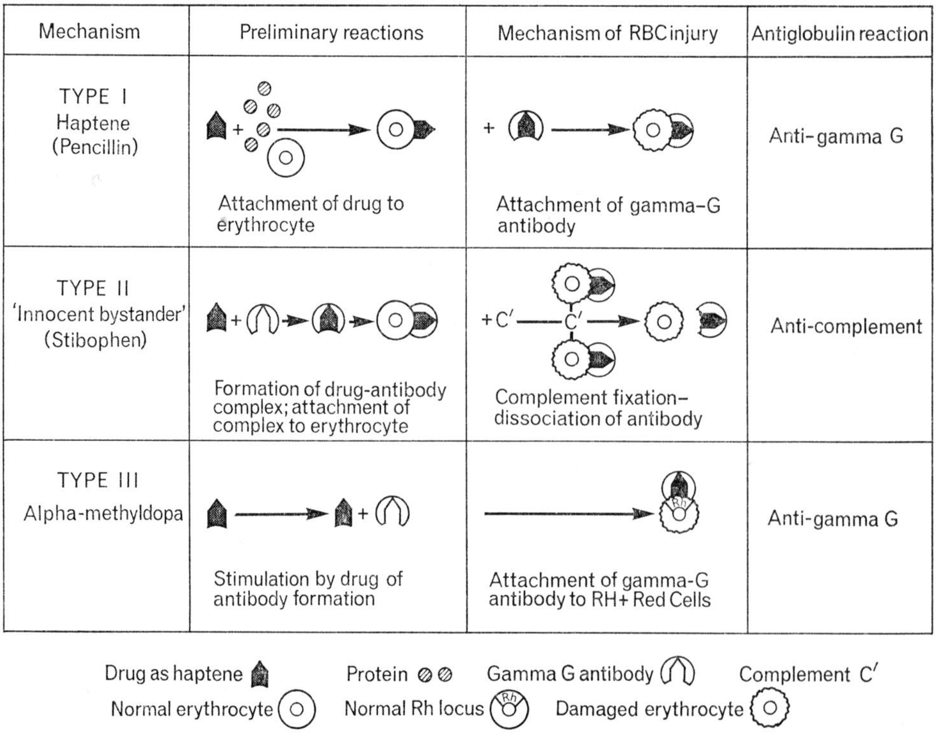

Mechanism	Preliminary reactions	Mechanism of RBC injury	Antiglobulin reaction
TYPE I Haptene (Pencillin)	Attachment of drug to erythrocyte	Attachment of gamma–G antibody	Anti-gamma G
TYPE II 'Innocent bystander' (Stibophen)	Formation of drug-antibody complex; attachment of complex to erythrocyte	Complement fixation– dissociation of antibody	Anti-complement
TYPE III Alpha-methyldopa	Stimulation by drug of antibody formation	Attachment of gamma-G antibody to RH+ Red Cells	Anti-gamma G

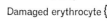

Drug as haptene   Protein   Gamma G antibody   Complement C′

Normal erythrocyte (○)   Normal Rh locus   Damaged erythrocyte

Methyldopa: Drug-induced Haemolytic Anaemia with Positive Direct Coombs Test and IgG Antibodies

In 1965 Carstairs and colleagues found that three patients on methyldopa therapy had developed 'idiopathic' warm-antibody (IgG) auto-immune haemolytic anaemia (Carstairs *et al.*, 1966*b*). In January 1966 the Committee on Safety of Drugs issued a warning about the association of methyldopa treatment and haemolytic anaemia based on nine cases reported by doctors or by the manufacturers of the drug (Cahal, 1966). Subsequently some 30 cases were notified to the Committee.

Carstairs *et al.* (1966*a*) investigated this problem further and examined a consecutive series of hypertensive patients on methyldopa treatment who had no symptoms of haemolytic anaemia. Forty-one (20 per cent) of 202 unselected patients gave a positive direct Coombs test (D.C.T.) of the IgG type. Of a control group of 76 hypertensive patients on other antihypertensive therapy, none had a positive Coombs reaction of the pure IgG type, although two had a positive test of the non-IgG type. No patient on methyldopa had overt haemolytic anaemia, but of the patients with a positive D.C.T., six had raised reticulocyte counts and in a further six there was a possible slight depression of the platelet count. Red cell survival was measured in four patients, and in one there was a shortened survival time.

The incidence of a positive D.C.T. was dose-dependent; 9 per cent of those taking 1 gram or less a day were affected and between 1–2 grams daily the figure was 19 per cent. Above 2 grams per day, 36 per cent had a positive D.C.T. The duration of treatment was also important, and in most cases the test became positive between 6 and 12 months after commencement of therapy.

Worlledge and her colleagues (1966) summarized the clinical, haematological and serological data of the 30 cases who had developed auto-immune haemolytic anaemia whilst on methyldopa therapy, and had been reported to the Committee on Safety of Drugs. Twenty-five of these cases were studied in detail; 24 had overt haemolytic anaemia. The patients had been treated for periods varying from 3 to 37 months, but 10 had been on treatment for one year or less; the majority of patients were receiving 1 gram or less of methyldopa per day.

The initial symptoms which led to the discovery of haemolytic anaemia were extremely variable. It is not known whether the direct Coombs test was positive before A.I.H.A. developed. In some patients the onset of the disease was acute, but in most it was insidious. Although two patients dated the onset of their symptoms from an influenza-like illness, there was no obvious correlation between the incidence of upper-respiratory-tract infection and the development of overt haemolysis.

Enlargement of the liver and lymph glands was not reported; there was, however, a variable degree of splenomegaly in 13 out of the 25 cases; this was definite in only three. The severity of the anaemia varied and was unrelated to the total dose of methyldopa. In all the anaemic patients the peripheral blood films showed spherocytosis and polychromasia; the Coombs antiglobulin reaction was positive in all cases and was entirely of the IgG ('warm antibody') type.

In most patients the anaemia responded rapidly to withdrawal of the methyldopa or to administration of corticosteroids. Seven patients were treated by stopping the methyldopa and recovered rapidly; the remaining 18 patients were given prednisone, and, of these, two died while still anaemic, one of multiple pulmonary emboli (perhaps directly attributable to the haemolytic process) and the other of the complications of duodenal ulceration, perhaps exacerbated by the steroid treatment. Methyldopa was continued in six of these patients, one died of a cerebrovascular accident after recovery from haemolytic anaemia, three developed a recurrence of haemolysis when the prednisone was reduced or stopped, and two were maintained on large doses of steroids.

The prognosis for anaemia seemed to be good in most of the patients. All those who continued on methyldopa treatment had a positive direct Coombs test. The first reversion to a negative Coombs test occurred seven months after methyldopa was withdrawn in a patient who had been only mildly anaemic and who had not received prednisone.

Many drugs have been shown to be capable of initiating red cell destruction by provoking the appearance of antibodies that destroy red-blood cells; these include quinidine, quinine, phenacetin, certain insecticides, stibophen, *p*-aminosalicylic acid, sulphasalazine (salicylazosulphapyridine) and dipyrone. More than one mechanism is known, but the antibody formed is directed against the drug, or a drug fragment, not against inherited intrinsic red cell antigens, and can only be demonstrated in the presence of the drug. In an excellent review, given in The Lilly Lecture in 1968, Wintrobe (1969) has discussed and explained the three types of drug-induced Coombs-positive haemolytic anaemias; reference should be made to this publication for further data regarding the mechanisms involved.

The antibody associated with methyldopa treatment is unique in that it can be easily eluted from the patient's cells and both the eluted antibody and antibody in the serum can sensitize normal cells. Worlledge *et al.* (1966) have suggested some possible explanations for this and for the curious delay before the antibody appears. It is improbable that the antibody these patients form is directed against the drug; all attempts to demonstrate a drug specificity *in vitro* have failed. The drug or a derivative may become incorporated into the red cells, possibly at the formative normoblast or reticulocyte stage, and by doing so causes some subtle alteration of the red cell antigens, so that an antibody which cross-reacts with normal red cell antigen is produced against them. This could explain the delay in development of A.I.H.A., since the changed red cell antigen would not reach the antibody-producing cells until the end of its normal life-span of about 120 days, as there is no reason to suppose that such subtly altered cells would have a reduced life-span.

An alternative hypothesis suggested was that the drug might act directly on the immune mechanism and by doing so increase its responsiveness to self-antigens.

The possibility that a metabolite of methyldopa might be responsible for the haemolytic anaemia can be inferred from the work of Wurzel and Silverman (1966). Methyldopa, in a final concentration of 5 mg/ml, sensitized normal group O, Rh-positive, donor red cells *in vitro* at room temperature. However, in a final concentration of one-tenth of that amount (0·5 mg/ml), seven out of ten metabolites or closely related catecholamines sensitized the red cells more rapidly.

Methyldopa is a useful hypotensive agent and certainly there are not so many good hypotensives that this one can be spared; however, Carstairs *et al.* (1966a) estimated that over 100,000 patients were receiving regular treatment with the drug at that time. The level of use of this drug is still considerable and this must be a matter of some concern since Carstairs *et al.* (1966a) found a 20 per cent incidence of positive direct Coombs reaction in their patients, and Louis *et al.* (1967) observed a comparable incidence. Therefore if this percentage incidence is extrapolated to the total number of patients involved, then some 25,000 patients could be at risk from haemolytic anaemia.

A leading article in *The Lancet* (1966) has reviewed the situation and has recommended that, since the danger period is the second six months of treatment, blood should be sent for a Coombs test in the seventh, and after the twelfth month of treatment. If a positive test is found, the patient should, if possible, be given an alternative hypotensive agent.

The presence of a positive Coombs test may make the matching of blood for transfusion difficult: it is recommended therefore that patients who are pregnant, or in need of surgical operations should also be tested.

Apart from the publications discussed in this section, other investigators have also described haemolytic anaemia associated with methyldopa; they include:

Brandt and Lund, 1966; Cramond, 1966; Darnborough, 1966; Hamilton *et al.*, 1966; Hay, 1966; Hayes, 1966; O'Shea, 1966; Paton, 1966; Schwartz and Dige-Peterson, 1966. Other groups have reported positive direct Coombs test but no overt haemolytic anaemia; they include:

Buchanan *et al.*, 1966; Cotton, 1966; Frezzine, 1966; Weiner and Paton, 1966; Wurzel and Silverman, 1966; Cantor and Barnetts, 1967; Weinreich and Rohr, 1967.

Stibophen: Drug-induced Haemolytic Anaemia with Positive Direct Coombs Test ('Innocent Bystander' Type)

In the 'innocent bystander type', the red cell is injured during the interaction of an antibody with an extraneous antigen (i.e. drug). Stibophen, quinine, quinidine and phenacetin produce this type of response.

When the drug is oxidized metabolically it probably combines with some body protein. This drug-protein complex serves as an antigen and leads to the formation of an antibody. The antibody shows strong affinity for the red cell [see Fig. 4.1] and, by binding to the cell, is able to activate the complement mechanism at the cell surface. This is detectable by the anti-complement antiglobulin reaction. Such cells, if heavily coated with complement, may be subjected to premature destruction in the reticulo-endothelial system. The antigen-antibody complex appears to dissociate spontaneously from the damaged cell, and the antigamma Coombs reaction is thus negative. The 'innocent bystander' terminology is very appropriate since the immune reaction is directed not against autologous tissue components but against the drug, the blood cell is injured as an innocent bystander (Wintrobe, 1969).

Penicillin: Drug-induced Haemolytic Anaemia with Positive Direct Coombs Test ('Haptene' Type) with IgG Antibodies

In 1959, Ley *et al.* reported that penicillin may cause an immune haemolytic anaemia and during the next 9 years 13 further cases were recorded (Strumia and Raymond, 1962; Beardwell, 1964; Van Arsdel and Gilliland, 1965; Clayton *et al.*, 1965; Dawson and Segal, 1966; Lai *et al.*, 1966; Petz and Fudenberg, 1966; Nesmith and Davis, 1968, and White *et al.*, 1968). With the exception of two, these reports appeared in American literature. Reports of penicillin-induced haemolytic anaemia are fewer in Great Britain probably because lower doses of penicillin are used. It is possible, however, that immune haemolysis may go unrecognized, since high doses of penicillin are usually given to patients suffering from subacute bacterial endocarditis and septicaemia in whom increasing anaemia is part of the clinical picture.

White and colleagues (1968) have analysed data from all reported cases. Nine patients received penicillin for subacute bacterial endocarditis, three had other infections, in one case the antibiotic was used as a post-operative cover, and in one case no diagnosis was given. Thirteen of the patients had been given 20 mega units of penicillin per day at some stage of treatment and one patient had received 10 mega units daily for 26 days. In six cases there was evidence of drug allergy before haemolytic anaemia developed; five patients developed a rash and one had pyrexia and malaise.

In all 14 reported cases, there was a positive direct antiglobulin reaction at the time the haemolysis was first diagnosed; this reaction was detected as early as two days and as late as 26 days after commencing penicillin therapy. Four patients who had initially received small doses of penicillin some days or weeks before larger doses were given, developed a sudden brisk haemolysis which contrasted with the slow onset seen with constant high dosage. The peripheral blood picture did not help diagnosis; spherocytosis was seen in one case and auto-agglutination was not reported.

There was an eosinophilia in peripheral blood or bone marrow in eight patients, and in one there was a leucopenia at the height of haemolysis, accompanied by a marked left shift in granulopoiesis.

No patient died as a result of uncontrolled haemolysis, although in one case the haemoglobin fell from 12·6 to 3 grams/100 ml in 9 days accompanied by a reticulocytosis of 66 per cent. Six patients had an anaemia severe enough to require blood transfusion. In all cases haemolysis stopped when penicillin was withdrawn; corticosteroids were given to three patients without any apparent beneficial effects.

The antigen is a hapten-protein complex formed by penicillin combined covalently with proteins on the red cell membrane and in the serum. It is not known how many molecules of penicillin must combine with red cell protein before the antibody can cause immune destruction. Haemolytic anaemia does not seem to occur in patients receiving low doses of penicillin and penicillin has only been found on the surface of red cells in patients on at least 10 mega units per day (Clayton et al., 1965; White et al., 1968 and others). Levine and Redmond (1966) have investigated this point in detail, and using specific haemagglutination techniques and a specific benzylpenicilloyl from rabbits, found that 100 per cent of patients on 10–30 mega units per day gave a very strong reaction and that 33 per cent on 1·2–2·4 mega units per day gave only weak reactions. In the latter group, the reaction was linked with high total dose.

In most patients the antibody was IgG, although in the cases reported by Van Arsdel and Gilliland (1965) and Swanson and colleagues (1966) a minor IgM component was also detected. The fact that relatively few patients treated with high doses of penicillin develop a haemolytic anaemia suggests that only certain patients are capable of producing sufficient IgG penicillin antibody.

Cross-reaction of the IgG penicillin antibody with red cells sensitized with ampicillin, methicillin, cephaloridine, or any other member of the penicillin or cephalosporin families is likely because of the very close similarities in chemical structure of these antibiotics. White et al. (1968) have warned that these agents do not therefore offer a rational alternative to any specific penicillin therapy if the latter has to be stopped on account of haemolysis.

OTHER COMMONLY USED DRUGS ASSOCIATED WITH HAEMOLYTIC ANAEMIA

Dapsone (diaminodiphenylsulphone)

Dapsone, a sulphone, was introduced in 1943 and is still the standard treatment for lepromatous or tuberculoid (neural) leprosy; its main advantage over newer agents like thiambutosine and clofazimine is that leprologists are used to it and that it costs only a few shillings for a year's course of treatment, a factor of no

mean importance in the developing countries in which it is used.

Although dapsone has been definitely implicated in haemolytic anaemia, it occurs rarely and it is fair to comment that this has usually been associated with high dosage. Most leprologists keep the initial dosage low in the treatment of lepromatous leprosy, for example 100 mg per week for the 1st month increasing stepwise over 6 months to 600 mg per week. This not only avoids the danger of haemolytic anaemia but also the erythema nodosum reaction (lepra reaction) on the skin when the patient becomes sensitive to the products of the mycobacteria that are being destroyed in his tissues. With the tuberculoid type of disease dosage is also cautious and is started low and increased slowly to avoid reaction in, and destruction of, nerve tissue. In such cases a typical dosage regime would be 50 mg of dapsone per week for the 1st month rising stepwise to 400 mg per week during the 5th month. There may also be frequent rest periods in both regimes (Morgan, 1967).

It is not surprising therefore to note that Garrett and Corcos (1952), in a report on about 10,000 lepers receiving dapsone did not mention the occurrence of haemolytic anaemia. Smith and Alexander (1959) noted Heinz bodies in the red cells of four patients but here the dosage of dapsone was 100–200 mg per day. Pengelly (1963) studied the survival of red cells labelled with Cr^{51} in four patients on dapsone treatment for dermatitis herpetiformis. All four patients showed a reduced erythrocyte survival time on a dosage of 50–150 mg daily. In only two patients was there any previous suggestion of a haemolytic state. Glucose-6-phosphate dehydrogenase activity and glutathione stability was normal in all four cases.

A normal volunteer was given Cr^{51} labelled red cells and the Cr^{51} loss was followed by blood samples taken every 2 or 3 days. Dapsone was then given for a further 19 days and the total dosage was high—2,050 mg. The Cr^{51} curve remained within normal limits for the first 22 days and then fell below the normal range indicating that dapsone caused haemolysis of mature red cells.

Nalidixic Acid

There are two reports of haemolytic anaemia due to nalidixic acid in infants. The first case was reported by Belton and Jones (1965) in a newborn child who developed a haemolytic anaemia attributed to nalidixic acid in the breast milk.

The mother had received nalidixic acid 1 gram q.d.s. and amylobarbitone sodium 65 mg t.d.s. from the 9th post-partum day. Lactation was established by the 3rd day and was maintained; on the 16th day the infant appeared pale and jaundiced and haematological examination indicated a drug-induced haemolytic anaemia; the direct Coombs test was negative. On the same day, the infant was transfused with 150 ml of blood and bottle-feeding was started. The reticulocyte count gradually fell to 1 per cent in 10 days (previously 20 per cent of red cells), by which time no Heinz bodies could be seen (previously 50 per cent of the red cells contained one or more Heinz bodies).

Thereafter recovery was uneventful and 7 months after birth the child was perfectly normal. The concentration of nalidixic acid in breast milk was calculated to be about 4 μg/ml, which, assuming a milk intake of 500 ml per day, would correspond to a foetal dose of 2 mg per day of the drug, a very small amount to account for the haemolytic anaemia. The authors, however, suggested that reduced maternal urinary excretion of the drug due to reduced glomerular filtration associated with the raised blood-urea may have raised the serum level in the mother and hence the amount of the drug present in the milk. However, other studies cited by Belton and Jones (1965) have shown that patients with chronic renal failure treated with nalidixic acid show little difference in serum levels of the drug from those in normal subjects, although occasionally higher levels have been encountered.

The second case, an 18-month old boy with urinary infection, was reported by Vargas and González (1967). The child was treated with nalidixic acid, 60 mg/kg per day divided into four doses; the course of infection was favourable but on the 20th day of treatment, the boy became very pale and results of blood and bone-marrow examination suggested a haemolytic process. The direct Coombs test was negative.

Nalidixic acid was discontinued and 11 days afterwards the results of blood and urine examination were satisfactory, and the child was discharged; he did not receive treatment for this anaemia because it was not significant and did not produce dyspnoea or other symptoms.

Belton and Jones (1965) cited two other cases known to the manufacturers of the drug. The first was in a grossly glucose-6-phosphate dehydrogenase deficient Negro and haemolytic anaemia was almost certainly associated with the use of nalidixic acid. In a second patient, who had uraemia and prostatic carcinomatosis, the role of the drug was uncertain.

Mefenamic Acid

Mefenamic acid, an anti-arthritic agent, has been reported by Scott *et al.* (1968) to be associated with auto-immune haemolytic anaemia in three patients. In each case the auto-immune haemolytic anaemia was of the warm antibody γG type, and the antibodies had some rhesus specificity. The patients had received 1·5 grams of mefenamic acid daily for between 1 and 2 years; all three patients recovered when the drug was withdrawn; two patients were given prednisone treatment (40 or 60 mg per day) and one received azathioprine 200 mg per day when the mefenamic acid was stopped. The direct antihuman globulin test remained positive for respectively 5, 9 and 3 months, and then became negative.

No inhibition of antibody activity was detected after pre-incubation of the patient's serum with mefenamic acid or its derivatives. Similarly, pre-incubation with normal cells with these compounds did not enhance the antibody activity. No Heinz bodies were found in normal red cells after 6 hours' incubation with mefenamic acid or its derivatives.

Direct antihuman globulin tests were done on the red cells of 36 patients (25 rheumatoid arthritis, 4 osteoarthritis, 7 miscellaneous rheumatic conditions, including Reiter's syndrome, systemic lupus erythematosus, and psoriatic arthritis) who had been treated with mefenamic acid continuously for at least 3 months. The average daily dose was 1·5 grams (range 0·75–2 grams) and the mean duration of treatment was 13 months (range 3–31 months).

Only one patient (rheumatoid arthritis) gave a positive antihuman globulin test, using broad-spectrum antihuman globulin serum, on one occasion, but this was subsequently negative despite continuing mefenamic acid therapy.

In all therapy, the relative importance of complications depends on the usefulness and value of the therapeutic agent. With mefenamic acid Cahill *et al.* (1965), Barnardo *et al.* (1966) and Myles *et al.* (1967) have suggested that it is of comparable value to aspirin and phenylbutazone. It does, however, have a very low incidence of upper intestinal side-effects, which are common with the majority of drugs used in chronic rheumatic diseases. Scott *et al.* (1968) have therefore recommended that mefenamic acid be used with caution in long-term therapy and that patients should be watched carefully for evidence of haemolysis.

DRUG-INDUCED APLASTIC ANAEMIA

A number of drugs have been incriminated in the development of aplastic anaemia; among these are chloramphenicol, propylthiouracil, indomethacin, mepacrine, cyclophosphamide, salicylates and *Thorotrast*.

Elucidation of the mechanism by which these compounds induce aplastic anaemia is complicated by a

TABLE 4.4

DRUGS AND AGENTS ASSOCIATED WITH APLASTIC ANAEMIA (PANCYTOPENIA) AND ERYTHROID HYPOPLASIA

(based on Huguley, 1966; Wintrobe, 1969)

CLASS OF DRUG	MEMBERS
Analgesics and anti-arthritics	phenylbutazone, acetylsalicylic acid, gold salts (sodium aurothiomalate)
Antibacterial agents	chloramphenicol, sulphonamides
Non-antibacterial sulphonamide derivatives	tolbutamide, carbutamide
Anticonvulsants	phenytoin sodium (diphenylhydantoin sodium), methoin (mephenytoin), troxidone (trimethadione)
Insecticides and pesticides	gamma benzene hexachloride, chlorophenothane (DDT), chlordan
Solvents and other chemicals	benzene, potassium perchlorate
Antimalarials	mepacrine (quinacrine)

number of unexplained facts. Firstly, there is no facet of chemical structure common to these incriminated compounds. Secondly, many of these agents are used widely with comparative safety, and it is only in the minority of cases that aplastic anaemia develops, and thirdly, there does not appear to be any readily discernible metabolic defect to explain the selectivity of this iatrogenic effect on certain patients. In summary, it is not possible to predict which chemical structures are likely to induce aplastic anaemia nor is it possible to predict which patients are likely to develop aplastic anaemia.

CHLORAMPHENICOL

Although chloramphenicol is a broad-spectrum antibiotic whose effectiveness has been established in a variety of infections due to Gram-positive and Gram-negative organisms, its toxic effects may be extremely serious and it should not be used when alternative antibiotics are effective. The specific indications for the use of chloramphenicol are restricted to severe salmonella infections, especially typhoid fever, and *H. influenzae* meningitis.

Blood dyscrasias were reported even in the early days of clinical use and today the association between chloramphenicol dosage and serious blood dyscrasias such as aplastic anaemia or thrombocytopenia or granulocytopenia is well recognized. Many hundreds of cases, the majority with fatal outcome, have been reported in the United Kingdom and in the United States. Among all drugs chloramphenicol ranks first as the cause of severe iatrogenic blood disorders; Ory and Yow (1963), and Manten (1968) have reviewed the literature. Bone-marrow arrest and aplastic anaemia are the most common and serious toxic effects associated with chloramphenicol therapy. This toxicity may occur after the administration of small doses for short periods or may appear only after prolonged therapy. If the aplastic anaemia is detected early, and the antibiotic is discontinued, the bone-marrow may recover, but often the disease ends fatally. Cases have been reported as occurring after the administration of only a few grams, often tragically enough, for some trivial indication (*British Medical Journal*, 1963).

The toxic effects of chloramphenicol may occur at any age but are commonest in older children and more so in females than in males. Premature and newborn infants are particularly susceptible, and there have been several deaths reported (Hodgman, 1961); a symptom complex the 'grey syndrome' developed in these infants, all of whom received doses larger than 100 mg/kg of body weight daily. The symptoms which have been described in detail by Ory and Yow (1963) appeared after 3 or 4 days of treatment, and deaths occurred within 24–48 hours of onset of symptoms. Post-mortem studies did not reveal the cause of death and no characteristic changes were found. However, it is very likely that death was due to the abnormally progressive

accumulations of chloramphenicol, and some of its degradation metabolites, since in the newborn infant the immature liver is deficient in conjugation mechanisms and there is a decrease in the renal tubular secretion of the chloramphenicol glucuronide.

Early in the development of chloramphenicol toxicity, vacuoles appear in the erythroid and myeloid cell precursors in the bone-marrow (Rosenbach *et al.*, 1960; Saidi and Wallerstein, 1960; McCurdy, 1961; Saidi *et al.*, 1961). These lesions are reversible and their relation to later more serious bone-marrow depression is unknown.

Ingall and others (1965) observed vacuoles in erythroid-cell and myeloid-cell cytoplasm in the bone-marrows of five out of eight children treated with short courses of chloramphenicol for a variety of infections. These changes were morphologically identical with vacuolization seen in phenylalanine deficiency. Treatment of these patients with 100 mg/kg/day of laevo-phenylalanine by mouth caused the vacuoles to disappear in two children after 48 and 96 hours, and in a third child the size and number of vacuoles were markedly diminished. All three children had continued to receive chloramphenicol in the same dosage.

Ingall *et al.* (1965) therefore suggested that chloramphenicol might act on the bone-marrow by affecting phenylalanine metabolism. Chloramphenicol has also been shown to block the incorporation of alanine into protein moieties (Gale, 1958), thus chloramphenicol could block phenylalanine utilization as a primary effect or secondarily as a result of interference with alanine metabolism.

It has also been suggested that genetic factors might influence the susceptibility of patients to chloramphenicol-induced aplastic anaemia. Nagao and Mauer (1969) reported the clinical courses of aplastic anaemia in identical twins. The first twin was treated with chloramphenicol for an upper respiratory tract infection at the age of 5 months; at 6 months the symptoms recurred and treatment was continued. At 8 months, he was admitted to hospital with ecchymoses of 5 days' duration. On admission, his haemoglobin was 6·2 grams/100 ml and his white cell count was 6,250/cu mm, the platelet count was 0. Aspirated bone-marrow was hypoplastic and a diagnosis of aplastic anaemia due to chloramphenicol therapy was made.

The second twin suffered from the same respiratory tract infections and also received chloramphenicol at the same time and doses as his twin. At the time of diagnosis of aplastic anaemia on his twin, he was admitted to hospital in the hope that he could be a source of bone-marrow transfusion. On admission, the second twin had a haemoglobin of 8·6 grams/100 ml and a white cell count of 14,500 cu mm with 19 per cent neutrophils and 79 per cent lymphocytes. The platelet count was 8,500 cu mm. The bone-marrow aspirate was cellular but contained 77 per cent lymphocytes. Gradually a pancytopenia developed and the bone-marrow became hypoplastic. He was treated with packed red cells and platelet transfusions were given, and complete recovery ensued.

There have been other suggested mechanisms of how chloramphenicol induces blood dyscrasias. Inhibition of iron uptake has been suggested as also sensitization of bone-marrow on the basis of an allergy. These studies have been well reviewed by Manten (1968).

The incidence of serious blood dyscrasias associated with chloramphenicol has been variously estimated as aplasia of bone-marrow, 1 in 500 to 1 in 100,000 treated cases (*British Medical Journal*, 1963), aplasia of bone-marrow with consequent aplastic anaemia and agranulocytosis, 1 in 58,000 (Kahler, 1965), and 1 in 75,000 (Girdwood, 1964). The lethality of this irreversible effect has been estimated as 1 in 76,000 (Kahler, 1965).

In the United Kingdom, the Committee on Safety of Drugs announced that during the two-year period prior to 1967, it had received reports of 24 fatal cases of blood dyscrasias following the administration of chloramphenicol. These reports accounted for 80 per cent of all fatal cases of blood dyscrasias reported to have occurred in patients who received an antibiotic.

The Committee considered that chloramphenicol should never be used for the treatment of trivial infections and that it should not be used except when careful clinical assessment, usually supplemented by laboratory studies, indicated that no other antibiotic would suffice.

The Committee recognized that chloramphenicol was a highly effective agent in typhoid fever and in *H. influenzae* meningitis, and in such cases they were of the opinion that the advantages of chloramphenicol greatly outweighed its hazards (*British Medical Journal*, 1967).

OTHER AGENTS

Propylthiouracil

The antithyroid drug propylthiouracil has commonly been reported to cause leucopenia during treatment and less commonly agranulocytosis (see Dalderup, 1968). However, two cases of propylthiouracil-induced aplastic anaemia have been reported, the first by Martelo and associates (1967) and the second by Aksoy and Erdem (1968) from Istanbul.

The first case showed spontaneous clinical and haematological improvement after withdrawal of propylthiouracil but the second had more serious consequences. The patient, a 39-year-old man, was admitted to hospital with weakness, fatigue, palpitation, weight loss, pallor, epistaxis and petechiae. Two months before he had been diagnosed as having Graves' disease and was treated with propylthiouracil. In a period of 3 weeks he received a fairly moderate course of treatment with 80 × 50 mg tablets of this drug. A week after propylthiouracil was stopped, the patient began to complain of epistaxis and weakness; blood transfusions were given without much success.

Haematological and bone-marrow examinations led to a diagnosis of aplastic anaemia due to propylthiouracil. Aksoy and Erdem (1968) reported that the condition of this patient was still critical 2 months after the propylthiouracil had been stopped in spite of treatment with whole blood transfusions (seven in 3 weeks), 250 mg of methyltestosterone weekly and dexamethasone, 6 mg per day. The clinical picture at that time was dominated by haemorrhagic manifestations (epistaxis, bleeding from the gums, and widespread purpuric spots); the R.B.C. increased only to 2,130,000 per cu mm (1,350,000 before treatment), the haemoglobin rose to 5·6 grams/100 ml (3·5 before treatment) and platelets increased to 100,000 per cu mm (10,800 before treatment).

The authors thought that the patient had some personal susceptibility to propylthiouracil which might possibly involve some essential metabolic process; they were not, however, prepared to suggest the nature of the metabolic process involved. An alternative possibility of an immune mechanism being involved was not supported by experimental evidence.

Indomethacin

The anti-arthritic agent indomethacin occasionally produces mild to moderately severe anaemia, and leucopenia, thrombocytopenia, pancytopenia and agranulocytosis have been observed infrequently (see Prescott, 1968). However, one case of indomethacin-induced aplastic anaemia was reported by Canada and Burka (1968).

The patient was a 42-year-old woman who had been in good health with the exception of a proved carcinoma of the breast 6 years earlier. A radical mastectomy and bilateral oophorectomy had been performed at that time. There had been no recurrence of the tumour.

Ten days before admission to hospital, she was treated with indomethacin 75 to 100 mg daily, for osteoarthritis. She had been taking aspirin periodically for several years for this condition. There was no indication that she had ever been given phenylbutazone.

Three days after she began taking the indomethacin she developed a petechial rash starting on the legs and spreading to her entire body. The rash was not painful and did not itch.

The haemoglobin was normal on admission to hospital but fell to 8·4 grams/100 ml four days later; the white cell count, initially 3,300, fell to 800 within one week. There was an absolute and relative neutropenia. Bone-marrow examination showed a complete absence of nucleated elements. The platelet count varied between 30,000 and 80,000 per cu mm. There was a constant fever (101°F) during the hospital course.

During her stay in hospital her illness was complicated by continual episodes of internal bleeding; she was treated with prednisolone, 80 mg daily and testosterone enanthate. Three weeks after admission she began showing increasing unresponsiveness and began coughing up blood. Acute respiratory distress followed with cardiac arrest, and attempts to resuscitate failed. Permission for autopsy was not granted.

The authors concluded that, in this case, drug-induced or drug-triggered blood dyscrasia must be considered, although the diagnosis of aleukaemic leukaemia could not be eliminated.

Mepacrine

Custer (1946) has reviewed the medical literature on mepacrine up to that time; he revealed the relatively high incidence of aplastic anaemia among soldiers who took mepacrine as a suppressant antimalarial (100 mg/day) during the Second World War. The incidence reached a peak of 2·84 cases per 100,000 soldiers. Schindel (1968) has reviewed more recent literature.

Mepacrine is now obsolete in antimalaria suppression or treatment since better and less toxic drugs have become available; however, it is of considerable value in the eradication of tapeworms and may occasionally be used for its anti-inflammatory properties. Tapeworm eradication requires relatively high dosage (10 × 100 mg tablets) at single administration while the anti-inflammatory usage, as for example in chronic discoid lupus erythematosus, is with lower dosage (100–200 mg daily) for long periods of time. Aplastic anaemia could be a potential hazard with this latter use.

Cyclophosphamide

The antineoplastic agent cyclophosphamide has been implicated in aplastic anaemia although the occurrence is rare (Meyler, 1966b).

Salicylates

Cases of aplastic anaemia and other blood dyscrasias associated with analgesic abuse have been reviewed by Prescott (1968). The degree of analgesic (aspirin or phenacetin) abuse has recently been revealed by Murray and others (1970) in a survey of psychiatric patients. Of 181 patients interviewed, 16 had consumed a total of more than 1 kg of analgesic; a further 26 patients admitted to a daily ingestion of analgesic during the previous six months. These data give an idea of the type of problem involved in this abuse, an abuse largely possible because of the ready availability of these analgesics.

Although out of context in this section, it is of interest to note that Williams and associates (1969) reported a case of megaloblastic anaemia in a patient who had habitually ingested large quantities of an analgesic containing aspirin, salicylamide and caffeine for relief of headache. This case is of particular interest since prior to diagnosis of drug involvement there was a pattern of remission of anaemia in the hospital and recurrence at home. It was only when more intensive inquiry into medications taken was made that the chronic ingestion of the analgesic preparation was uncovered. The authors reported that the patient had remained normal during a period of 12 months after stopping the analgesic. This case serves as another example of the type of problem involved in analgesic abuse.

Thorotrast (232-Thorium Dioxide)

In Portugal, Da Silva Horta et al. (1965) checked records of 2,377 individuals who had received injections of Thorotrast between 1930 and 1952. A total of 1,107 cases were traced; of these 699 had died and 408 were still living; certified cause of death was obtained for the former group.

Sixteen fatal blood dyscrasias had occurred; eight of these were leukaemias, six aplastic anaemias (pancytopenia) and two were purpuras.

The authors considered that the toxicity of Thorotrast was such that its use was never justified in people with life expectation of more than two years.

This agent is no longer used in the United Kingdom; it was banned in France in 1936 and in 1964 the United States Commissioner of Food and Drugs advised that it was unsafe for administration to man. Other aspects of Thorotrast toxicity have been reviewed in CHAPTER 9.

Chlorpropamide plus Methyldopa

Both chlorpropamide and alpha-methyldopa are known to give rise to blood dyscrasias, but neither has been reported singly as causing aplastic anaemia. However, a single case thought to have been caused by this combination of drugs was reported by McMurdoch et al. (1968).

Nitrofurantoin plus Prednisolone

McDuffie (1965) reported that a 14-year-old girl with lupus erythematosus was treated with daily doses of prednisolone; she also received nitrofurantoin and subsequently died of aplastic anaemia.

DRUG-INDUCED MEGALOBLASTIC ANAEMIA

The development of megaloblastic anaemia in patients receiving anticonvulsant drugs, notably phenytoin, primidone, and phenobarbitone is well recognized (Hawkins and Meynell, 1954, 1958; Rhind and Varadi, 1954; Ryan and Forshaw, 1955; Fuld and Moorhouse, 1956; Klipstein, 1964; Reynolds et al., 1966a).

Nitrofurantoin is chemically related to phenytoin (diphenylhydantoin) and has also been reported as causing megaloblastic anaemia (Bass, 1963). The structure-activity and structure-toxicity relationship between these compounds is very clear; this is shown on FIGURE 4.2.

All four compounds are thought to induce anaemia by causing a disturbance in folic acid metabolism. Hoffbrand and Necheles (1968) have investigated the effect of phenytoin on folic acid metabolism and shown that the drug inhibited folate absorption from folate polyglutamates, which are major components of food glutamates. They also showed in in vitro studies that phenytoin inhibited the activity of folate conjugase from

FIG. 4.2. *Structural relationship between the anticonvulsant drugs known to cause megaloblastic anaemia*

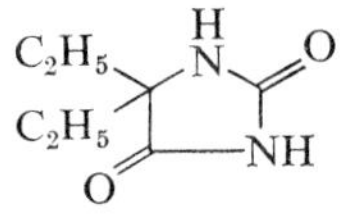

Phenytoin (Diphenylhydantoin)

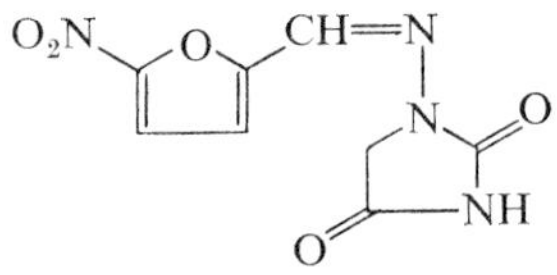

Nitrofurantoin

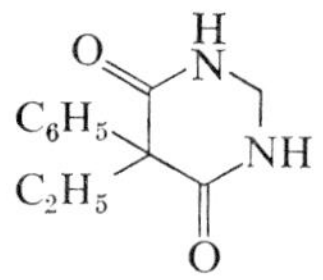

Primidone (Primaclone)

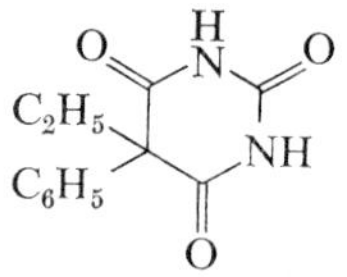

Phenobarbitone (Phenobarbital)

human jejunal mucosa. The important link between these two findings is that folate conjugase is responsible for the splitting of folate polyglutamates in the diet into simpler folate monoglutamates prior to absorption. Thus phenytoin is thought to reduce the formation of folate monoglutamates, which prevents the effective absorption of folate monoglutamate and thus leads to folate deficiency.

Rosenberg and colleagues (1968) confirmed that phenytoin inhibited the activity of folate conjugase *in vitro* and showed that, in patients, phenytoin reduced folate absorption from folate polyglutamates although the absorption of free folates was not affected.

Treatment of anticonvulsant-induced megaloblastic anaemia with folic acid has been successful in some cases (Reynolds *et al.*, 1966*b*).

Of interest in the general spectrum of phenytoin-induced iatrogenic effects is the well known unsightly manifestation of gum hyperplasia seen in children under treatment for epilepsy with this anticonvulsant. The cause of this hyperplasia is unknown; there is no evidence to suggest that it is related to a folic acid deficiency although obviously with such cases a full

investigation should be made of the haematological status of the child.

DRUG-INDUCED LEUCOPENIA AND AGRANULOCYTOSIS

Drug-induced leucopenia and agranulocytosis may occur as part of a general pancytopenia such as can be caused by any of the drugs listed in TABLE 4.4. More specifically drugs causing leucopenia or agranulocytosis are listed in TABLE 4.5. These tables are from the American Medical Association, Registry of Blood Dyscrasias (Huguley, 1966; Wintrobe, 1967*a*).

The antimitotic drugs such as busulphan, chlorambucil, vinblastine, vincristine, the nitrogen mustards and other drugs of related activity have been intentionally excluded from the catalogue of drugs causing leucopenia or agranulocytosis since this action of these drugs is part of their therapeutic purpose.

TABLE 4.5

DRUGS ASSOCIATED WITH LEUCOPENIA AND AGRANULOCYTOSIS

CLASS OF DRUG	MEMBERS
Analgesics and anti-arthritics	aminopyrine, dipyrone (methampyrone), phenylbutazone, acetylsalicylic acid
Antibacterial agents	chloramphenicol, penicillin, sulphonamides
Non-antibacterial sulphonamide derivatives	various hypoglycaemics and diuretics
Anticonvulsants	phenindione, phenytoin soluble (diphenylhydantoin sodium)
Tranquillizers, non-phenothiazine	meprobamate, imipramine
Phenothiazines	chlorpromazine, promazine, pecazine (mepazine), prochlorperazine
Antithyroid agents	thiouracil propylthiouracil, methimazole

Drugs that produce leucopenia or agranulocytosis do so relatively frequently and estimates of 1 in 100 to 1 in 1,000 have been made for patients who receive conventional treatment for several weeks. Together leucopenia and agranulocytosis accounted for about 40 per cent of the reports on blood dyscrasias received by the Registry of Blood Dyscrasias (Huguley, 1966).

There appear to be at least two mechanisms by which drugs produce agranulocytosis. Certain drugs, especially amidopyrine (aminopyrine) and its more popular derivative, dipyrone, usually produce agranulocytosis by an immune mechanism. This can be demonstrated *in vitro*. Also clinically the administration of a very small challenging dose of aminopyrine to a patient who had recovered from an attack of agranulocytosis was followed within 6–10 hours by disappearance of all the neutrophils from the blood (Dameshek and Colmes, 1936). Furthermore it was shown that the transfusion of blood, withdrawn from a sensitive patient three hours after administration of aminopyrine, produced in normal subjects significant granulocytopenia within 40 minutes, and recovery in 4 hours. The patient's serum was also shown to cause *in vitro* lysis of granulocytes in the presence of the drug (Moeschlin and Wagner, 1952). The possible immunological mechanisms involved in this reaction have been discussed in detail by Wintrobe (1969).

The phenothiazine tranquillizers, together with the hydantoins, sulphonamides, chloramphenicol and antithyroid drugs have been responsible for the major proportion of drug-induced agranulocytosis reported. Immune mechanisms have not been demonstrated and just how these drugs induce agranulocytosis is not known. In this type of granulocytopenia, there is a latent period of varying duration. After 20 or more days, a sharp drop in the leucocyte count occurs in association with what appears to be a hypofunction of the bone-marrow. DNA synthesis has been shown to be impaired by chlorpromazine and it has been suggested that the normal person who shows no ill effect from chlorpromazine administration overcomes the delay in DNA synthesis because the proliferative potentiality of his marrow cells is sufficiently great to compensate for the drug-induced delay. However, the person who has a limited proliferative potential would show ill effects when treated with the drug.

Whether the agranulocytosis induced by phenothiazines other than chlorpromazine, and whether that due to the other agents mentioned, follow a similar pattern of cause, is not known. Possibly other mechanisms are involved and possibly combinations of mechanisms occur. Certainly, according to published reports, some of the drugs associated with agranulocytosis appear to produce this by one mechanism in certain cases and by another in other instances. In some cases the iatrogenic effect is seen soon after the drug has been given and bears no relation to the amount of dosage; in other cases large doses and long latent periods seem to be characteristic.

Awareness of the possible production of agranulocytosis by a drug should lead the physician to warn the patient to watch for fever or any symptoms of infection. If symptoms do develop, the patient should stop taking the drug immediately and should report to the physician. If this procedure is followed, early diagnosis and, usually, rapid recovery will result. The fall in leucocyte count, once it begins, is rapid. Routine blood cell counts may detect the disorder before infection develops, which greatly improves the chance of rapid recovery. Once the drug is discontinued, recovery usually begins within a week. The mortality rate can be more than 20 per cent because of the frequency and severity of the infections, which characteristically complicate agranulocytosis.

DRUG-INDUCED THROMBOCYTOPENIA

CHLORAMPHENICOL

Thrombocytopenia is a relatively common manifestation with drugs that cause a severe pancytopenia, i.e.

anaemia, leucopenia and thrombocytopenia. Chloramphenicol will induce pancytopenia and the commonest presenting symptom in a series of 40 cases reported by Sharp (1963) was epistaxis, purpura or menorrhagia, all manifestations of haemorrhagic diathesis. A similar complication as part of a pancytopenic condition has been reported with phenylbutazone.

RIFAMPICIN

Rifampicin is a new oral antitubercular antibiotic of considerable therapeutic promise and together with ethambutol is probably the combination of choice in the treatment of tuberculosis resistant to the 'main-line' agents. Blajchman and associates (1970) have reported two cases of severe thrombocytopenia associated with rifampicin treatment. It is pertinent to draw attention to these reports here since hitherto rifampicin has been considered to have remarkably low toxicity.

In the first case severe thrombocytopenia occurred during administration and readministration of the antibiotic. The patient's erythrocytes gave a positive direct antiglobulin test due to complement on the red cell surface; in the serum, complement-fixing antibodies were detected which were directed against the drug. In the initial administration of rifampicin, ethambutol was given as well but, as shown by the immunological studies, the latter was not incriminated in the thrombocytopenia.

Immunological studies showed antibodies, of both IgG and IgM type, capable of fixing complement to both normal and the patient's platelets, but only in the presence of rifampicin. In addition, the IgM type of antibody, but not the IgG, was capable of fixing complement to normal red cells; again only in the presence of the drug.

The second patient was on an intermittent high dose regimen for 4 months, preceded by 3 months of daily treatment. He did not receive ethambutol.

The direct antiglobulin test was weakly positive owing to complement on the red cell surface. Antirifampicin antibodies were found in the serum before a

TABLE 4.6

DRUGS ASSOCIATED WITH THROMBOCYTOPENIA
(based on Huguley, 1966; Wintrobe, 1969)

CLASS OF DRUG	MEMBERS
Analgesics	phenylbutazone, acetylsalicylic acid
Antibacterial agents	sulphonamides, rifampicin, penicillin, chloramphenicol
Non-antibacterial sulphonamide derivatives	chlorothiazide, chlorpropamide, tolbutamide, acetazolamide, carbutamide
Cinchona alkaloids	quinine, quinidine
Tranquillizers	meprobamate

dose of rifampicin, and were not detectable 6 hours later when thrombocytopenia was observed.

A list of drugs, recognized by the American Medical Association Registry on Blood Dyscrasias, as being associated with thrombocytopenia is given in TABLE 4.6 (Huguley, 1966; Wintrobe, 1969).

Thrombocytopenia is a less frequent adverse drug reaction than granulocytopenia and has usually been less serious in its consequences. Wintrobe (1969) has calculated that about 17 per cent of cases reported to the AMA Registry were of this type.

In most instances the reaction would appear to be caused by an immunological mechanism.

DRUGS INTERFERING WITH BLOOD GROUP AND COM-PATABILITY TESTING

Although such drugs are not of themselves directly iatrogenic they may set in motion a sequence of events which can have a serious effect on the patient; for this reason mention of these drugs and their effects are made in this context.

Drugs may interfere with blood group and compatability testing either by producing rouleaux formation or by causing a direct positive antiglobulin test (Coombs test). Some drugs therefore may be a potential source of error in correct blood grouping and cross matching and lead to transfusion mismatching with its attendant hazards.

ROULEAUX FORMATION

The most common cause of a marked degree of rouleaux formation is the infusion of high-molecular-weight dextrans, e.g. dextran 150 or dextran 110, that have a mean molecular weight of 110,000 or higher. Low-molecular-weight dextrans such as *Rheomacrodex* are less likely to cause rouleaux formation.

Rouleaux formation may give the appearance of agglutination with both anti-A and anti-B sera and cause misidentification of blood group AB. If the patient's cells are washed with saline before grouping the problem is minimized. The presence in serum of high-molecular-weight dextran may also give a false appearance of agglutination in the added donor cells. Diluting the recipient's serum 1 in 2 or 1 in 4 with saline is recommended since this will have little adverse effect on true agglutination.

POSITIVE COOMBS TEST

Drugs which give a positive direct antiglobulin test are of two types: drugs that cause an immune haemolytic anaemia in which the antibody works only in the presence of the drug (e.g. penicillin, sulphonamides, sodium aminosalicylate, quinine, quinidine, phenacetin, and antazoline hydrochloride). This group of drugs rarely interferes with compatability tests.

However, of much greater importance are the drugs that cause auto-immune haemolytic anaemia where the antibody reacts in the absence of the drug and is thus active against normal red cells. Examples of these are methyldopa and mefenamic acid.

In practice (Ali, 1970) those drugs which have been found to be particularly likely to give rise to problems of blood grouping and compatability are:

  i. High-molecular-weight dextrans
  ii. Methyldopa
  iii. Mefenamic acid
  iv. Penicillin in doses greater than 20 mega units/day.

The blood transfusion laboratory should always be informed if patients are receiving these drugs.

DRUG-INDUCED METHAEMOGLOBINAEMIA AND SULPHAEMOGLOBINAEMIA

Methaemoglobin is formed when the iron in the haemoglobin molecule is oxidized from the ferrous to the ferric state. In this form it cannot be oxygenated and is, therefore, useless for oxygen transport. This oxidation is reversible and methaemoglobin is readily reduced to haemoglobin by appropriate reducing substances.

The precise chemical structure of sulphaemoglobin has not been determined; it is produced by the action of hydrogen sulphide on oxyhaemoglobin. Sulphaemoglobin cannot be oxygenated, nor can it be reconverted to haemoglobin.

The effect of the presence of methaemoglobin or sulphaemoglobin is two-fold. Firstly, that portion of haemoglobin that is converted to methaemoglobin or sulphaemoglobin is not available for oxygen transport. Secondly, Darling and Roughton (1942) demonstrated that the presence of methaemoglobin in the circulation altered the dissociation curve of the remaining oxyhaemoglobin in such a way that tissue oxygen tensions must fall to lower levels than normal before the remaining oxyhaemoglobin yields its oxygen.

In mild cases, cyanosis is the cardinal sign. In more severe cases this is accompanied by the syndrome of acute hypoxia, with exertional dyspnoea, headache, dizziness and deterioration of mental functions. In extreme instances this syndrome may progress to stupor or even coma (Cecil and Loeb, 1959).

In the first quarter of the twentieth century a great interest was expressed in a small ill-defined group of cases. They were characterized by cyanosis with the presence of methaemoglobinaemia and sulphaemo-globinaemia. Bowel dysfunction was found in the majority and headache was a frequent symptom. This disorder was thought to be caused by the absorption of an enterogenous oxidant from the gut. Shortly after 1925 it was demonstrated that phenacetin could produce both sulphaemoglobin and methaemoglobin. From this date the clinical entity of enterogenous cyanosis disappeared and a new hazard of drug therapy was discovered.

Drug-induced methaemoglobinaemia has been demonstrated to be caused by phenacetin, sulphonamides, bismuth subnitrate, nitrites, nitrates, pamaquin, primaquine, sulphones, acetanilide, phenazone, chlorates, aniline and nitrobenzene. Administration of a reducing substance is needed to convert the methaemoglobin back to oxyhaemoglobin. Ascorbic acid is non-toxic, but is less effective than methylene blue. Methylene blue, 250 mg per day in divided doses with ascorbic acid 400–500 mg per day is effective treatment; however, if there is urgency in treatment methylene blue 1–2 mg per kg, i.v. or ascorbic acid 0·5–1 gram, i.v. can be given.

Sulphaemoglobinaemia is caused predominantly by phenacetin and acetanilide; sulphaemoglobin cannot be reconverted to normal haemoglobin (Cecil and Loeb, 1959; Laurence, 1963).

RECOMMENDED FURTHER READING

BEUTLER, E. (1959) The hemolytic effect of primaquine and related compounds: A review, *Blood*, **14**, 103–39.

HAMPTON, J. R. (1970) Platelet abnormalities induced by the administration of oestrogens, *J. clin. Path.*, **23**, Suppl. (Ass. Clin. Path.), **3**, 75–80.

HORSFIELD, G. I., and CHALMERS, J. N. M. (1963) Megaloblastic anaemia associated with anticonvulsant therapy, *Practitioner*, **191**, 316–21.

HUGULEY, C. M., JR., (1966) Hematological reactions, *J. Amer. med. Ass.*, **196**, 408–10.

MEYER, M. C., and GUTTMAN, D. E. (1968) The binding of drugs by plasma proteins, *J. pharm. Sci.*, **57**, 895–918.

WADE, O. L. (1966) Prescribing of chloramphenicol and aplastic anaemia, *J. roy. Coll. gen. Practit.*, **12**, 277–86.

WALLERSTEIN, R. O., CONDIT, P. K., KASPER, C. K., BROWN, J. W., and MORRISON, F. R. (1969) Statewide study of chloramphenicol therapy and fatal aplastic anemia, *J. Amer. med. Ass.*, **208**, 2045–50.

WINTROBE, M. M. (1969) The therapeutic millennium and its price: A view from the haematopoietic system, The Lilly Lecture, 1968, *J. roy. Coll. Phycns Lond.*, **3**, 99–119.

WITTS, L. J. (1961) Some aspects of the pathology of anaemia, *Brit. med. J.*, **2**, 325–8, 404–10.

REFERENCES

AKSOY, M., and ERDEM, S. (1968) Aplastic anaemia after propylthiouracil, *Lancet*, **i**, 1379.

ALI, M. A. (1970) Drugs interfering with blood grouping and compatability tests, *Prescribers' J.*, **10**, 60–2.

BARNARDO, D. E., CURREY, H. L. F., MASON, R. M., FOX, R. W., and WEATHERALL, M. (1966) Mefenamic acid and flufenamic acid compared with aspirin and phenylbutazone in rheumatoid arthritis, *Brit. med. J.*, **2**, 342–3.

BASS, B. H. (1963) Megaloblastic anaemia due to nitrofurantoin, *Lancet*, **i**, 530–1.

BEARDWELL, C. G. (1964) Acute haemolytic anaemia with antipenicillin antibodies complicating subacute bacterial endocarditis, *Proc. roy. Soc. Med.*, **57**, 332–3.

BELTON, E. M., and JONES, R. V. (1965) Haemolytic anaemia due to nalidixic acid, *Lancet*, **ii**, 691.

BEUTLER, E. (1957) The glutathione instability of drug-sensitive red cells; a new method for the *in vitro* detection of drug sensitivity, *J. Lab. clin. med.*, **49**, 84–95.

BEUTLER, E. (1959) The hemolytic effect of primaquine and related compounds: A review, *Blood*, **14**, 103–39.

BEUTLER, E., DERN, R. J., and ALVING, A. S. (1954) The hemolytic effect of primaquine, IV. The relationship of cell age to hemolysis, *J. Lab. clin. Med.*, **44**, 439–42.

BEUTLER, E., DERN, R. J., FLANAGAN, C. L., and ALVING, A. S. (1955) The hemolytic effect of primaquine, VII. Biochemical studies of drug-sensitive erythrocytes, *J. Lab. clin. Med.*, **45**, 286–95.

BEUTLER, E., YEH, M., and FAIRBANKS, V. F. (1962) The normal human female as a mosaic of X-chromosome activity: Studies using the gene for G-6-PD-deficiency as a marker, *Proc. nat. Acad. Sci. (Wash.)*, **48**, 9–16.

BLAJCHMAN, M. A., LOWRY, R. C., PETTIT, J. E., and STRADLING, P. (1970) Rifampicin-induced immune thrombocytopenia, *Brit. med. J.*, **3**, 24–6.

BRANDT, N. J., and LUND, J. (1966) Methyldopa and haemolytic anaemia, *Lancet*, **i**, 771.

BREWER, G. J., TARLOV, A. R., and ALVING, A. S. (1960) Methaemoglobin reduction test, *Bull. Wld Hlth Org.*, **22**, 633–40.

BREWER, G. J., TARLOV, A. R., and KELLERMEYER, R. W. (1962) The hemolytic effect of primaquine, XII. Shortened erythrocyte life span in primaquine sensitive male Negroes in the absence of drug administration, *J. Lab. clin. Med.*, **58**, 217–33.

BRITISH MEDICAL JOURNAL (1963) Broad-spectrum antibiotics, in Today's Drugs, *Brit. med. J.*, **1**, 1276–77.

BRITISH MEDICAL JOURNAL (1967) Toxicity of chloramphenicol, leading article, *Brit. med. J.*, **1**, 649.

BUCHANAN, J. G., RUSH, B., and DE ERUNCHY, G. C. (1966) Methyldopa and acquired haemolytic anaemia, *Med. J. Aust.*, **2**, 700–1.

CAHAL, D. A. (1966) Methyldopa and haemolytic anaemia, *Lancet*, **i**, 201.

CAHILL, W. J., HILL, R. D., JESSOP, J., and KENDALL, P. H. (1965) Trial of mefenamic acid, *Ann. phys. Med.*, **8**, 26–9.

CANADA, A. T., JR., and BURKA, E. R. (1968) Aplastic anemia after indomethacin, *New Engl. J. Med.*, **278**, 743–4.

CANTOR, S., and BARNETTS, A. J. (1967) Haematological effects of methyldopa, *Lancet*, **i**, 625.

CARSON, P. E., FLANAGAN, C. L., ICKES, C. E., and ALVING, A. S. (1956) Enzymatic deficiency in primaquine-sensitive erythrocytes, *Science*, **124**, 484–5.

CARSON, P. E., SCHRIER, S. L., and KELLERMEYER, R. W. (1959) Mechanism of inactivation of glucose 6-phosphate dehydrogenase in human erythrocytes, *Nature (Lond.)*, **184**, 1292–3.

CARSTAIRS, K. C., BRECKENRIDGE, A., DOLLERY, C. T., and WORLLEDGE, S. M. (1966a) Incidence of a positive direct Coombs test in patients on α methyldopa, *Lancet*, **ii**, 133–5.

CARSTAIRS, K. C., WORLLEDGE, S., DOLLERY, C. T., and BRECKENRIDGE, A. (1966b) Methyldopa and haemolytic anaemia, *Lancet*, **i**, 201.

CECIL, R. L., and LOEB, R. F. (1959) *Textbook of Medicine*, 10th ed., Philadelphia, pp. 505–7.

CLAYTON, E. M., ALTSHULER, J., and BOVE, J. R. (1965) Penicillin antibody as a cause of positive direct antiglobulin tests, *Amer. J. clin. Path.*, **44**, 648–53.

COTTON, S. G. (1966) Methyldopa and haemolytic anaemia, *Lancet*, ii, 165.

CRAMOND, E. H. (1966) Haemolytic anaemia and alpha-methyldopa, *Med. J. Aust.*, 1, 995.

CUSTER, R. P. (1946) Aplastic anemia in soldiers treated with Atabrine (quinacrine), *Amer. J. med. Sci.*, 212, 211–24.

DALDERUP, C. B. M. (1968) Antithyroid drugs, in *Side Effects of Drugs*, Vol. VI, eds. Meyler, L., and Herxheimer, A., Excerpta Medica Foundation, Amsterdam, pp. 433–5.

DAMESHEK, W., and COLMES, A. (1936) The effect of drugs in the production of agranulocytosis with particular reference to amidopyrine hypersensitivity, *J. clin. Invest.*, 15, 85–97.

DARLING, R. C., and ROUGHTON, F. J. W. (1942) The effect of methaemoglobin on the equilibrium between oxygen and haemoglobin, *Amer. J. Physiol.*, 137, 56–68.

DARNBOROUGH, J. (1966) Methyldopa and haemolytic anaemia, *Lancet*, i, 262.

DA SILVA HORTA, J., ABBATT, J. D., DA MOTTA, L. C., and RORIZ, M. L. (1965) Malignancy and other late effects following administration of Thorotrast, *Lancet*, ii, 201–5.

DAWSON, R. B., JR., and SEGAL, B. L. (1966) Penicillin-induced immunohemolytic anemia, *Arch. intern. Med.*, 118, 575–9.

DERN, R. J., BEUTLER, E., and ALVING, A. S. (1954a) The hemolytic effect of primaquine, II. The natural course of the hemolytic anemia and the mechanism of its self-limited character, *J. Lab. clin. Med.*, 44, 171–6.

DERN, R. J., WEINSTEIN, I. M., LEROY, G. V., TALMAGE, D. W., and ALVING, A. S. (1954b) The hemolytic effect of primaquine, I. The localisation of the drug-induced hemolytic defect in primaquine-sensitive individuals, *J. Lab. clin. Med.*, 43, 303–9.

FLANAGAN, C. L., SCHRIER, S. L., CARSON, P. E., and ALVING, A. S. (1958) The hemolytic effect of primaquine, VIII. The effect of drug administration on parameters of primaquine sensitivity, *J. Lab. clin. Med.*, 51, 600–8.

FREZZINE, C. (1966) Anemia emolitica autoimmune da alfa-metildopa, *Clin. ter.*, 36, 263.

FULD, H., and MOORHOUSE, E. H. (1956) Observations on megaloblastic anaemias after primidone, *Brit. med. J.*, 1, 1021–3.

GALE, E. F. (1958) Mode of action of chloramphenicol, in *Ciba Foundation Symposium on Amino Acids and Peptides with Antimetabolic Activity*, ed. Wolstenholme, G. E. W., and O'Connor, C. M., London, pp. 19–33.

GARRETT, A. S., and CORCOS, M. G. (1952) Dapsone treatment of leprosy, *Leprosy Rev.*, 23, 106–8.

GIRDWOOD, R. H. (1964) Drug induced blood disorders, *Brit. J. clin. Pract.*, 18, 701–7.

GLOCK, G. E., and McLEAN, P. (1953) Further studies on the properties of glucose-6-phosphate dehydrogenase and 6-phosphogluconate dehydrogenase of rat liver, *Biochem. J.*, 55, 400–8.

HAMILTON, M., JENKINS, G. C., and TURNBULL, A. L. (1966) Methyldopa and haemolytic anaemia, *Lancet*, i, 549.

HAWKINS, C. F., and MEYNELL, M. J. (1954) Megaloblastic anaemia due to phenytoin sodium, *Lancet*, ii, 737–8.

HAWKINS, C. F., and MEYNELL, M. J. (1958) Macrocytosis and macrocytic anaemia caused by anticonvulsant drugs, *Quart. J. Med.*, 27, 45–63.

HAY, J. (1966) Haemolytic anaemia and alpha-methyldopa, *Med. J. Aust.*, 1, 1090.

HAYES, D. (1966) Methyldopa and haemolytic anaemia, *Lancet*, i, 365.

HOCKWALD, R. S., ARNOLD, J., CLAYMAN, C. B., and ALVING, A. S. (1952) Status of primaquine, IV. Toxicity of primaquine in Negroes, *J. Amer. med. Ass.*, 149, 1568–70.

HODGMAN, J. E. (1961) Chloramphenicol, *Pediat. Clin. N. Amer.*, 8, 1027–42.

HOFFBRAND, A. V., and NECHELES, T. F. (1968) Mechanism of folate deficiency in patients receiving phenytoin, *Lancet*, ii, 528–30.

HUGULEY, C. M., JR. (1966) Hematological reactions, *J. Amer. med. Ass.*, 196, 408–10.

INGALL, D., SHERMAN, J. D., COCKBURN, F., and KLEIN, R. (1965) Amelioration by ingestion of phenylalanine of toxic effects of chloramphenicol on bone-marrow, *New Engl. J. Med.*, 272, 180–5.

KÄHLER, H. J. (1965) Chloramphenicol: Ein vielseitiges und zeitloses Antibiotikum, *Med. Klin.*, 60, 2005–11.

KILPSTEIN, F. A. (1964) Subnormal serum folate and macrocytosis associated with anticonvulsant drug therapy, *Blood*, 23, 68–86.

KIRKMAN, H. N. (1959) Glucose-6-phosphate dehydrogenase and human erythrocytes, *Nature (Lond.)*, 184, 1291–2.

KORNBERG, A. (1950) Enzymic synthesis of triphosphopyridine nucleotide, *J. biol. Chem.*, 182, 805–13.

LAI, M., ROSNER, F., and RITZ, N. D. (1966) Hemolytic anemia due to antibodies to penicillin, *J. Amer. med. Ass.*, 198, 483–4.

LANCET (1966) Methyldopa and haemolytic anaemia, leading article, *Lancet*, ii, 151–2.

LAURENCE, D. R. (1963) *Clinical Pharmacology*, 2nd ed. London, pp. 453–4.

LEVINE, B. B., and REDMOND, A. (1966) Information Exchange Group No. 5, cited by White *et al.* (1968) *Brit. med. J.*, 2, 26–8.

LEY, A. B., CAHAM, A., and MAYER, K. (1959) in *Proceedings of the Seventh Congress of the International Society of Blood Transfusion*, Basel, p. 539.

LOUIS, W. J., DOYLE, A. E., JERUMS, G., and KINCAID-SMITH, P. (1967) Methyl-dopa and haemolytic anaemia, *Med. J. Aust.*, 2, 104–6.

MANTEN, A. (1968) Antibiotic drugs, in *Side Effects of Drugs*, Vol. VI, eds. Meyler, L., and Herxheimer, A., Excerpta Medica Foundation, Amsterdam, pp. 263–314.

MARKS, P. A., and GROSS, R. T. (1959) Further characterisation of the enzymic defect in glucose-6-phosphate deficiency, *J. clin. Invest.*, 38, 1023–4.

MARKS, P. A., SZEINBERG, A., and BANKS, J. (1961) Erythrocyte glucose 6-phosphate dehydrogenase of normal and mutant human subjects: Properties of purified enzymes, J. biol. Chem., 236, 10–17.

MARTELO, O. J., KATIMS, R. B., and YUNIS, A. A. (1967) Bone marrow aplasia following propylthiouracil therapy. Report of a case with complete recovery, *Arch. intern. Med.*, 120, 587–90.

McCURDY, P. R. (1961) Chloramphenicol bone marrow toxicity, *J. Amer. med. Ass.*, 176, 588–93.

McDUFFIE, F. C. (1965) Bone-marrow depression after drug therapy in patients with systemic lupus erythematosus, *Ann. rheum. Dis.*, 24, 289–92.

McMURDOCH, J. McC., SPEIRS, C. F., and MACE, M. (1968) Fatal marrow aplasia after chlorpropamide and methyldopa, *Lancet*, i, 207.

MEYLER, L. (1966a) Chemotherapeutic drugs, in *Side Effects of Drugs*, Vol. V, eds. Meyler, L., *et al.*, Excerpta Medica Foundation, Amsterdam, pp. 256–83.

MEYLER, L. (1966b) Cytostatic drugs, in *Side Effects of Drugs*, Vol. V, eds. Meyler, L., *et al.*, Excerpta Medica Foundation, Amsterdam, pp. 472–94.

MOESCHLIN, S., and WAGNER, K. (1952) Agranulocytosis due to occurrence of leukocyte-agglutinins, *Acta. haemat. (Basel)*, **8**, 29–41.

MORGAN, H. V. (1967) personal communication.

MURRAY, R. M., TIMBURY, G. C., and LINTON, A. L. (1970) Analgesic abuse in psychiatric patients, *Lancet*, i, 1303–5.

MYLES, A. B., BACON, P. A., and WILLIAMS, K. A. (1967) Mefenamic acid in rheumatoid arthritis, *Ann. rheum. Dis.*, **26**, 494–8.

NAGAO, T., and MAUER, A. M. (1969) Concordance for drug-induced aplastic anemia in identical twins, *New Engl. J. Med.*, **281**, 7–11.

NESMITH, L. W., and DAVIS, J. W. (1968) Hemolytic anemia caused by penicillin, *J. Amer. med. Ass.*, **203**, 27–30.

ORY, E. M., and YOW, E. M. (1963) The use and abuse of the broad spectrum antibiotics, *J. Amer. med. Ass.*, **185**, 273–9.

O'SHEA, R. F. (1966) Haemolytic anaemia and alpha methyldopa, *Med. J. Aust.*, **1**, 816.

PARR, C. W. (1962) Drug-induced haemolytic anaemia, *Lond. Hosp. Gazette*, **65**, (Clin. Sci. Suppl.), iii–viii.

PATON, A. (1966) Methyldopa and haemolytic anaemia, *Lancet*, i, 549.

PENGELLY, C. D. R. (1963) Dapsone induced haemolysis, *Brit. med. J.*, **2**, 662–4.

PETZ, L. D., and FUDENBERG, F. D. (1966) Coombs-positive hemolytic anemia caused by penicillin administration, *New Engl. J. Med.*, **274**, 171–8.

PRESCOTT, L. F. (1968) Antipyretic and analgesic drugs, in *Side Effects of Drugs*, Vol. VI, eds. Meyler, L., and Herxheimer, A., Excerpta Medica Foundation, Amsterdam, pp. 101–39.

REYNOLDS, E. H., HALLPIKE, J. F., PHILLIPS, B. M., and MATTHEWS, D. M. (1966b) Reversible absorptive defects in anticonvulsant megaloblastic anaemia, *J. clin. Path.*, **18**, 593–8.

REYNOLDS, E. H., MILNER, G., MATTHEWS, D. M., and CHANARIN, I. (1966a) Anticonvulsant therapy, megaloblastic haemopoiesis and folic acid metabolism, *Quart. J. Med.*, **35**, 521–37.

RHIND, E. G., and VARADI, S. (1954) Megaloblastic anaemia due to phenytoin sodium, *Lancet*, ii, 921.

ROSENBACH, L. M., CAVILES, A. P., and MITUS, W. J. (1960) Chloramphenicol toxicity: Reversible vacuolisation of erythroid cells, *New Engl. J. Med.*, **263**, 724–8.

ROSENBERG, I. H., GODWIN, H. A., STREIFF, R. R., and CASTLE, W. B. (1968) Impairment of intestinal deconjugation of dietary folate, *Lancet*, ii, 530–2.

RYAN, G. M. S., and FORSHAW, J. W. B. (1955) Megaloblastic anaemia due to phenytoin sodium, *Brit. med. J.*, **2**, 242–3.

SAIDI, P., and WALLERSTEIN, R. O. (1960) Effect of chloramphenicol on erythropoiesis, *Clin. Res.*, **8**, 131.

SAIDI, P., WALLERSTEIN, R. O., and AGGELER, P. M. (1961) Effect of chloramphenicol on erythropoiesis, *J. Lab. clin. Med.*, **75**, 247–56.

SCHINDEL, L. (1968) Antiprotozoal drugs, in *Side Effects of Drugs*, Vol. VI, eds. Meyler, L., and Herxheimer, A., Excerpta Medica Foundation, Amsterdam, pp. 320–34.

SCHWARTZ, M., and DIGE-PETERSON, H. (1966) Methyldopa and haemolytic anaemia, *Lancet*, i, 434.

SCOTT, G. L., MYLES, A. B., and BACON, P. A. (1968) Autoimmune haemolytic anaemia and mefenamic acid therapy, *Brit. med. J.*, **3**, 534–5.

SHARP, A. A. (1963) Chloramphenicol-induced blood dyscrasias: Analysis of 40 cases, *Brit. med. J.*, **1**, 735–6.

SMITH, R. S., and ALEXANDER, S. (1959) Heinz-body anaemia due to Dapsone, *Brit. med. J.*, **1**, 625–7.

STRUMIA, P. V., and RAYMOND, F. D. (1962) Acquired hemolytic anemia and antipenicillin antibody, *Arch. intern. Med.*, **109**, 603–8.

SWANSON, M. A., CHANMOUGAN, D., and SCHWARTZ, R. S. (1966) Immunohemolytic anemia due to antipenicillin antibodies, *New Engl. J. Med.*, **274**, 178–81.

TARLOV, A. R., BREWER, G. J., CARDON, P. E., and ALVING, A. S. (1962) Primaquine sensitivity, *Arch. intern. Med.*, **109**, 209–34.

VAN ARSDEL, P. P., JR., and GILLILAND, B. C. (1965) Anemia secondary to penicillin treatment. Studies on two patients with 'non-allergic' serum hemagglutins, *J. Lab. clin. Med.*, **65**, 277–85.

VARGAS, L. P., and GONZALEZ, C. S. (1967) Haemolytic anaemia after nalidixic acid, *Lancet*, ii, 97–8.

VELLA, F., and IBRAHIM, S. A. (1962) Erythrocyte glucose-6 phosphate deficiency in Khartoum, *Sudan med. J.*, **1**, 136–7.

WEINER, W., and PATON, A. (1966) Methyldopa and haemolytic anaemia, *Lancet*, ii, 860–1.

WEINREICH, J., and ROHR, R. (1967) Autoimmunhämolytische Anämie als mögliche Komplikation einer Langzeittherapie mit α Methyl-Dopa, *Dtsch. med. Wschr.*, **92**, 161–3.

WHITE, J. M., BROWN, D. L., HEPNER, G. W., and WORLEDGE, S. M. (1968) Penicillin-induced haemolytic anaemia, *Brit. med. J.*, **2**, 26–8.

WILLIAMS, J. O., MENGEL, C. E., SULLIVAN, L. W., and HAQ, A. S. (1969) Megaloblastic anemia associated with chronic ingestion of an analgesic, *New Engl. J. Med.*, **280**, 312–13.

WINTROBE, M. M. (1967) *Clinical Hematology*, 6th ed., Philadelphia.

WINTROBE, M. M. (1969) The therapeutic millennium and its price: A view from the haematopoietic system, The Lilly Lecture, 1968, *J. roy. Coll. Phycns Lond.*, **3**, 99–119.

WORLEDGE, S. M., CARSTAIRS, K. C., and DACIE, J. V. (1966) Autoimmune haemolytic anaemia associated with α methyldopa therapy, *Lancet*, ii, 135–9.

WURZEL, H. A., and SILVERMAN, J. L. (1966) Methyl-Dopa and haemolytic anaemia, *Lancet*, i, 1158.

5

CARDIAC DYSFUNCTION

DRUG-INDUCED ABNORMALITIES OF MYOCARDIAL FUNCTION WITH CHARACTERISTIC ECG CHANGES

DIGITALIS

A recent survey of hospital in-patients in Belfast (Hurwitz and Wade, 1969) showed that 19·8 per cent of patients treated with digoxin suffered an adverse reaction to it, and that reactions to digitalis accounted for one-third of all drug reactions monitored.

The four principal actions of digitalis on the heart are summarized below. The major facets of digitalis toxicity are enumerated together with indications of how these may be avoided or counteracted.

Direct Stimulation of the Myocardium with Increased Force of Contraction

Digitalis increases the work done by the dilated, failing ventricle without increasing its oxygen consumption. The dilated failing heart is reduced in size simultaneously with the increased work efficiency. This is most likely due to active shortening of myocardial fibres (increased diastolic tone) and also to reduction of the distending force (venous pressure). Reduction in the diastolic size alone is a considerable advantage since this results in lower oxygen consumption for equivalent work.

This increased cardiac output leads to reduction in the reflex venoconstriction, characteristic of low output heart failure, and venous pressure is lowered. Secondly, there is a reduction in plasma volume due to improved renal blood flow and the resulting diuresis.

Increased Myocardial Excitability

This has no therapeutic benefit. High dosage of digitalis causes ventricular ectopic beats and these give rise to the classic digitalis-induced pulsus bigeminus, when each normal beat is closely followed by a ventricular ectopic beat which is then followed by a compensatory pause.

Ventricular ectopic beats may show complexes of different shapes on the same ECG. This suggests that there is more than one focus in the ventricular initiating impulses and that there is an increased risk of ventricular tachycardia and fibrillation.

Because digitalis causes increased myocardial excitability, careful thought must be given to the choice of any concommitant therapy, since other agents, for example sympathomimetic amines and aminophylline,

may also increase cardiac excitability in their own right, and a combination of one of these with digitalis could precipitate arrhythmias in the digitalized patient. Reserpine is another example of a drug that could precipitate digitalis arrhythmia under these circumstances.

Any therapy that reduces the serum potassium level in a digitalized patient will increase the risk of digitalis-induced cardiac arrhythmias. Diuretics, particularly the thiazide group and adrenal steroids, may precipitate digitalis toxicity by depleting the body of potassium.

Intravenous glucose may lower the serum potassium since the passage of glucose into the skeletal muscle is coupled with movement of potassium ions in the same direction.

Digitalis-induced arrhythmia may demand the administration of potassium chloride orally (5–7 grams) which acts in 30 minutes. Since toxic effects are liable to last for several days, 1 gram of potassium chloride may have to be given orally three times a day for two to three days. Serum potassium should not, however, be allowed to exceed normal limits and it should be remembered that potassium by any route is dangerous in the presence of renal failure.

The β-adrenergic blocker, propranolol, can abolish digitalis-induced arrhythmias and it is probably safer than potassium in unskilled hands. Procainamide and quinidine have been used to treat digitalis-induced arrhythmias but they increase markedly the block of conducting tissue and the heart may stop; however, in an emergency, when the serum potassium has not been estimated, it may be necessary to use these cardiac depressants cautiously.

Calcium increases digitalis actions in animals and the administration of intravenous calcium to digitalized patients requires caution. Reduction in ionized calcium in the blood by means of a chelating agent, e.g. trisodium edetate, is sometimes used in therapy for digitalis poisoning.

Depression of Conducting Tissue

The refractory period of the A-V node and the bundle of His are increased and conduction time is increased; this is shown by an increase in the P-R intervals on the ECG. In therapeutic doses this effect has little or no effect on heart rate, but it is used therapeutically in the treatment of auricular fibrillation to protect the ventricle from the too numerous impulses which would otherwise cause the ventricle to contract before diastolic filling was complete.

Toxic doses of digitalis may cause complete heart block; indeed this was first recorded by Withering

(1785) who described 'slow pulse, even as slow as 35 in a minute, cold sweats, syncope, convulsions, death'.

Therapeutically, the main warning in remembering that digitalis causes A-V block is that this pharmacological action may summate with that of quinidine or procainamide which may be given as cardiac depressants to treat digitalis-induced cardiac arrhythmias and which also cause A-V block.

Increased Vagal Activity on the Heart

There are some doubts about the locus of action of digitalis in producing increased vagal activity; it may be the vagus centre, the afferent nerve endings or on effectors in the myocardium. There are, however, no doubts about the outcome: there is a decreased auricular refractory period converting flutter to fibrillation, a delayed A-V conduction, and bradycardia.

Some skill and considerable practice are needed to use digitalis to best advantage and Withering's comments are still fully valid: 'it is better the world should derive some instruction, however imperfect, from my experience, than the lives of men should be hazarded by its unguarded exhibition, or that a medicine of so much efficacy should be condemned and rejected as dangerous and unmanageable'.

The effects of digitalis on the ECG may be summarized as follows:

(i) The T-wave becomes smaller, disappears, or may even invert.
(ii) The S-T segment sags below the isoelectric line.
(iii) The P-R interval is prolonged (delayed A-V conduction).
(iv) The Q-T interval is shortened (shorter ventricular systole).

The character of the S-T segment and T-wave changes cannot be used as an index of adequate digitalis therapy. With small digitalizing doses significant digitalis effects may be seen on the ECG; however, in other instances in the presence of a therapeutically adequate dosage, the effect on the ECG may be minimal. Similarly, digitalis toxicity cannot be judged on the basis of S-T segment, T-wave or Q-T interval variations. Digitalis toxicity may produce prolongation of the P-R interval or other symptoms of A-V block and may, at the same time, be associated with increased frequency of ventricular ectopic contractions from one or more foci. Paroxysmal atrial tachycardia with A-V block has received much attention as a manifestation of digitalis intoxication, but this may occur in a digitalized patient with no other evidence of digitalis intoxication. Thus, even the presence of this arrhythmia alone does not warrant the assumption that excessive digitalis has been given.

Laurence (1963) has written what is perhaps the best phrase to conclude such a summary of the adverse effects of digitalis—'digitalis, like most potent therapeutic agents can be a potent poison if misused'.

QUINIDINE AND QUININE

Quinidine, the dextro-isomer of quinine, is one of the natural alkaloids found in cinchona bark; it is a cardiac depressant and has been recognized as an agent for the treatment of arrhythmias for over 100 years. Quinidine has four principal actions: depression of excitability of cardiac muscle, prolongation of effective refractory period, depression of cardiac conducting tissue and reduction of vagal nerve activity.

The earliest and most readily observed ECG disturbances are a prolongation of the P-R interval, a prolonged QRS complex and Q-T interval. Quinidine may also produce atrial flutter.

Quinidine is a cumulative drug and the effects of large doses on the heart include extrasystoles, atrioventricular and intraventricular block, ventricular tachycardia and fibrillation, and cardiac asystole (*British Medical Journal*, 1969).

The incidence of death due to the use of quinidine in the treatment of chronic atrial arrhythmias has been reported as being between 3–4 per cent, and systemic embolism and toxic effects on the myocardium and CNS have been blamed for sudden death during quinidine therapy (Thomson, 1956; Selzer and Wray, 1964). Rokseth and Storstein (1963) reported cardiac complications in 57 out of 274 patients when quinidine was used in the conversion of atrial fibrillation. These complications included premature beats, nodal rhythm, and A-V block. In 12 patients there was sudden loss of consciousness. The authors warned that constant supervision was necessary during quinidine therapy since the syncope usually occurred without warning and was frequently associated with small doses of quinidine. This complication would seem to occur predominantly in patients with auricular fibrillation of long standing, large hearts and congestive heart failure.

The loss of consciousness was usually due to arrhythmia with failing cardiac output but respiratory depression also probably played a part. All patients recovered. Artificial respiration, and if necessary treatment of cardiac arrest, were recommended. The electrocardiograms showed ventricular premature beats, bradycardia, total A-V block, and nodal rhythm. Besides artificial respiration, 50 mg ephedrine intramuscularly seemed to be useful.

In rare instances quinidine has been connected with sudden death; the mechanism is unknown, but ventricular fibrillation may have been responsible, whilst the possibility of respiratory arrest (due to central action) has also been mentioned. Davies et al. (1965) presented case-reports of six cases of syncope following the use of quinidine for atrial fibrillation; one of the six cases was fatal, necropsy did not reveal any evidence of embolism, and the authors considered the attacks to be due to ventricular asystole or fibrillation. They commented that precautions regarding quinidine therapy, including hospitalization, a test dose, prior digitalization and cathode-ray oscilloscope monitoring, may all be carried out and yet the patient may suddenly die from the effects of quinidine therapy.

Selzer and Wray (1964) reported that 'quinidine syncope' was a common event in their experience after modest doses of quinidine and was usually due to paroxysmal ventricular fibrillation. It was suggested, and this has been subsequently confirmed by others, that the ventricular fibrillation was due to myocardial sensitivity to quinidine and not to the toxic effect of high blood levels of the alkaloid as implied by earlier investigators. Thus the importance of a test dose of quinidine and of never initiating quinidine therapy without there being adequate monitoring and resuscitative equipment close at hand has been stressed (*British Medical Journal*, 1969).

Within this general context of complications of therapy it must be recalled that quinidine is a cumulative drug and large doses give rise to cinchonism, characterized by tinnitus, headache, nausea, abdominal pain, skin rashes, disturbed vision, and amaurosis. The drug should be withheld if toxic effects more serious than nausea or diarrhoea occur. Quinidine is contraindicated in the aged and it is dangerous in patients with severe infections or cardiac damage.

Quinine (the one-time antimalarial and antipyretic) is not used clinically as a cardiac depressant; however, in a recent communication Lupovich and colleagues (1970) from Pittsburg have reported that it is now common practice for 'dope dealers' to adulterate heroin with quinine. To these connoisseurs quinine is superior to the other common adulterant, lactose, since firstly, its bitter taste mimics the taste of heroin itself making it difficult to detect the adulteration, and secondly, when injected 'main line' the quinine causes a vasodilation which mimics certain vascular effects of heroin sufficiently to help confound the naive purchaser.

Thus many addicts are currently injecting themselves intravenously with relatively large amounts of quinine. The authors cite details of two cases in which there was a clinically apparent depression of myocardial excitability.

The first case arrived at hospital in a coma; within 10 minutes heart and respiration ceased. Closed chest cardiac massage and endotracheal intubation with ventilation were successful in restoring the heart beat. After intravenous administration of 2 mg of nalorphine spontaneous respiration resumed and the patient became alert and responsive. Cardiac evaluation disclosed no clinical, radiologic, electrocardiographic or chemical evidence of underlying heart disease. Thin-layer chromatography detected quinine and morphine (deacetylated metabolite of heroin) in the urine. On questioning, the patient related that he had injected heroin intravenously but did not experience the expected results. Two hours later he self-administered another dose purchased from the same dealer and lost consciousness.

The second patient had requested treatment of heroin addiction of 15 years' duration; he had been taking four to five 'bags' of heroin daily for the previous 8 months. At a previous routine pre-employment medical examination he had been told he had an 'irregular heart beat'. Electrocardiogram at admission showed second-degree A-V block with Wenkebach phenomena; a urine sample taken on the following day was positive for quinine. During the next 3 days the patient had first-degree A-V block with a P-R interval of 0.21 seconds. On the 5th hospital day, the second-degree block with Wenkebach phenomena was again noted; exercise reverted the rhythm to a normal sinus mechanism with the P-R interval gradually increasing from 0.18 to 0.22 seconds within 30 seconds. A Valsalva manoeuvre then induced second-degree block. The next day the urine was negative for quinine. On the 7th hospital day, exercise again abolished the second-degree block but a Valsalva manoeuvre failed to reinduce it. The patient was discharged on the 11th hospital day with a normal sinus rhythm and a P-R interval of 0.17 seconds; at this point a Valsalva manoeuvre failed to induce any degree of A-V block.

This form of quinine cardiotoxicity has hitherto not been appreciated as a complication of intravenously administered narcotics.

EMETINE (EMETINE HYDROCHLORIDE, EMETINE BISMUTH IODIDE)

Emetine is a toxic drug; it is highly active against extra-intestinal amoebiasis and against the symptoms of amoebic dysentery. Although the importance of its toxicity may have been exaggerated (Adams, 1960) it is certainly true that toxicity has precluded its administration in the high doses necessary to treat severe amoebic infections.

The most important toxic effects of emetine are cardiovascular. Tachycardia and electrocardiographic abnormalities, myocarditis, pericarditis and hypotension have occurred. The ECG offers a sensitive and early index of cardiotoxicity and various changes have been described. They include lowering and inversion of T-waves, deformation of S-T segments, deformation of QRS complexes, and prolongation of P-R and Q-T time; atrial tachycardia, premature beats or both may occur (Wagner, 1964). Excretion and detoxification are slow. Therefore, the cumulative action of the drug is one of the hazards involved.

The incidence of these electrocardiographic changes is fairly high. They were observed, for example, in 43 out of 49 cases treated with 60 mg emetine per day intramuscularly for 10–15 days. In another report ECG changes were found in all 25 cases studied. In 23 (92 per cent) cardiographic effects were present by the time the course of emetine was completed; in two patients there was a delay of 8 days and of 17 days after stopping treatment, respectively (Turner, 1963). In two patients the ECG became so grossly abnormal as to suggest myocardial infarction.

It has been recommended that emetine should be

discontinued if either tachycardia or an abnormal ECG occurs because of the danger of cardiac arrest.

Work aimed at the elucidation of the chemical structure of natural emetine opened up the route to the synthesis of possibly less toxic derivatives and in the early and mid-1960s one of these compounds, dehydro-emetine, was subjected to extensive clinical investigation. It was shown to be as active as emetine but considerably better tolerated. Transient ECG changes, mainly T-wave changes, have been observed following treatment. These changes, rarely associated with clinical symptoms, were less frequent and of shorter duration than under therapy with emetine. When dehydroemetine was given orally as resinate, side-effects were reduced and in most instances were limited to nausea, diarrhoea and weakness; Schindel (1968) has reviewed the literature on this emetine derivative.

AMITRIPTYLINE

In a series of 65 patients given the antidepressant amitriptyline orally in a dosage of 75–225 mg daily, 12 showed definite ECG changes and 21 showed less clear changes. The ECG changes included isoelectric T_1 and T_2 waves or both, depression of S-T interval and flattening of the T-waves in the I and II leads, inversion of the T-waves in lead III, ventricular extrasystoles and tachycardia. In two patients left bundle branch block developed during the treatment, and disappeared when amitriptyline was withdrawn (Rasmussen and Krist-jansen, 1963).

IMIPRAMINE

Marked ECG changes have been reported following administration of the antidepressant imipramine. Kristiansen (1961), in order to study the alteration in the ECG during treatment with imipramine, took ECG recordings before and after the performance of work on Master's steps, together with measurement of blood pressure in the supine and standing position, plasma potassium and potassium urinary excretion in 23 patients. All patients received imipramine; the highest dose given was 200 mg daily.

In 15 cases there were ECG changes comprising of flattening or inversion of the T-waves in leads I and II, which were first manifested on or were aggravated by physical exertion. These changes were independent of variations in plasma potassium or urinary excretion of potassium. Hypotension could only have played any part in five of these cases.

The frequency of hypotension with imipramine therapy may be of importance, but there does appear to be a direct myocardial effect which, with the usual dose in healthy subjects, is reversible. A direct toxic effect on the heart by imipramine is supported by the fact that imipramine tends to accumulate in myocardial tissue.

The effects of imipramine on the myocardium have been demonstrated even more clearly in cases of imipramine poisoning, where there was supraventricular tachycardia, with ventricular complexes widened by conduction delay; runs of ventricular tachycardia and considerable variation in rate; alternating T-waves, extrasystoles, broadening of the QRS complexes, S-T depression and flattening of the T-waves. Ventricular flutter, atrial fibrillation and A-V block have also occurred.

These abnormal ECG changes can persist up to 80 hours after an overdose of imipramine (Edwards, 1964).

These changes induced by imipramine in therapeutic dosage do not appear significant or serious in healthy persons, but in other circumstances there may be an increased risk of myocardial disease.

THIORIDAZINE

In a number of patients changes in ECG have been noticed to occur during therapy with the phenothiazine tranquillizer, thioridazine. In one report by Kelly *et al.* (1963) a total of 28 ECGs were presented in which changes were seen during treatment with thioridazine at doses as low as 200 mg daily. Inverted or flattened T-waves and convex S-T segments were observed. In two fatal cases, alternation of heart block and ventricular tachycardia occurred prior to death. A 51-year-old man receiving thioridazine, 1,500 mg daily, died following collapse with ventricular tachycardia. A 46-year-old woman receiving thioridazine, 3,600 mg daily, collapsed and died within 24 hours. A ventricular tachycardia was present with a bizarre combination of heart block and ectopic beats.

GUANETHIDINE

Griffiths (1968) describes a case in which bradycardia (rate 52/min) occurred in a 65-year-old woman who was being re-treated with guanethidine for hypertension, and who had previously suffered subjective intolerable side-effects from this drug. The ECG showed complete A-V block. The prescribed dose of guanethidine (50 mg daily) was within therapeutic limits. Suppression of catecholamine excitation in the bundle of His was thought to have caused this complication. Guanethidine therapy was discontinued and oral isoprenaline restored a normal rhythm after 3 weeks' treatment. Guanethidine is retained in tissues for some days and this is probably the reason for the delay in return of a normal rhythm.

FRUSEMIDE (FURSEMIDE, FUROSEMIDE)

Three cases of sudden death following intravenous or intramuscular frusemide have appeared in the literature in recent years. In two cases, a 62-year-old man (Machtey, 1968) and a 7-year-old boy (Rance, 1969), sudden collapse occurred within one minute of injection of the diuretic. The ECG in both cases showed ventricular asystole. In the child the heart was restarted but he died 48 hours later from a further cardiac arrest.

The third patient, 94 years old, also died one minute after intramuscular injection of frusemide; the final

ECG in this case was reported as showing ventricular tachycardia (Machtey, 1968).

All three cases had impaired renal function. The child was being treated for nephrotic syndrome, and the two men had markedly raised blood urea and grossly raised blood glucose levels.

CARDIOTOXICITY OF ISO-PRENALINE AND OTHER SYMPATHOMIMETIC AMINES

The epidemiological association between the increase in death rate in the young asthmatic and the abuse of pressurized aerosols containing symphthomimetic amines has stimulated considerable interest in the way in which isoprenaline (isoproterenol) and other symphthomimetic amines could cause these sudden deaths (Grant et al., 1968; Gresham and Calder, 1968).

It has been well documented that isoprenaline can cause myocardial necrosis in rats (Chappel et al., 1959a, 1959b; Rona et al., 1959a, 1959b; Selye and Bajusz, 1959; Beznak, 1962; Handforth, 1962; Ferrans et al., 1964; Wexlar et al., 1968). Potentiation of the cardiotoxic effect of isoprenaline by steroids was described by Selye and Bajusz (1959) and Chappel et al. (1959a) and by thyroxine by Chappel et al. (1959b). Despite these findings of myocardial necrosis caused by isoprenaline in the rat, no such toxicity has been described in man.

Lockett (1965) found that in cats doses of isoprenaline fifteen times smaller than those tolerated by healthy heart-lung preparations, were sufficient to stop a heart experimentally embarrassed by an increased work-load caused by overventilation of the lung. She suggested therefore that isoprenaline and orciprenaline might be dangerous when given to a patient with a failing overloaded myocardium.

Collins et al. (1969) studied the cardiotoxicity of isoprenaline in dogs during hypoxic conditions. In dogs breathing room air, isoprenaline caused an increase in heart rate, increased cardiac output and increased rate of left ventricular ejection, and slight fall in both systolic and diastolic blood pressure. However, isoprenaline given to dogs under hypoxic conditions caused a reduction in heart rate and cardiac contractility and a much larger fall in systolic and diastolic blood pressures. Dogs that died from isoprenaline overdosage in room air, died in ventricular fibrillation, with doses of isoprenaline of up to 250 micrograms per kg i.v. but under hypoxic conditions death occurred in ventricular asystole with doses as low as 10 micrograms per kg i.v.

It is of considerable interest to note, in this respect, that in three cases of sudden death following isoprenaline usage, in which ECG recordings showed that cardiac arrest was preceded by a progressive bradycardia and finally resulted in asystole, no ventricular fibrillation was observed (Grant et al., 1968). However, Gresham and Calder (1968) believed that ventricular

fibrillation was the cause of death in six young asthmatics, but only on the basis of post-mortem findings!

The increased cardiotoxicity of isoprenaline in hypoxic conditions may be relevant clinically, particularly in view of the findings that isoprenaline and other bronchodilator agents cause a worsening in ventilation perfusion ratio in the lungs due to vasodilation in poorly ventilated regions of lung and increasing ventilation of the already well ventilated areas of the lung, and that this is associated with a fall in arterial paO_2 (Chapman and Hughes, 1966; Field, 1967; Knudson and Constantine, 1967; Palmer and Diament, 1967a, 1967b; Rees et al., 1967; Chapman and Dowd, 1969).

Chapman and Hughes (1966) described eight consecutive cases of chronic non-specific lung disease in seven of which there was an average fall in paO_2 of 9·9 mmHg following inhalation of isoprenaline. Field

FIG. 5.1. *Comparison of structural formulae of some sympathomimetic bronchodilators*

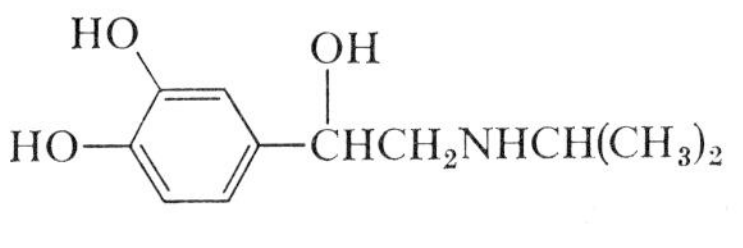

Isoprenaline (Isoproterenol)

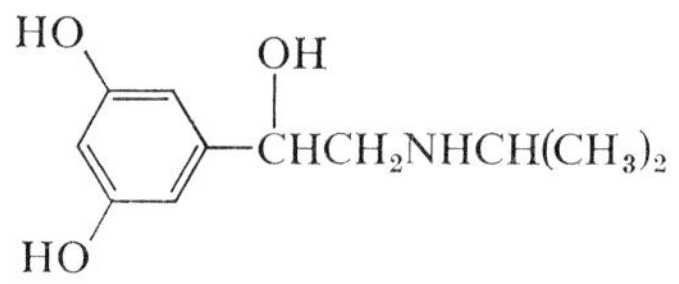

Orciprenaline (Metaproterenol)

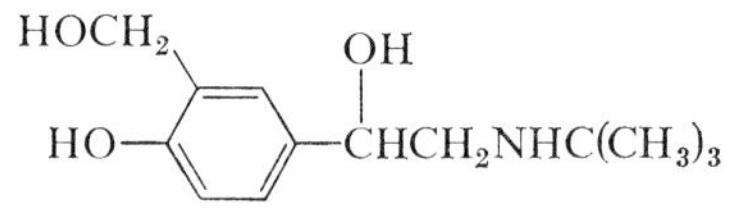

Salbutamol

(1967) described 26 asthma patients in whom the ventilation perfusion ratio was worsened by isoprenaline. Knudson and Constantine (1967) described a further 10 cases in which FEV_1 increased following isoprenaline but the paO_2 fell and the ventilation perfusion ratio was worsened. It is important to note that similar effects of increased FEV_1 and fall in paO_2 have been described following intravenous aminophylline (Halmagyi and Cotes, 1959), and also after atropine methonitrate (Field, 1967), and after salbutamol and orciprenaline (metaproterenol) (Chapman, 1969).

The fall of paO_2 caused by alteration of the ventilation perfusion ratio might, therefore, be clinically relevant if the patient's paO_2 is initially coincident with the steep portion of the oxygen dissociation curve for haemoglobin, where a small change in paO_2 can produce a large fall in oxygen carrying ability.

The only bronchodilator agent that has been tested by Chapman that does not cause a worsening of ventilation perfusion ratio is *Medihaler-Duo*, in which a mixture of isoprenaline and phenylephrine is used. It is believed that the isoprenaline and the phenylephrine summate in their action to produce bronchodilation and exert opposing α and β actions on the pulmonary vasculature so that increased perfusion of under-ventilated lung does not occur.

The structural formulae of the sympathomimetic amines discussed in this section are compared in FIGURE 5.1.

DRUG-INDUCED MYOCARDITIS

Clinical observations have shown that the heart is involved more frequently as a shock organ in cases of drug allergy than has hitherto been realized. There are those relatively rare conditions which clinically resemble the myocardial infarction characteristic of patients with arteriosclerosis but which can now be recognized as forming part of an allergic drug reaction. These clinical signs of myocardial infarction, together with the typical ECG changes, are often associated with skin changes and eosinophilia, and it is precisely the latter manifestations that indicate the probability of an association with drug treatment.

Meyler (1968) reported 11 cases of drug-induced myocarditis; the drugs incriminated were *p*-amino-salicylic acid, acetylsalicylic acid, sulphonamides, phenylbutazone, methylthiouracil and benzathine penicillin G.

In Meyler's cases nine of the patients showed simultaneous cutaneous lesions of urticaria, angioneurotic oedema, rash or purpura; two cases developed jaundice; two cases had arthritis, and two cases nephritis. All 11 of Meyler's cases showed signs of drug hypersensitivity in addition to their myocarditis and all cases showed ECG changes involving the S-T segment, and/or inverted T-waves.

Four of the 11 cases were symptom free and ECG changes were discovered during investigation; five of the cases complained of dyspnoea alone.

MacSearraigh and Patel (1968) from Kampala reported the case of a 12-year-old African boy who developed a fulminating skin lesion 2 days after sulphadimidine therapy (for otitis media—6 grams of sulphadimidine over two days), and acute cardiomyopathy 28 days later. These authors rightly drew attention to the fact that in developing countries, where the budget for drugs is limited and infectious disease rampant, sulphonamides are used as first-line treatment. In their experience the use of sulphonamides was fraught with major hazard on rare occasions.

There is no clear cut information regarding the background of cardiotoxicity and sulphonamide therapy. A direct toxic effect on cellular (myocardial) enzymes was discussed by Goodman and Gilman (1955). They also suggested a hypersensitivity vasculitis such as periarteritis nodosa or disseminated lupus erythematosus, which is in agreement with Schonholzer (1940), Rich (1942), and Rich and Gregory (1943). A necropsy report which stated that death was due to periarteritis nodosa, with findings of diffuse eosinophylic myocarditis 30 days after sulphathiazole therapy (Simon, 1943), seems to have authenticated this. General concensus of opinion supports the hypersensitivity hypothesis, and we find this acceptable, but do not agree with the refutation of Fawcett (1948) that sulphonamides do not cause cardiomyopathy, since there is convincing necropsy evidence of focal myocarditis after sulphonamides (Blanchard and Mertens, 1958; Simon, 1943; French and Weller, 1942).

In connexion with the hypersensitivity hypothesis it is of considerable importance that one of Meyler's (1968) cases who had a muscle biopsy showed histological changes of arteries. Van Rijseel and Meyler (1948) described seven fatal cases of proven arteritis following sulphonamide treatment, and one other similar case after methylthiouracil.

From a structure-activity relationship, it is of interest that in a number of patients who received sulphonylureas, focal myocarditis and microgranulomata of the viscera (liver, heart and kidneys) have been found at autopsy. There were no apparent clinical features attributable to these lesions (Bloodworth, 1963).

An elderly woman with diabetes received tolbutamide (a sulphonylurea) for over three years. After a short illness associated with symptoms of weakness, vomiting and congestive heart failure she died. At autopsy focal necrotizing angiitis of the kidneys, uterus and peri-adrenal vessels was found, as well as a diffuse interstitial and perivascular infiltration by eosinophils and mononuclear cells in the myocardium. Acute arteriolitis and periarteritis with fibrinoid necrosis was present in a number of organs (Kline *et al.*, 1963).

Fatal myocarditis after vaccination against smallpox can occur although it is probably a rare complication. Electrocardiographic evidence of myocarditis may perhaps be more frequently obtainable; it seems likely that this adverse effect is not always noticed and is indeed often not even looked for.

ENDOCARDIAL FIBROSIS INDUCED BY METHYSERGIDE

Methysergide was introduced into the therapy of migraine in 1959 because of its anti-serotonin activity and a current theory that serotonin (5-HT) played a role in the migrainous process. The structural relationship between these two molecules is shown in FIGURE 5.2.

The retroperitoneal fibrosis arising during methysergide therapy is practically identical clinically and pathologically with the 'idiopathic' form of that disease. The pulmonary aortic complications are very similar to those seen in rheumatoid disorders and the endocardial lesions bear a strong resemblance to those found in the carcinoid syndrome. Since each of these conditions is rare their rather sudden repeated emergence in one group of patients, all taking the same drug over a relatively short period of time, lends credence to perhaps more than a casual association between drug

FIG. 5.2. *Structural relationship between methysergide and serotonin*

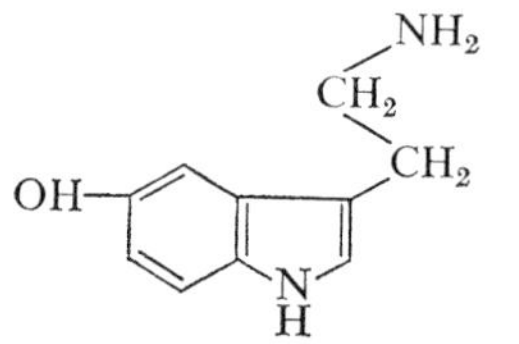

Serotonin (5-hydroxytryptamine)

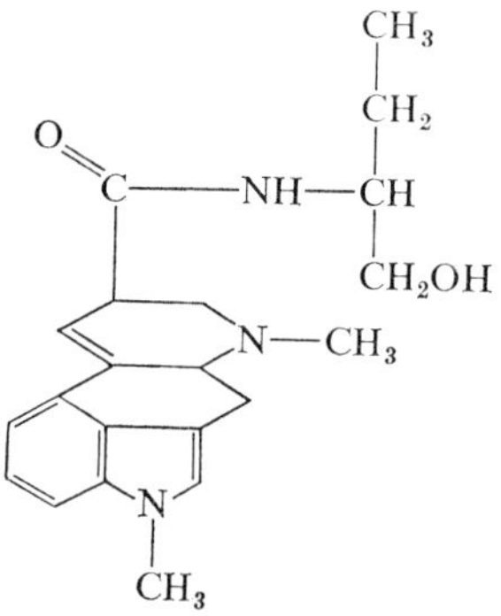

Methysergide

and disease. The association is strengthened by the fact that the spontaneous form of the disease is usually progressive, but the drug-induced form shows some regression on cessation of treatment and recrudescence of the disease on readministration of the drug. The latter relation is now well documented in the case of retroperitoneal fibrosis and the drug-induced association seems well founded (Graham, 1964; Utz *et al.*, 1965). In the case of pleuro-pulmonary fibrosis and

endocardial fibrosis, the evidence is certainly pointing in this direction; but the number of examples is less, the possibilities of other factors as aetiologic agents are greater, and the examples of regression on withdrawing the drug are less dramatic.

It is pertinent therefore in this context to mention in brief detail the relationship between methysergide and retroperitoneal fibrosis since this obviously has a bearing on the incidence of endocardial fibrosis. Graham (1964) presented experience with methysergide in 500 cases and judged that, of all the drugs available, this was the best for preventing vascular headaches of the migraine type. In his series, 20 per cent of patients encountered side-effects so unpleasant or disabling that the use of the drug was discontinued. Two of these patients developed retroperitoneal fibrosis following severe infections of the leg and thrombophlebitis. Utz and his colleagues at the Mayo Clinic (Utz *et al.*, 1965) reported retroperitoneal fibrosis, confirmed at surgery, in three patients after methysergide was administered for periods longer than a year. They admitted that a direct causal relationship between the drug and retroperitoneal fibrosis had not been established by their cases but pointed out that none of the other common precipitating causes of the condition was present.

Graham (1968) reviewed the first 27 cases with methysergide-induced retroperitoneal fibrosis and found that seven patients had significant cardiac murmur; in four of these cases the murmurs were known to have developed during methysergide therapy. In three cases the murmurs regressed significantly after discontinuing methysergide therapy.

In a prospective study involving careful recording of cardiac findings, in patients before and after they took methysergide, Graham (1968) found 23 cases who developed significant murmurs; 14 patients had murmurs of aortic insufficiency; five disappeared several months after stopping methysergide. Fifteen patients had systolic murmurs, some basal, some apical, some both; three of these disappeared after ceasing therapy.

MacNeal (quoted by Graham, 1968) reported that he had seen 13 cases of methysergide-induced murmurs; nine with mitral insufficiency and four with aortic insufficiency. The aortic murmurs disappeared after stopping therapy but the mitral murmurs remained unchanged.

In the reported cases of pericardial fibrosis there was a preponderance of five females to one male.

RECOMMENDED FURTHER READING

BRITISH MEDICAL JOURNAL (1969) Digitalis and the cardiac glycosides, in Today's Drugs, *Brit. med. J.*, **2**, 744–6.
BRITISH MEDICAL JOURNAL (1969) Is quinine outdated?, leading article, *Brit. med. J.*, **1**, 331–2.
KOO-YOUNG CHUNG (1968) Cardiac failure from digitalis intoxication, in *Drug-Induced Diseases*, Vol. 3, eds. Meyler, L., and Peck, H. M., Excerpta Medica Foundation, Amsterdam, pp. 53–93.
MCMICHAEL, J. (1963) The heart and digitalis, *Brit. med. J.*, **2**, 73–9.

REFERENCES

ADAMS, A. R. D. (1960) Amoebiasis and amoebic dysentery, *Brit. med. J.*, **1**, 956–7.

BEZNAK, M. (1962) Hemodynamics during the acute phase of myocardial damage caused by isoproterenol, *Canad. J. Biochem.*, **40**, 25–30.

BLANCHARD, A. J., and MERTENS, G. A. (1958) Hypersensitivity myocarditis occurring with sulphamethoxypyridazine therapy, *Canad. med. Ass. J.*, **79**, 627–30.

BLOODWORTH, J. M. B., JR. (1963) Morphologic changes associated with sulphonylurea therapy, *Metabolism*, **12**, 287–301.

BRITISH MEDICAL JOURNAL (1969) Is quinine outdated?, leading article, *Brit. med. J.*, **1**, 331–2.

CHAPMAN, T. T. (1969) Bronchodilator aerosols, *Brit. med. J.*, **4**, 557.

CHAPMAN, T. T., and DOWD, D. (1969) Bronchodilator combinations and arterial oxygen tensions in chronic non-specific lung disease, *Pharmacol. Clin.*, **1**, 107–9.

CHAPMAN, T. T., and HUGHES, D. T. D. (1966) Increasing hypoxia in chronic lung disease following administration of a bronchodilator, *J. Irish. med. Ass.*, **59**, 184–9.

CHAPPEL, C. I., RONA, G., and GAUNDRY, R. (1959a) Relationship between thyroid function and cardiotoxic properties of isoproterenol, *Endocrinology*, **65**, 208–14.

CHAPPEL, C. I., RONA, G., and GAUNDRY, R. (1959b) The influence of adrenal-cortical steroids on cardiac necrosis produced by isoproterenol, *Acta endocr. (Kbh.)*, **32**, 419–24.

COLLINS, J. M., MCDEVITT, D. G., SHANKS, R. G., and SWANTON, J. G. (1969) The cardiotoxicity of isoprenaline during hypoxia, *Brit. J. Pharmacol.*, **36**, 35–45.

DAVIES, P., LEAK, D., and ORAM, S. (1965) Quinidine-induced syncope, *Brit. med. J.*, **2**, 517–20.

EDWARDS, A. C. (1964) Imipramine myocardial toxicity, *N.Y. St. J. Med.*, **64**, 1979–82.

FAWCETT, R. M. (1948) Myocardium after sulfonamide therapy, *Arch. Path.*, **45**, 25–35.

FERRANS, V. J., HIBBS, R. G., BLACK, W. C., and WEIL-BAECHER, D. G. (1964) Isoproterenol-induced myocardial necrosis, *Amer. Heart J.*, **68**, 71–90.

FIELD, G. B. (1967) The effects of posture, oxygen, isoproterenol and atropine on ventilation perfusion relationships in the lung in asthma, *Clin. Sci.*, **32**, 279–88.

FRENCH, A. J., and WELLER, C. V. (1942) Interstitial myocarditis following clinical and experimental use of sulfonamide drugs, *Amer. J. Path.*, **18**, 109–21.

GOODMAN, L. S., and GILMAN, A. (1955) *Pharmacological Basis of Therapeutics*, 2nd ed., New York, p. 1300.

GRAHAM, J. R. (1964) Methysergide for prevention of headache: Experience in five hundred patients over three years, *New Engl. J. Med.*, **270**, 67–72.

GRAHAM, J. R. (1968) Fibrosis associated with methysergide therapy, in *Drug-Induced Diseases*, Vol. 3, eds. Meyler, L., and Peck, H. M., Excerpta Medica Foundation, Amsterdam, pp. 249–69.

GRANT, I. W. B., KENNEDY, W. P. V., and MALONE, D. N. (1968) Deaths from asthma, *Brit. med. J.*, **2**, 429–30.

GRESHAM, G. A., and CALDER, I. M. (1968) Sudden death in young asthmatics, *Brit. med. J.*, **3**, 186–7.

GRIFFITHS, H. J. L. (1968) A case of complete heart block produced by guanethidine, *Amer. Heart J.*, **75**, 371–4.

HALMAGYI, D. R., and COTES, J. E. (1959) Reduction in systemic blood oxygen as a result of procedures affecting pulmonary circulation in patients with chronic pulmonary disease, *Clin. Sci.*, **18**, 475–89.

HANDFORTH, C. P. (1962) Isoproterenol-induced myocardial infarction in animals, *Arch. Path.*, **73**, 161–5.

HURWITZ, N., and WADE, O. L. (1969) Intensive hospital monitoring of adverse reactions to drugs, *Brit. med. J.*, **1**, 531–6.

KELLY, H. G., FAY, J. E., and LAVERTY, C. S. (1963) Thioridazine hydrochloride (Melloril): Its effect on the electrocardiogram and a report of two fatalities with electrocardiographic abnormalities, *Canad. med. Ass. J.*, **89**, 546–54.

KLINE, I. K., KLINE, T. S., and SAPHIR, O. (1963) Myocarditis in senescence, *Amer. Heart J.*, **65**, 446–57.

KNUDSON, R. J., and CONSTANTINE, H. P. (1967) An effect of isoproterenol on ventilation perfusion ratios in asthmatic versus normal subjects, *J. appl. Physiol.*, **22**, 402–6.

KRISTIANSEN, E. S. (1961) Cardiac complications during treatment with imipramine (Tofranil), *Acta psychiat. (Kbh.)*, **120**, 1125–6.

LAURENCE, D. R. (1963) *Clinical Pharmacology*, 2nd ed., London, p. 317.

LOCKET, M. F. (1963) Dangerous effects of isoprenaline in myocardial failure, *Lancet*, **ii**, 104–6.

LUPOVICH, P., PILEWSKI, R., SAPIRA, J. D., and JUSELIUS, R. (1970) Cardiotoxicity of quinine as adulterant in drugs, *J. Amer. med. Ass.*, **212**, 1216.

MACHTEY, I. (1968) Sudden death after intramuscular frusemide, *Lancet*, **ii**, 1301.

MACSEARRAIGH, E. T. M., and PATEL, K. M. (1968) Cardiomyopathy as a complication of sulphonamide therapy, *Brit. med. J.*, **3**, 33.

MEYLER, L. (1968) Myocarditis due to drugs, in *Drug-Induced Diseases*, Vol. 3, eds. Meyler, L., and Peck, H. M., Excerpta Medica Foundation, Amsterdam, pp. 152–7.

PALMER, K. N. V., and DIAMENT, M. L. (1967a) Spirometry and blood-gas tensions in bronchial asthma and chronic bronchitis, *Lancet*, **ii**, 383–4.

PALMER, K. N. V., and DIAMENT, M. L. (1967b) Effect of aerosol isoprenaline on blood-gas tensions in severe bronchial asthma, *Lancet*, **ii**, 1232–3.

RANCE, C. P. (1969) Cardiac arrest after intramuscular frusemide, *Lancet*, **i**, 1265–6.

RASMUSSEN, E. B., and KRISTJANSEN, P. (1963) ECG changes after amitriptyline, *Amer. J. Psychiat.*, **119**, 781–2.

REES, H. A., BORTHWICK, R. C., MILLAR, J. S., and DONALD, K. W. (1967) Aminophylline in bronchial asthma, *Lancet*, **ii**, 1167–9.

RICH, A. R. (1942) Role of hypersensitivity in periarteritis nodosa as indicated by seven cases developing during serum sickness and sulfonamide therapy, *Bull. Johns Hopk. Hosp.*, **71**, 123–40.

RICH, A. R., and GREGORY, J. E. (1943) Experimental demonstration that periarteritis nodosa is manifestation of hypersensitivity, *Bull. Johns Hopk. Hosp.*, **72**, 65–88.

RIJSEL, T. G. VAN, and MEYLER, L. (1948) Necrotizing generalized arteritis due to use of sulfonamide drugs, *Acta. med. scand.*, **132**, 251–64.

ROKSETH, R., and STORSTEIN, O. (1963) Quinidine therapy of chronic auricular fibrillation, *Arch. intern. Med.*, **111**, 184–9.

RONA, G., CHAPPEL, C. I., BALAZS, T., and GAUNDREY, R. (1959a) An infarct-like myocardial lesion and other toxic manifestations produced by isoproterenol, *Arch. Path.*, **67**, 443–55.

RONA, G., ZOSTER, T., CHAPPEL, C. I., and GAUNDRY, R. (1959*b*) Myocardial lesions, circulatory and electrocardiographic changes produced by isoprenaline in the dog, *Rev. canad. Biol.*, **18**, 83–94.

SCHINDEL, L. (1968) Antiprotozoal drugs, in *Side Effects of Drugs*, Vol. VI, eds. Meyler, L., and Herxheimer, A., Excerpta Medica Foundation, Amsterdam, pp. 320–34.

SCHONHOLZER, G. (1940) Die bindung von Prontosil un die bluteiweisskörper, *Klin. Wschr.*, **19**, 790–1.

SELYE, H., and BAJUSZ, E. (1959) Conditioning by corticoids for the production of cardiac lesions with noradrenaline, *Acta endocr. (Kbh.)*, **30**, 183–7.

SELZER, A., and WRAY, H. W. (1964) Quinidine syncope. Paroxysmal ventricular fibrillation occurring during treatment of chronic atrial arrhythmias, *Circulation*, **30**, 17–26.

SIMON, M. A. (1943) Pathologic lesions following administration of sulfonamide drugs, *Amer. J. med. Sci.*, **205**, 439–54.

THOMSON, G. W. (1956) Quinidine as a cause of sudden death, *Circulation*, **14**, 757–65.

TURNER, P. P. (1963) The effects of emetine on the myocardium, *Brit. Heart J.*, **25**, 81–8.

UTZ, D. C., ROOKE, E. D., SPITTELL, J. A., JR., and BARTHOLOMEW, L. G. (1965) Retroperitoneal fibrosis in patients taking methysergide, *J. Amer. med. Ass.*, **191**, 983–5.

WAGNER, L. (1964) Toxische Wirkung des Emetins in Electrocardiogramm, *Wien med. Wschr.*, **114**, 180–6.

WEXLAR, B. C., JUDD, J. T., and KITTINGER, G. W. (1968) Myocardial necrosis induced by isoproterenol in rats, *Angiology*, **19**, 665–82.

WITHERING, W. (1785) *An Account of the Foxglove*, London.

6

INTRAVASCULAR CLOTTING

Blood coagulation is a specific safety device of the body. A normal function of coagulation factors, blood platelets and circulation is essential to haemostasis. The complicated interplay of these components together with the interplay of the walls of the blood vessels and their contents obviously presents a variety of ways in which a drug can disturb this physiological equilibrium. In clinical practice the most common, but not the only, symptoms of a disturbed clotting mechanism are either haemorrhagic diathesis or thrombosis and embolism. Corticosteroids, oestrogens and oral contraceptive combinations of oestrogen and progestogen are all implicated in iatrogenic intravascular clotting, although with corticoids the incidence relative to total use, and the publicity that has been received is very small when compared with oral contraceptives.

CORTICOSTEROIDS

Treatment with corticosteroids and corticotrophin (ACTH) may predispose to intravascular thrombosis and thrombophlebitis especially if the duration of medication is prolonged. Goodman *et al.* (1964) reported fatal pulmonary artery thrombosis in two children aged 4 years and 5 years who had been treated for nephrosis with prednisone 25–80 mg daily and chlorothiazide for many months.

A number of other investigators have included thrombosis and thrombophlebitis among the complications occurring with long-term treatment; for example Turiaf and colleagues (1962) reported seven cases of venous thrombosis, and two cases of cerebral accident, among 268 patients on long-term cortisone therapy for asthma. Saxena and Crawford (1965) treated 60 children with nephrosis with corticosteroids or ACTH for 1 or 2 years; there were two cases of cerebrovascular thrombosis. Bock (1966) reported on the side-effects of corticosteroid treatment in 412 patients with neurological disorders; 11 patients (3 per cent) developed thrombosis and embolism. Huriez and Agache (1966) surveyed 2,000 patients treated with ACTH and corticosteroids for dermatological disorders; there was a 1 per cent incidence of thrombosis with ACTH, 1 per cent with prednisone and 0·2 per cent with cortisone. Cardiovascular accidents occurred in 3 per cent of patients on ACTH, 3 per cent on cortisone, 2 per cent on dexamethasone and 0·4 per cent on prednisone. Zuckner *et al.* (1967) listed side-effects of intramuscular treatment with corticosteroids in 77 patients with rheumatoid arthritis over periods of treatment from 3 months to 5 years; 3 patients suffered thrombophlebitis. A Polish report (Florkiewicz and Klamut, 1966) described thrombophlebitis of the major veins attributed to prednisone therapy in 3 cases. Kornell (1966) reported on a patient with generalized scleroderma in whom treatment with prednisolone coincided with an acceleration of involvement of the myocardium.

ORAL CONTRACEPTIVES

Synthetic progestogens [FIG. 6.1] are effective oral contraceptive agents in women, but added oestrogen [FIG. 6.1] is needed to enhance reliability as well as to prevent 'breakthrough' bleeding. It is due to this oestrogen content that problems have arisen regarding an increased risk of thrombo-embolic disease in the otherwise young and healthy woman. Oral contraceptives that contain progestogens alone are not so effective as the combined oestrogen-progestogen preparations and their use is liable to lead to a greater risk of pregnancy and disturbances of menstruation. Such progestogen-only oral contraceptives, were in fact withdrawn from the United Kingdom market at the end of January 1970.

The literature reporting adverse effects of oral contraceptives continues to proliferate; however, recently there have been a number of authoritative statements and publications on the suspected increase in thrombosis and thrombo-embolic phenomena in women taking oral contraceptives. It is with these latter reports that this chapter is primarily concerned; references to the extensive studies that have led to these statements can be found in the list of publications recommended for further reading.

EPIDEMIOLOGY OF THROMBO-EMBOLIC DISEASE FROM ORAL CONTRACEPTIVES

Oestrogen therapy is known to be associated with an increased incidence of thrombo-embolic disorders and cases have been described by Daniel *et al.* (1967) following the use of oestrogens to suppress lactation and by Bailar (1967) following oestrogen treatment in prostatic cancer. Since most oral contraceptives have an oestrogen component it is not surprising, therefore, that shortly after the introduction of oestrogen-progestogen combinations as oral contraceptive agents their

FIG. 6.1. *Comparison of structural formulae of oestrogens and progestogens in combined oral contraceptive preparations*

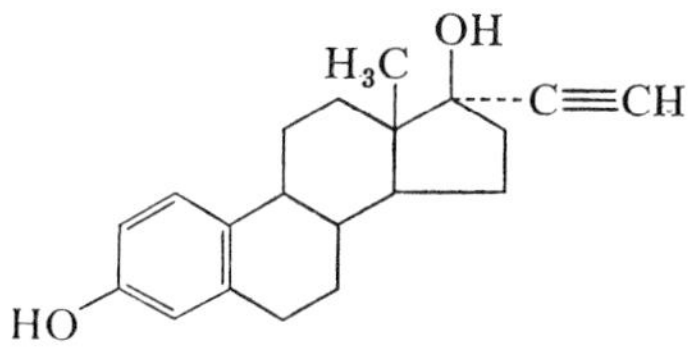

OESTROGEN
Ethinyloestradiol (Ethinylestradiol)

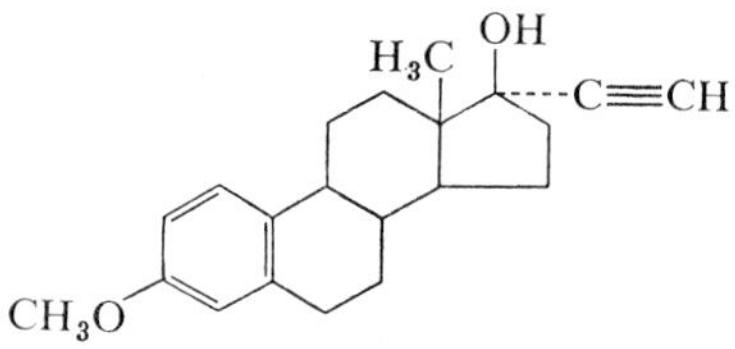

OESTROGEN
Mestranol

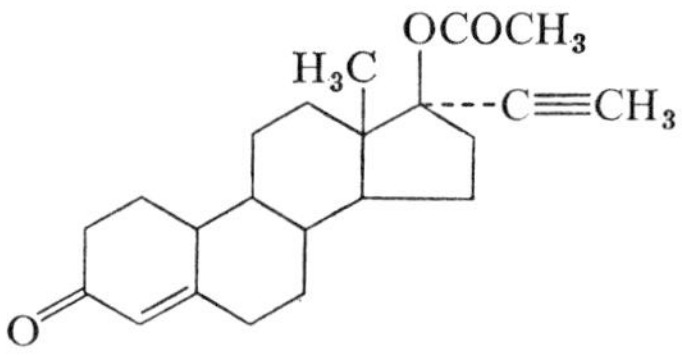

PROGESTOGEN
Norethisterone acetate (Norethindrone acetate)

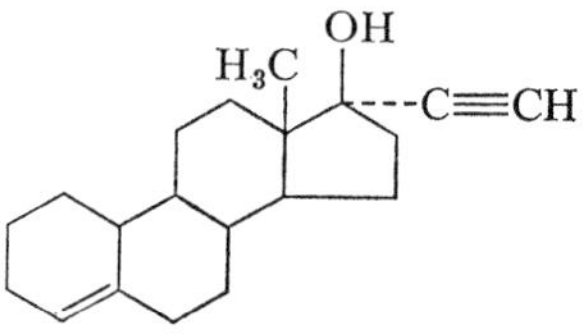

PROGESTOGEN
Lynoestrenol (Lynestrenol)

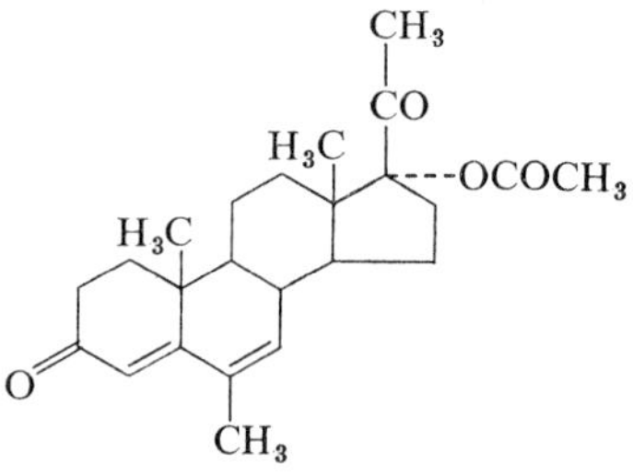

PROGESTOGEN
Megestrol acetate

usage was linked with thrombo-embolic phenomena. These fears were initially assuaged by assurances from interested bodies that the number of reported deaths from thrombo-embolism in the United States and in Britain had shown no increase in the years after these agents had become popular. Nevertheless, a sufficient number of cases was observed to prompt an independent inquiry into the matter in the United Kingdom by the Royal College of General Practitioners, by the Medical Research Council, and by the Committee on Safety of Drugs. These studies by Vessey and Doll (1968, 1969) and Inman and Vessey (1968) have now been completed and published.

In assembling the material for study particular care was taken to include all cases of death from thrombosis or embolism in women of child-bearing age. Cases where the disease was a terminal event, or occurred in a woman not exposed to pregnancy, were eliminated, as well as deaths in pregnancy and in the postnatal period. The cases were sub-divided into those in which a predisposing cause for thrombo-embolism could be identified, e.g. prolonged immobility, a recent surgical operation, hypertension or diabetes, and those where no such cause was evident. Accuracy of diagnosis was reasonably assured, since an autopsy was performed in 83 per cent of the patients in whom no predisposing cause was present. Nothing was left undone to ensure accuracy and completeness of the investigation, for previous studies have been criticized because of the likelihood of incomplete reporting.

Inman and Vessey (1968) investigated 334 deaths from pulmonary, coronary and cerebral thrombosis in women of child-bearing age, and from this study they concluded that there was a highly significant correlation between pulmonary embolism and the use of oral contraceptives, and a possible association with cerebral embolism. Vessey and Doll (1968, 1969) investigated the admissions to hospital of married women aged 16–40 for deep vein thrombosis or pulmonary embolism. Their analysis suggested that 1 woman in every 2,000 on oral contraceptives is admitted annually with these conditions against 1 in 20,000 not taking the pill.

The conclusion of the Committee on Safety of Drugs is that a strong association between the use of oral contraception and death from pulmonary embolism in previously healthy women has been established. The same is probably true for death from cerebral thrombosis, but the number of cases is admitted to be very small. The relationship to coronary thrombosis is less distinct; the production by oral contraceptives of abnormalities of carbohydrate and lipid metabolism similar to those of diabetes is known and the association between diabetes and coronary thrombosis is well established. The risk of a fatal outcome from the use of oral contraception, from pulmonary embolism or cerebral thrombosis, in the age group 20–34 is estimated at 1·5 annually per 100,000 healthy married non-pregnant women whereas the expected figure for non-users is of the order of 0·2. For the age group 35–44 the corresponding figures are appreciably higher, being 3·9 for users and 0·5 for non-users.

Meanwhile, the size of the problem increases in Britain; it is estimated that in 1963 there were only 58,000 users of contraceptive pills in the country and that by 1967 this had grown to 700,000 and in 1970 even with a conservative estimate, the number of users must exceed one and a half million per year in the United Kingdom.

In December 1969, the Committee on Safety of Drugs issued a warning statement (No. 9 in the Adverse Reaction Series) on the use of oral contraceptives containing oestrogens. They stated that approximately half the oral contraceptives prescribed in the United Kingdom contained 75 micrograms or more of oestrogen in the form of either mestranol or ethinyloestradiol; the remainder contained only 50 micrograms. Reports of suspected adverse reactions received by the Committee provided evidence that the incidence of thromboembolism was higher among women taking preparations containing larger doses of oestrogen than among those taking preparations containing the smaller dose.

The Committee had no evidence that oral contraceptives containing 50 micrograms of oestrogen were less effective than the others and thus recommended that oral contraceptives containing the smaller dose of oestrogen should normally be prescribed. TABLE 6.1 lists the low oestrogen-containing (0·05 mg) products available in the United Kingdom.

TABLE 6.1

ORAL CONTRACEPTIVES: COMBINED PREPARATIONS WITH LOW OESTROGEN CONTENT
(i.e. 50 micrograms oestrogen)

PROPRIETARY NAME	OESTROGEN CONTENT		PROGESTOGEN CONTENT	
		micrograms		milligrams
Anovlar 21	E	50	N	4
Gynovlar 21	E	50	N	3
Minilyn	E	50	L	2.5
Minovlar	E	50	N	1
Minovlar ED	E	50	N	1
Norinyl-1	M	50	N	1
Norlestrin 21	E	50	N	2.5
Orlest 28	E	50	N	1
Orthonovin 1/50	M	50	N	1
Ovulen 50	M	50	N	1
Volidan 21	E	50	Mg	4

E = Ethinyloestradiol   N = Norethisterone acetate
M = Mestranol   L = Lynoestrenol
Mg = Megestrol acetate

In February 1970, Vessey, writing in the *Prescribers' Journal*, gave emphasis to this warning of the Committee on Safety of Drugs and reviewed 'Thrombosis and the Pill' with special reference to the results of the three studies started in 1966 in the United Kingdom (Vessey and Doll, 1968, 1969; Inman and Vessey, 1968) and one in the United States (Jick *et al.*, 1969).

One of the British studies was concerned only with illness seen by the general practitioner. Most of the data related to the common disorder, superficial thrombophlebitis, and the risk of developing this condition was found to be about three times greater among women using oral contraceptives than among those not doing so. The other two British studies dealt with hospital admissions and fatalities; they were concerned with deep vein thrombosis, pulmonary embolism and cerebral and coronary thrombosis. In neither study was there any significant evidence that oral contraceptives were a cause of coronary thrombosis, but both indicated a six- to eight-fold increase in the risk of venous thromboembolism and of cerebral thrombosis among women using the preparations. Vessey (1970) combined the results for venous thrombo-embolism and cerebral thrombosis into a single table [see TABLE 6.2].

TABLE 6.2

MORBIDITY AND MORTALITY FROM THROMBOEMBOLIC DISEASE: RATES PER 100,000 WOMEN IN USERS AND NON-USERS OF ORAL CONTRACEPTIVES (VESSEY, 1970)

	AGE IN YEARS	ORAL CONTRACEPTIVES	
		USERS	NON-USERS
Morbidity* (General Practice)	15–49	450	130
Morbidity† (Hospital Admissions)	16–40	50	6
Mortality†	20–34	1.5	0.2
Mortality	35–44	3.9	0.5

* Venous thrombo-embolism (predominantly superficial thrombophlebitis)
† Venous thrombo-embolism (deep vein thrombosis and pulmonary embolism) and cerebral thrombosis

With regard to the preparation and duration of use, Vessey (1970) concluded that none of the four studies (three British, one American) gave any indication that the risk of thrombo-embolism was any greater early in the course of medication, as might be expected if it was an idiosyncratic effect, nor that the risk increased with increasing duration of use. Data from the British studies did not incriminate any particular oral contraceptive formulation with the risk of thrombo-embolism although results of the American study suggested that sequential preparations (i.e. oestrogen alone for 7, 14, 15 or 16 days followed by combined oestrogen and progestogen for respectively 15, 7, 5 and 5 days) might be more hazardous than combined preparations of oestrogen and progestogen.

With regard to genetic factors, Vessey (1970) commented that venous thrombo-embolism in association with the use of oral contraceptives was only about one-third as great among women of blood group O as among those belonging to other groups. There was no comparable data available for cerebral thrombosis.

Concerning the significance of the thrombo-embolic risks of oral contraception, Vessey (1970) has very neatly summarized the situation by concluding that the risk of dying from thrombo-embolism as a result of one year's medication with oral contraceptives is of the same order as the risk of dying from thrombo-embolism as a result of bearing one child.

In April 1970, Professor Scowen, Chairman of the Committee on Safety of Drugs, precirculated all doctors informing them that the full analysis of the data on which the Committee based its previous warning statement (December 1969) was to appear in the *British Medical Journal* (Inman *et al.*, 1970). In his letter he emphasized that the detailed evidence available to the Committee confirmed and strengthened the earlier conclusion of the Committee that the number of adverse reaction reports relating to thrombo-embolic complications was 30 per cent higher with oral contraceptives containing 100 micrograms or more of oestrogen and 20 per cent lower with those containing less than 100 micrograms than would be expected from the known risk of those preparations. The available results also demonstrated that a change to oral contraceptives of lower oestrogen dose could reduce the total deaths by 50 per cent and the morbidity from major thrombosis by at least 25 per cent; results also demonstrated that

the trend in all forms of thrombotic hazard was related to the dose of oestrogen. Doctors were recommended to prescribe combined preparations (i.e. oestrogen plus progestogen) which contained the lower dose of oestrogen.

In their paper Inman and his colleagues (1970) analysed reports of thrombo-embolism, following the use of oral contraceptives, received by drug safety committees in the United Kingdom, Sweden and Denmark to investigate possible differences in the risks associated with the various preparations. For this purpose the numbers of reports of thrombo-embolism attributed to each product were compared with the distribution that would have been expected from market research estimates of sales, assuming that all products carried the same risk.

A positive correlation was found between dose of oestrogen and the risk of pulmonary embolism, deep vein thrombosis, cerebral thrombosis, and coronary thrombosis in the United Kingdom, and a similar association was found for venous thrombosis and pulmonary embolism in Sweden and Denmark. An excess of cases of thrombo-embolism occurred at the highest dose of oestrogen.

This finding of a positive correlation between the dose of oestrogen and risk of coronary thrombosis is especially important since all previous studies reported have failed to provide clear evidence of such a relationship.

FIG. 6.2. *Stages in process of blood coagulation, showing known influence of oral contraceptives in increasing levels of specific factors.*
International nomenclature of blood coagulation factors is shown together with synonyms (based on Bell et al., 1968)

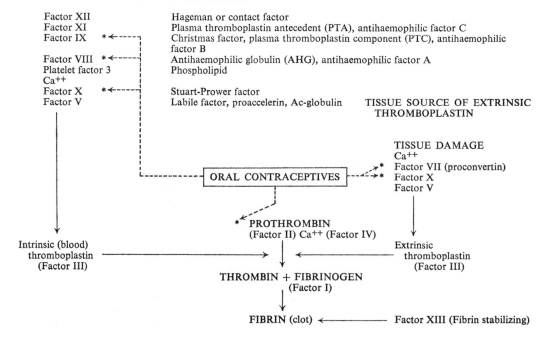

PLASMA SOURCE OF INTRINSIC THROMBOPLASTIN

Factor XII	Hageman or contact factor
Factor XI	Plasma thromboplastin antecedent (PTA), antihaemophilic factor C
Factor IX	Christmas factor, plasma thromboplastin component (PTC), antihaemophilic factor B
Factor VIII	Antihaemophilic globulin (AHG), antihaemophilic factor A
Platelet factor 3	Phospholipid
Ca++	
Factor X	Stuart-Prower factor
Factor V	Labile factor, proaccelerin, Ac-globulin

TISSUE SOURCE OF EXTRINSIC THROMBOPLASTIN

TISSUE DAMAGE
Ca++
Factor VII (proconvertin)
Factor X
Factor V

ORAL CONTRACEPTIVES

* PROTHROMBIN
(Factor II) Ca++ (Factor IV)

Intrinsic (blood) thromboplastin (Factor III)

Extrinsic thromboplastin (Factor III)

THROMBIN + FIBRINOGEN
(Factor I)

FIBRIN (clot) ◄──────── Factor XIII (Fibrin stabilizing)

No significant differences were detected between risks from sequential and combined preparations which contained the same dose of oestrogen, nor between the two oestrogens ethinyloestradiol and mestranol.

There were certain discrepancies in the data which suggested that oestrogen dosage might not be the only factor related to the risk from thrombo-embolism. For example there was a significant deficit of reports associated with the combination of mestranol 100 micrograms with norethynodrel 2·5 mg, and there was a significant excess of reports associated with the combination of ethinyloestradiol 50 micrograms with megestrol acetate 4 mg, and other combined products containing megestrol acetate. These results suggest that, although the oestrogen content of oral contraceptives is likely to be the most important factor in determining the risk of thrombo-embolism, the progestogen content may, in some preparations, influence this as well.

The sum of evidence is now so strong that there can be no reasonable doubt that thrombo-embolic disorders are associated with the use of oral contraceptives and that this effect is dose-related to the oestrogen content of these agents. Medication with a combined progestogen-oestrogen preparation is safer than with a sequential preparation especially when the oestrogen content does not exceed 50 micrograms. Medication with a progestogen alone is not so reliable and the greater risk of unwanted pregnancy and the disturbance of menstruation that occurs may well offset any advantages gained from the avoidance of possible oestrogen-induced thrombo-embolic disorder.

However, although the end-result is clear and the official recommendations have been made on this basis, the precise mechanism by which the thrombo-embolic disorders are induced has not been established. There are, however, good indications of the adverse role of oral contraceptives both on the clotting mechanisms of the blood [FIG. 6.2] and on haemodynamic factors. There is, in addition, a suggestion that genetic factors may be involved.

POSSIBLE MECHANISMS OF ORAL CONTRACEPTIVE-INDUCED THROMBO-EMBOLISM

Changes in the Clotting Mechanism

During pregnancy various changes which favour thrombo-embolic disorders have been reported to take place in the plasma clotting components. There is an increase in factor VII (stable factor, proconvertin, serum prothrombin conversion accelerator), factor VIII (antihaemophilic globulin), factor IX (plasma thromboplastin antecedent, PTA) and factor X (Stuart-Prower factor) and also in fibrinogen and platelets. Possibly, there are also changes in prothrombin and fibrinolytic components. It is not surprising therefore that there are also changes in some of the clotting components during oral contraceptive therapy.

In a relatively small series of women, Egeberg and Owren (1963) found an increase in factor VIII and a less marked increase in factor VII during contraceptive medication. Rutherford and co-workers (1964) demonstrated increased levels of prothrombin and factors VII, IX, and X. Poller and associates (1968) demonstrated an increase in factors VII and X in women taking oral contraceptives and showed that even with low-dose oral contraceptive agents there was a significant rise in the level of both factors VII and X from the third month onwards; but these changes did not appear to be dose-dependent.

Bolton et al. (1968) studied the electrophoretic activity of platelets in women on oral contraceptives; platelet mobility showed an increase in sensitivity to adenosine diphosphate but not to noradrenaline, a result that was very similar to that of patients with occlusive arterial disease. Only those contraceptives with an oestrogen component changed the sensitivity, this apparently being related to an oestrogen-induced change in platelet lecithin. In contrast, under normal conditions the mobility of platelets was sensitive to the presence of both adenosine diphosphate and noradrenaline. In pregnant women the situation was rather inconsistent although, in some cases, there was an increased sensitivity to both agents.

Influence on Haemodynamic Factors

Oral contraceptive medication has an influence on haemodynamic factors (Goodrich and Wood, 1964; Tausk, 1968; Walters and Lim, 1969) and without doubt one mechanism involved is hypervolaemia since oral contraceptives are well known to cause Na^+ and fluid retention [see CHAPTER 12]. It is the resulting slowing or stagnation of the blood that favours thrombosis.

Goodrich and Wood (1964) studied peripheral venous distensibility and venous blood flow in 60 women of whom 20 had been pregnant, 20 were in the third trimester of pregnancy and 20 were on oral contraceptives.

A small but significant increase in venous distensibility was found in the calf in both pregnant and 'pill' groups together with some decrease in the velocity of venous blood flow. In contrast in the forearm a comparable increase in distensibility (mean venous volume) was accompanied by increased velocity of flow.

The authors concluded that leg vein distension in pregnancy was not primarily due to mechanical factors and that the increased incidence of venous thrombosis in pregnancy and in women on oral contraceptives was stasis.

Walters and Lim (1969) carried out a serial study of haemodynamic changes in six healthy young women taking oral contraceptives of the combined oestrogen-progestogen type. Significant increases in cardiac output, systolic and mean blood pressures and plasma-volume occurred during 2 to 3 months of therapy. Heart-rate and diastolic blood-pressure changes were not significant and increase in cardiac output was due mainly to a concomitant increase in stroke-volume. Body weight increased significantly in all subjects, probably due to fluid retention. In a very full discussion the authors concluded that the blood-pressure pattern in these subjects was determined by several factors involving a balance between increased cardiac output, the degree of peripheral vasodilatation, increased fluid retention, and an interplay between the renal and adrenal hormonal systems. Disruption of the balance, they emphasized, could involve hypertension. Logically one could also add to this conclusion that should this balance be disturbed stasis of blood and thrombosis might also occur.

Tausk (1968) has reviewed much of the literature on the influence of the 'pill' on haemodynamic factors and although haemodynamic studies have shown that a slowing down of blood flow may be demonstrable in the leg veins, they have not yet given the clue as to the very exceptional circumstances under which one 'pill' user suffers a thrombosis whilst others do not. Salt and water retention, hypervolaemia and stasis are certainly factors of prime importance in thrombosis but they occur in the majority of patients on the pill, whereas thrombosis does not. Tausk (1968) has perhaps summarized the real problem with his comment that the reason why the mechanism of possible facilitation of thrombosis by oral contraceptives was unknown was largely due to the fact that the causes of thrombosis in general were equally unknown.

Participation of Genetic Factors

There is strong evidence that the risk of venous thrombo-embolism in association with the use of oral contraceptives is only about one-third as great among women who belong to blood group O as among those who belong to the other three groups (Jick *et al.*, 1969; Vessey, 1970). There is as yet no available comparable data for cerebral thrombosis in women of blood group O on oral contraceptive medication, and, at this stage, there is no reason to believe that the same genetic factors affect the risk of this condition which involves arterial rather than venous thrombosis. It is, however, obviously a study worthy of investigation.

It is interesting to speculate whether this reduced risk of venous thrombo-embolism in blood group O women on the 'pill' can be explained by the relatively lower level of antihaemophilic globulin (factor VIII) in these women of blood group O. Factor VIII, as described

earlier, is increased during oral contraceptive medication, and it may well be that due to its initial lower leve in these women the influence of oral contraceptives does not raise the level to that necessary for participation in, or contribution towards, thrombo-embolic episodes. Preston and Barr (1964) have shown that subjects of blood group O have a lower level of antihaemophilic globulin than people of blood group A and Langman and Doll (1965) have shown that people of blood group O are more likely to bleed as a result of peptic ulceration than those of A, B or AB.

A prospective drug-surveillance programme, conducted in three Boston hospitals, revealed a deficit of patients of blood group O among those who received anticoagulants for venous thrombosis. This observation led to a co-operative study in the United States, Sweden and the United Kingdom to obtain the blood groupings of young women, who developed venous thrombosis while taking oral contraceptives or during pregnancy or the puerperium or at other times. These findings have been published by Jick and colleagues (1969) and are summarized in TABLE 6.3.

TABLE 6.3

RELATIVE RISK OF THROMBO-EMBOLISM A/O
AND (A+B+AB)/O IN EACH SERIES OF PATIENTS
(Jick *et al.*, 1969)

TYPE OF PATIENT WITH THROMBO-EMBOLISM	COMPARISON	POOL ESTIMATED RISK FROM U.S.A., SWEDEN, U.K.
Non-pregnant women not using oral contraceptives	A/O (A+B+AB)/O	1.8 1.8
Pregnant or puerperal women	A/O (A+B+AB)/O	2.1 2.1
Women using oral contraceptives	A/O (A+B+AB)/O	3.2 3.3
Control series	A/O (A+B+AB)/O	0.9 1.2

There was a conspicuous deficit of patients of blood group O in all the groups studied. This deficit was particularly prominent when the thrombo-embolism was associated with oral contraceptives or pregnancy.

RECOMMENDED FURTHER READING

ATKINSON, E. A., FAIRBURN, B., and HEATHFIELD, K. W. G. (1970) Intracranial venous thrombosis as complication of oral contraception, *Lancet*, i, 914–18.

BRITISH MEDICAL JOURNAL (1969) Strokes and the pill, leading article, *Brit. med. J.*, **1**, 733.

INMAN, W. H. W., and VESSEY, M. P. (1968) Investigation of deaths from pulmonary, coronary and cerebral thrombosis and embolism in women of child bearing age, *Brit. med. J.*, **2**, 193–9.

INMAN, W. H. W., VESSEY, M. P., WESTERHOLM, B., and

ENGELUND, A. (1970) Thromboembolic disease and the steroidal content of oral contraceptives. A report to the Committee on Safety of Drugs, *Brit. med. J.*, **2**, 203–9.

JICK, H., SLONE, D., WESTERHOLM, B., INMAN, W. B. W., VESSEY, M. P., SHAPIRO, S., LEWIS, G. P., and WORCESTER, J. (1969) Venous thromboembolic disease and ABO blood type: A cooperative study, *Lancet,*, i, 539–42.

TALBOT, S., WAKLEY, E. J., RYRIE, D., and LANGMAN, M. J. S. (1970) ABO blood-groups and venous thromboembolic disease, *Lancet*, i, 1257–9.

VESSEY, M. P., and DOLL, R. (1968) Investigation of relation between use of oral contraceptives and thromboembolic disease, *Brit. med. J.*, **2**, 199–205.

VESSEY, M. P., and DOLL, R. (1969) Investigation of relation between use of oral contraceptives and thromboembolic disease. A further report, *Brit. med. J.*, **2**, 651–7.

WALTERS, W. A. W., and LIM, Y. L. (1969) Cardiovascular dynamics in women receiving oral contraceptive therapy, *Lancet*, **ii**, 879–81.

REFERENCES

BAILAR, J. C. (1967) Thromboembolism and oestrogen therapy, *Lancet*, **ii**, 560.

BELL, G. H., DAVIDSON, J. N., and SCARBOROUGH, H. (1968) *Textbook of Physiology and Biochemistry*, 7th ed., Edinburgh, p. 450.

BOCK, H. E. (1966) Kortikosteroidtherapie neurologischer Erkrankungen mit besonderer Berücksichtigung der Nebenwirkungen, *Ther. Umsch.*, **23**, 112–19.

BOLTON, C. H., HAMPTON, J. R., and MITCHELL, J. R. A. (1968) Effect of oral contraceptive agents on platelets and plasma-phospholipids, *Lancet*, **i**, 1336–41.

DANIEL, D. G., CAMPBELL, H., and TURNBULL, A. C. (1967) Puerperal thromboembolism and suppression of lactation, *Lancet*, **ii**, 287–9.

EGEBERG, O., and OWREN, P. A. (1963) Contraception and blood coagulability, *Brit. med. J.*, **1**, 220–1.

FLORKIEWICZ, H., and KLAMUT, M. (1966) Thrombophlebitis as a consequence of prednisone administration, *Pol. Tyg. lek.*, **21**, 1932–4.

GOODRICH, S. M., and WOOD, J. E. (1964) Peripheral venous distensibility and velocity of venous blood flow during pregnancy or during oral contraceptive therapy, *Amer. J. Obstet. Gynec.*, **90**, 740–4.

GOOTMAN, N., GROSS, J., and MENSCH, A. (1964) Pulmonary artery thrombosis: A complication occurring with prednisone and chlorothiazide therapy in two nephrotic patients, *Pediatrics*, **34**, 861–8.

HURIEZ, C., and AGACHE, P. (1966) La gamme des corticotropes en dermatologie. Indications tirées de 2000 cas traités, *Concours méd.*, **88**, 4413–28.

INMAN, W. H. W., and VESSEY, M. P. (1968) Investigation of deaths from pulmonary, coronary and cerebral thrombosis and embolism in women of child bearing age, *Brit. med. J.*, **2**, 193–9.

INMAN, W. H. W., VESSEY, M. P., WESTERHOLM, B., and ENGELUND, A. (1970) Thromboembolic disease and the steroidal content of oral contraceptives, A Report to the Committee on Safety of Drugs, *Brit. med. J.*, **2**, 203–9.

JICK, H., SLONE, D., WESTERHOLM, B., INMAN, W. H. W., VESSEY, M. P., SHAPIRO, S., LEWIS, G. P., and WORCESTER, J. (1969) Venous thromboembolic disease and ABO blood type: A cooperative study, *Lancet*, **i**, 539–42.

KORNELL, S. (1966) Adverse effect of corticosteroid therapy in a patient with progressive systemic sclerosis (generalized scleroderma), *Manitoba med. Rev.*, **46**, 579–82.

LANGMAN, M. J. S., and DOLL, R. (1965) ABO blood group and secretor state in relation to clinical characteristics of peptic ulcers, *Gut*, **6**, 270–3.

POLLER, L., TABIOWO, A., and THOMPSON, J. M. (1968) Effects of low-dose oral contraceptives on blood coagulation, *Brit. med. J.*, **2**, 218–19.

PRESTON, A. E., and BARR, A. (1964) The plasma concentration of factor VIII in the normal population, *Brit. J. Haemat.*, **10**, 238–45.

RUTHERFORD, R. N., HOUGIE, C., BANKES, A. L., and COBURN, W. A. (1964) The effects of sex steroids and pregnancy on blood coagulation factors. Comparative study, *Obstet. and Gynec.*, **24**, 886–92.

SAXENA, K. M., and CRAWFORD, J. D. (1965) The treatment of nephrosis, *New Engl. J. Med.*, **272**, 522–7.

TAUSK, M. (1968) Oral contraceptives and the incidence of thrombosis, in *Drug-Induced Diseases*, Vol. 3, eds. Meyler, L., and Peck, H. M., Excerpta Medica Foundation, Amsterdam, pp. 183–209.

TURIAF, J., BASSET, G., GEORGES, R., JEANJEAN, Y., and BATTESTI, J. P. (1962) Advantages, disadvantages and complications, metabolic changes and hormono-secretory disorders, caused by long-term cortisone therapy for asthma with continuous dyspnea, *Rev. Tuberc. (Paris)*, **26**, 1212–67.

VESSEY, M. P. (1970) Thrombosis and the pill, *Prescribers' J.*, **10**, 1–7.

VESSEY, M. P., and DOLL, R. (1968) Investigation of relation between use of oral contraceptives and thromboembolic disease, *Brit. med. J.*, **2**, 199–205.

VESSEY, M. P., and DOLL, R. (1969) Investigation of relation between use of oral contraceptives and thromboembolic disease. A further report, *Brit. med. J.*, **2**, 651–7.

WALTERS, W. A. W., and LIM, Y. L. (1969) Cardiovascular dynamics in women receiving oral contraceptive therapy, *Lancet*, **ii**, 879–81.

ZUCKNER, J., UDDIN, J., and RAMSEY, R. H. (1967) Prolonged effect from intramuscular corticosteroids. Triamcinolone acetonide in rheumatoid arthritis, *Acta. rheum. scand.*, **12**, 307–17.

CLASSIFIED REFERENCES

In view of the magnitude of the literature on thromboembolic disease and intravascular clotting caused by oral contraceptives, additional references (in abbreviated form) to those already given have been assembled. These have been classified for ease of further reference into:

1. Venous thrombosis
2. Cerebrovascular accidents
3. Coronary infarction
4. Uncomplicated intravascular clotting
5. Altered blood coagulability

1. VENOUS THROMBOSIS WITH PULMONARY EMBOLISM

BRADFORD, D. E. (1965) *Lancet*, **ii**, 902.

CAHAL, D. A. (1965) *Brit. med. J.*, **1**, 993.

DORPH, S., and JORGENSEN, S. T. (1965) *Ugeskr. Laeg.*, **127**, 1621.

FERGUSON, J. M. (1967) *J. Amer. med. Ass.*, **200**, 560.

GOLDBERG, W. M. (1963) *New Engl. J. med.*, **269**, 1265.

GRASSET, J., and GAUTHER, R. (1965) *Obstet. and Gynec.*, **64**, 197.

HERSHFIELD, B. M. (1964) *N.Y. med. J.*, **64**, 302.
JORDAN, W. M. (1961) *Lancet*, **ii**, 1146.
LEATHER, H. M. (1965) *Lancet*, **i**, 270.
LINDENBOOM, G. A. (1967) *Ned. T. Geneesk.*, **111**, 161.
MENDES DE LEON, D. E., and LANKESTER, J. (1966) *Ned. T. Geneesk.*, **110**, 1226.
SCHATY, I. J., *et al.* (1964) *J. Amer. med. Ass.*, **188**, 493.
SHAFER, J., and BEHR, G. (1962) *Brit. med. J.*, **2**, 1543.
SHOSH, P., *et al.*, (1968) *Brit. med. J.*, **1**, 512.

2. CEREBROVASCULAR ACCIDENTS

BAINES, G. F. (1965) *Brit. med. J.*, **1**, 189.
BICKERSTAFF, E. R., and MacDONALD HOLMES, J. (1967) *Brit. med. J.*, **1**, 726.
BRADFORD, D. E. (1967) *Lancet*, **i**, 679.
BREHM, H. (1964) *Int. J. Fertil.*, **9**, 45.
CASPARY, E. A., and PEBERDY, M. (1965) *Brit. med. J.*, **1**, 1142.
COLE, M. (1967) *Arch. intern. Med.*, **120**, 551.
DE-GENNES, J. L., and THORVET, F. (1967) *Presse méd.*, **75**, 1709.
BRITISH MEDICAL JOURNAL (1967) Editorial, *Brit. med. J.*, **2**, 355.
EGBERG, O., and OWREN, P. A. (1963) *Brit. med. J.*, **1**, 220.
HALLER, J. (1964) *Fortschr. Geburtsh. Gynäk.*, **21**, 37.
ILLI, K., *et al.* (1965) *Brit. med. J.*, **2**, 1164.
KEEN, H., *et al.* (1965) *Lancet*, **ii**, 505.
KIRKCHHOFF, H., and POLIWODA, H. (1964) Anovular-Schering, in *Proceedings of the Seventh IPPF Conference, Singapore*, I.C.S. 72, Excerpta Medica Foundation, Amsterdam, p. 341.
NEVIN, N. C. (1967) *Brit. med. J.*, **1**, 1586.
OLIVER, M. F. (1967) *Lancet*, **ii**, 510.
PINCUS, G. (1961) in *Modern Trends in Endocrinology*, Ser. 2., ed. Gardiner-Hill, H., New York, p. 231.
SHAFEY, S., and SCHEINBERG, P. (1966) *Neurology (Minneap.)*, **16**, 205.
STEWART-WALLACE, A. M. (1964) *Brit. med. J.*, **2**, 1528.
THOMPSON, J. M., and POLLER, L. (1965) *Brit. med. J.*, **2**, 270.
WALSH, F. B., *et al.* (1965) *Arch. Ophthal.*, **74**, 628.
WHITTY, C. W. M., *et al.* (1966) *Lancet*, **i**, 856.
WINTER, I. C. (1965) *Metabolism*, **14**, 422.
WOLF, S. M., *et al.* (1967) *Bull. Los Angeles neurol. Soc.*, **32**, 141.
WYNN, V., and DOAR, J. W. H. (1966) *Lancet*, **ii**, 715.
WYNN, V., *et al.* (1966) *Lancet*, **ii**, 720.

3. CORONARY INFARCTION

BENDER, S. (1964) *Practitioner*, **192**, 359.
BOYCE, J., *et al.* (1963) *Lancet*, **i**, 111.
DORPH, S., and JORGENSEN, S. J. (1965) *Ugeskr. Laeg.*, **127**, 1621.
HOSTENG, T. O. (1965) *Norske Laeg.*, **85**, 1692.
LLOYD, G. (1965) *Brit. med. J.*, **1**, 587.
NAYSMITH, J. H. (1965) *Brit. med. J.*, **1**, 250.
OLIVER, M. F. (1965) *Brit. med. J.*, **1**, 315.
OLIVER, M. F. (1970) *Brit. med. J.*, **2**, 210.
OSBORN, G. R. (1965) *Brit. med. J.*, **1**, 1128.
ROBINSON, R. W., *et al.* (1963) *Ugeskr. Laeg.*, **125**, 155.
VISSIER, J. (1967) *Ned. T. Geneesk.*, **111**, 796.

4. UNCOMPLICATED INTRAVASCULAR CLOTTING

Hepatic Vein

ECKER, J. A., *et al.* (1966) *Amer. J. Gastroent.*, **45**, 429.
GRAYSON, M. J., and RULLY, M. C. (1968) *Brit. med. J.*, **1**, 512.
KRASS, I. (1968) *Brit. med. J.*, **1**, 708.
ROTHWELL-JACKSON, R. L. (1968) *Brit. med. J.*, **1**, 252.
SIGUIER, F., *et al.* (1967) *Bull. Soc. méd. Hôp. Paris*, **118**. 1235.
STEMP, K., and MOSBECK, J. (1967) *Brit. med. J.*, **4**, 660.

Pelvic and Leg Vessels

ALLEN, R. G. (1968) *Brit. med. J.*, **1**, 512.
BENDER, S. (1966) *Practitioner*, **197**, 119.
BOOMGAARD, J., and BURGERS, G. J. A. (1967) *Ned. T. Geneesk.*, **111**, 2332.
BROOK, M. H., and JACKSON, N. J. (1963) *Canad. med. Ass. J.*, **89**, 1094.
CASS, R. (1963) *New Engl. J. Med.*, **269**, 761.
MULLER, C. (1964) *Ther. Umsch.*, **21**, 512.
RYAN, G. M., *et al.* (1962) *Amer. J. Obstet. Gynec.*, **90**, 715.
TEN-HOLT, S. P. (1962) *Ned. T. Geneesk.*, **106**, 1703.

Other Sites, Carotid Arteries

BOHULT, J., *et al.* (1967) *Acta med. scand.*, **181**, 453.
GENNES, J. L., *et al.* (1967) *Bull. Soc. méd. Hôp. Paris*, **118**, 899.

Vertebral Artery

EHTISHAMUDDIN, M. (1965) *Brit. med. J.*, **1**, 921.

5. ALTERATION OF BLOOD COAGULABILITY

ASK-UPMARK, E. (1967) *Acta med. scand.*, **181**, 737.
BRITISH MEDICAL JOURNAL (1963) Editorial, *Brit. med. J.*, **1**, 207.
BRITISH MEDICAL JOURNAL (1964) Editorial, *Brit. med. J.*, **2**, 1089.
DANO, P. (1965) *Ugeskr. Laeg.*, **127**, 1577.
DRILL, V. A. (1965) *Metabolism*, **14**, Suppl., 295.
FESTE, J. R., and KAUFMAN, R. H. (1965) *Sth. med. J. (Bgham, Ala.)*, **58**, 945.
HALL, R. E. (1963) *Bull. Sloane Hosp. Wom. N.Y.*, **9**, 17.
LAMBLEY, D. G., and WARE, J. W. (1967) *Brit. J. Urol.*, **37**, 147.
McGOWAN, L. (1963) *Canad. med. Ass. J.*, **88**, 923.
McWILLIAM, R. S., *et al.* (1963) *Canad. med. Ass. J.*, **88**, 1032.
POLLER, L. (1970) *J. clin. Path.*, **23**, Suppl. (Ass. Clin. Path.), **3**, 67.
REED, D. L., and COEN, W. W. (1963) *New Engl. J. Med.*, **269**, 622.
RIVLIN, S., *et al.* (1967) *Brit. med. J.*, **3**, 864.
SCOREY, J. (1965) *Brit. med. J.*, **2**, 301.
SVENSK FARMACEUTISK TIDSKRIFT (1965) Editorial, *Svensk. farm. T.*, **69**, 851.
THOMSON, J. M., and POLLER, L. (1965) *Brit. med. J.*, **2**, 270.

PLATE 1

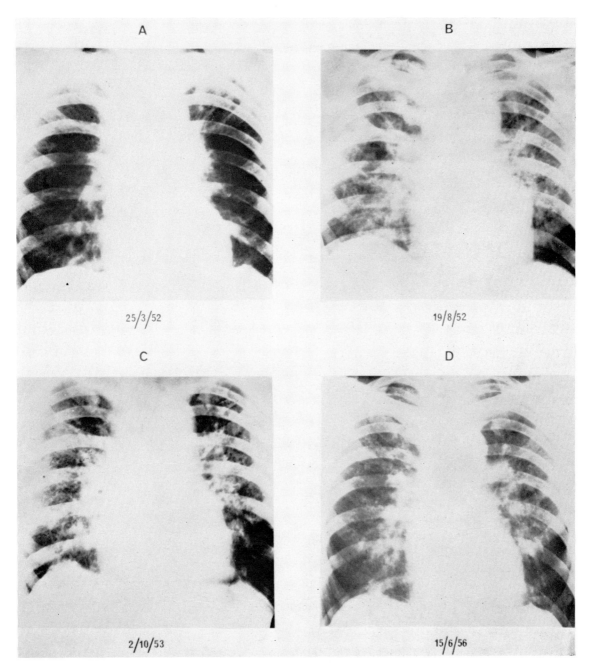

Hexamethonium lung. A series of anteroposterior X-rays in a man who had taken hexamethonium for control of his hypertension. A, shows a pretreatment X-ray and B, C and D show the pulmonary shadowing of fibrosis which is characteristic of this reaction. (Courtesy of Dr. F. J. Prime, Institute of Diseases of the Chest, Brompton Hospital, and Professor R. E. Steiner, Department of Diagnostic Radiology, Royal Postgraduate Medical School.)

PLATE 2

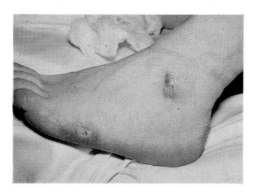

A. Bullae due to barbiturate overdosage.

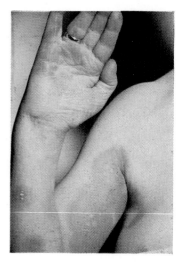

B. Eruption induced by phenolphthalein.

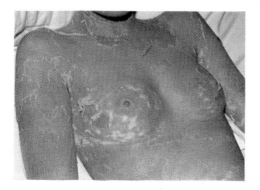

C. Toxic epidermal necrolysis due to sulphonamides.

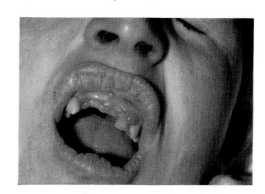

D. Gingival hyperplasia due to diphenylhydantoin.

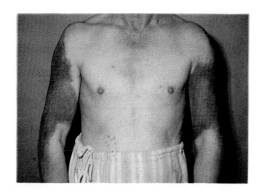

E. Bruising due to warfarin.

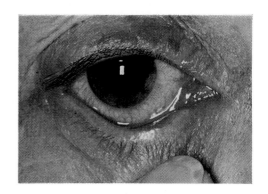

F. Eye reaction due to atropine.

DRUG-INDUCED SKIN REACTIONS

(Figures A–E, courtesy of Dr. A. McQueen.)

(Figure F, courtesy of Dr. P. Hansell, Director of A–V Communications, Institute of Ophthalmology, University of London.)

PLATE 3

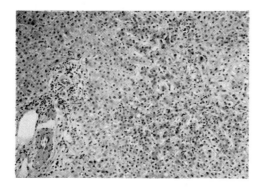

DRUG-INDUCED JAUNDICE

A. Chlorpromazine-induced jaundice. A woman aged 30 years was delivered of her first child by Caesarian section and subsequently developed puerperal mania and was treated with chlorpromazine, 50 mg. thrice daily for 14 days. She developed jaundice which persisted in spite of stopping treatment. Laparotomy was performed and a wedge section of the liver removed. The section shows the central vein and centrilobular cholestasis with pigment phagocytosis and inflammatory filtrate around the bile ducts.

DRUG-INDUCED DISORDERS OF THE EYE

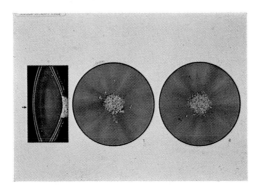

B. Posterior cortical cataract associated with oral
contraceptive medication.

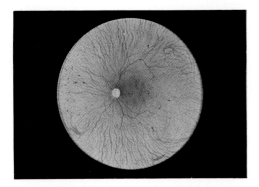

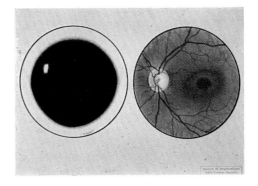

C. Chloroquine retinopathy.   D. Cornea and retina after chloroquine treatment.

(Figure A, courtesy of Dr. C. Brown, Institute of Pathology, The London Hospital.)
(Figures B–D, courtesy of Dr. P. Hansell, Director of A–V Communications, Institute of Ophthalmology, University of London.)

PLATE 4

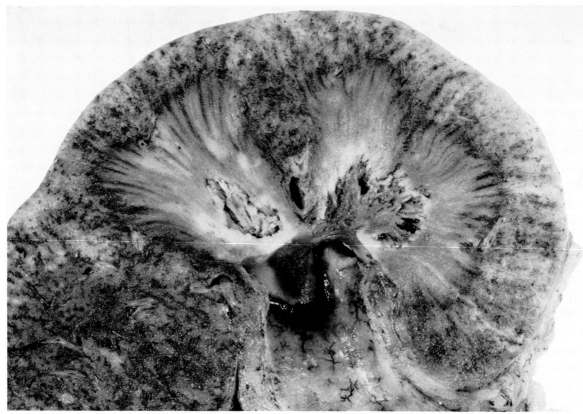

Analgesic papillary necrosis. Post-mortem specimen from a female patient aged 79 years; 8 Compound Codeine Tablets per day had been taken for many years for rheumatism and she was known to have suffered from analgesic nephropathy. The kidney shows complete loss of the renal papilla. (Courtesy of Dr. D. J. Pollock, Institute of Pathology, The London Hospital.)

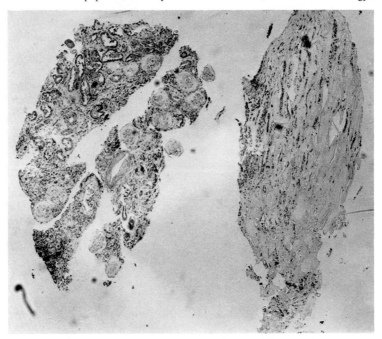

Analgesic papillary necrosis. Two pieces of renal biopsy from a male patient aged 45 years who had previously had a colectomy for ulcerative colitis. This patient had controlled his iliostomy by taking Compound Codeine Tablets for many years. The biopsy specimens show interstitial fibrosis and glomerular hyalinization. (Courtesy of Dr. D. J. Pollock, Institute of Pathology, The London Hospital.)

7

LUNG DISEASE

A variety of drugs may provoke adverse respiratory reactions of many different types. These reactions may so closely resemble respiratory disease due to other causes, that a causative drug factor may easily be overlooked. The problem of pulmonary reactions due to drugs was reviewed by Davies (1969) and this was followed by leading articles in *Lancet* (1969) and *British Medical Journal* (1969a and 1969b) which highlighted this problem.

In view of the similarity between drug-induced symptoms and diseases, and the wide variety of drugs causing identical conditions, the problem will be considered under pathological entities.

ASTHMA

Asthma is the commonest drug-induced respiratory disease, and may be allergic in some cases.

DRUG-INDUCED ALLERGIC ASTHMA

Asthma with or without generalized anaphylactic shock or urticaria is probably mediated by Type I (reaginic) allergic hypersensitivity. Type I hypersensitivity has been reported following the administration of the penicillins and tetracyclines, erythromycin, neomycin, streptomycin, griseofulvin, cephaloridine, ethionamide, monoamine oxidase inhibitors, radio-opaque organic iodides, local anaesthetics, mercurials, vitamin K, bromsulphthalein, suxamethonium, antisera, vaccines and allergenic extracts.

Asthma may also occur as part of a drug-induced serum sickness syndrome, the symptoms of which include fever, arthralgia, urticaria, maculopapular eruptions and lymphadenopathy; Type III hypersensitivity (Arthus type) may be involved in the mechanism of this syndrome.

Though the mechanisms of most drug-induced asthmas are poorly understood the comparatively rare pituitary-snuff-taker's lung is one in which the mechanism is known (Pepys, 1969). This syndrome consists of an extrinsic allergic alveolitis in which patients have dyspnoea with cough and widespread crepitations. Chest radiographs show extensive miliary mottling. Microscopically, the lungs show fibrosis in alveolar walls with collections of lymphocytes, plasma cells and scanty eosinophils. There is also an intra-alveolar exudate and formation of a hyaline membrane. The presence in these patients' sera of precipitins against bovine and porcine serum proteins and pituitary antigens suggests that this lung reaction is mediated by a Type III hypersensitivity. In addition, the inhalation of pituitary snuff may provoke rhinitis (Type I hypersensitivity) and allergic asthma (Type I and Type III hypersensitivity).

The commonest cause of drug-induced asthma is aspirin. Asthmatics who are sensitive to aspirin constitute a characteristic clinical group. They have generally suffered from rhinitis and nasal polyposis for several years before the onset of their asthma. The asthma usually starts in middle life and tends to become chronic shortly after its onset. Asthma symptoms precede the development of aspirin intolerance by months or years, though it is rare that aspirin itself causes the first asthmatic attack. Angioneurotic oedema and urticaria may also accompany these aspirin-induced asthma attacks. Aspirin-induced asthma is characterized by the onset of symptoms 20–30 minutes after the ingestion of the drug, it is usually severe and prolonged and occasionally fatal. Some workers think that patients with aspirin-induced asthma have a poor prognosis; however, long-term therapy with corticosteroids may control their disease.

Samter and Beers (1967 and 1968) have studied 182 aspirin-sensitive subjects and have found a low incidence of atopy. Few patients had positive skin tests to common allergens, and there was no correlation between exposure to allergens and symptoms. In these subjects, there were no adverse reactions with sodium salicylate, salicylic esters, choline salicylate, thioaspirin or N-acetyl-p-aminophenol. Therefore, intolerance to aspirin is not intolerance to salicylates generally. Moreover, several substances unrelated to aspirin can induce 'aspirin-like' asthma in these susceptible patients on first exposure; such substances include indomethacin, amidopyrine and the yellow dye tartrazine, which is a common colouring matter in foodstuffs. Their structural dissimilarity is such that an immunological cross reactivity is precluded. Samter and Beers have also pointed out that all these substances inducing aspirin-like reactions have one characteristic in common—namely, that they are peripheral analgesics. It was suggested that these reactions are mediated by non-immunological processes and that these peripheral analgesics act on receptors in the nasal and bronchial mucosa. These receptors initiate a series of pathological reflexes resulting in bronchoconstriction.

The diagnosis of aspirin sensitivity has to be made from the patient's history. Skin tests with aspirin are unhelpful and dangerous, serological tests are invariably negative, and aspirin provocation tests are hazardous. Whereas it is obvious that aspirin-intolerant patients must be warned to avoid taking aspirin, it is not so well known that these patients must also be warned about some drugs chemically unrelated to aspirin, and foods containing certain specific additives. Aspirin-induced asthma should be treated promptly and vigorously with corticosteroids.

Drug-induced asthma may result from the normal pharmacological action of drugs, for example the exacerbation of airway obstruction in asthmatic persons by propranolol acting by β-receptor blockade or by parasympathomimetic drugs such as acetyl-β-methyl-choline. Paradoxical pharmacological effects may be caused by bronchodilator drugs such as isoprenaline (isoproterenol), which, contrary to expectation, precipitate an asthmatic attack rather than relieve bronchospasm. Keighley (1966) described three patients with a personal or family history of atopy, all of whom developed severe refractory asthma. An analysis of the hospital records of these patients, showed that whereas their airway obstruction was controllable with conventional therapy, including corticosteroids in high doses, complete remission could not be obtained until all sympathomimetic-amine-containing pressurized aerosols were discontinued. In all three of these patients, subsequent challenge with isoprenaline aerosols precipitated severe and protracted airway obstruction. One of Keighley's patients showed a marked bronchoconstriction with small doses of isoprenaline, and this was associated with a marked and sustained eosinophilia. Another patient showed progressively more violent reactions with repeated challenging of isoprenaline. These two cases seemed to indicate an allergic component to the asthma, although, as Keighley admitted, the precise mechanism was unknown. One could postulate of course that the reaction was merely a normal pharmacological action of the drug on a susceptible patient; isoprenaline has an effect on β-receptors and causes bronchodilatation, but at the same time it causes vasodilatation in the bronchi and bronchioles, which may result in vascular congestion in the mucous membranes of the bronchioles with airway obstruction in the absence of any smooth muscle bronchoconstriction.

Kennedy (1965) noted that out of a group of 20 asthmatic patients, the bronchoconstriction worsened in four patients after the inhalation of deptropine citrate, and in one patient after atropine methonitrate. The latter patient also developed severe asthma 30 minutes after inhalation of isoprenaline combined with deptropine citrate. Thus it would seem that bronchodilators other than sympathomimetics can cause a paradoxical increase in airway resistance in susceptible patients.

DRUG-INDUCED PULMONARY EOSINOPHILIA

Drug-induced pulmonary eosinophilia is characterized clinically by a cough, fever and severe dyspnoea usually without wheeze. Widespread crepitations may be audible. On investigation oesinophilia may be noted and patchy transient pulmonary shadows and sometimes pleural effusions can be seen on chest radiographs. This syndrome is most commonly caused by nitrofurantoin, although other drugs may also produce a similar reaction. The mechanism of this hypersensitivity reaction is not known. It has been suggested that sensitivity reactions in the lungs are due to trapping of eosinophils in the alveoli.

In 1962, Israel and Diamond reported on 'recurrent pulmonary infiltration and pleural effusion due to nitrofurantoin sensitivity'. Their patient developed four separate episodes of fever, chills, cough, dyspnoea and cyanosis following the administration of nitrofurantoin. Chest X-rays revealed pulmonary infiltrations and small pleural effusions but peripheral eosinophilia was not present with the first attack, appearing only with later attacks and reaching a maximum of 19 per cent of the leucocyte count. With each succeeding episode the incubation period, which was initially about two weeks, became shorter reaching $8\frac{1}{2}$ hours at the fourth challenge. Following withdrawal of the drug, symptoms usually disappeared within 24 hours. Israel and Diamond deliberately challenged this patient with 100 mg of nitrofurantoin and noticed a rise in eosinophils from 650 to 1,625 per mm^3 over a 24-hour period.

Similar pulmonary complications with nitrofurantoin have also been reported by Luebbers (1962), Muir and Stanton (1963), Murray and Kronenberg (1965), and Bayer et al. (1965). Murray (1968) described a typical case of nitrofurantoin hypersensitivity. A 61-year-old man had a transurethral resection for benign prostatic enlargement. On a routine urinalysis one year later pyuria was noted, and nitrofurantoin therapy, 100 mg three times daily, was begun. Twenty-four hours later there was fever to 103°F (39·4°C), shaking chills, nonproductive cough and dyspnoea. Numerous fine râles were heard throughout both lung bases. The chest X-ray was negative but the white count rose to 13,800 with 86 per cent neutrophil polymorphonuclearcytes, but only 2 per cent eosinophils. The nitrofurantoin was stopped and twelve hours later the patient felt well and his lungs were clear. The next day he was given a challenge dose of 50 mg of nitrofurantoin and four hours later there was fever to 103°F (39·4°C) and numerous basal râles. Ten hours later the patient felt perfectly well and his lungs were clear.

In considering the differential diagnosis of pulmonary oedema and nitrofurantoin sensitivity a history of drug ingestion, fever, chills, aching pains, non-productive cough, absence of a gallop rhythm, normal circulation time and leucocytosis, with or without eosinophilia, bias the diagnosis in favour of drug reaction. The chest X-ray will not show pulmonary congestion but rather an infiltrate or pleural effusion and the chest electrocardiogram is usually normal except for sinus tachycardia. It is possible that the two syndromes may co-exist. Nitrofurantoin reaction may also be mistaken for pulmonary embolism, pneumonia or bronchitis. The history of administration of the drug in these situations should raise the suspicion of the syndrome.

The definite diagnosis of nitrofurantoin reaction can be made from the response to a challenge dose of nitrofurantoin if the circumstances warrant such a decision. A dose of 50 mg should be given 6-hourly until symptoms appear and then the drug should be stopped promptly. X-rays of the chest, white-cell count with differential counts and total eosinophil counts should be obtained just before administration of the drug and on appearance of the symptoms.

Pulmonary eosinophilia has also followed therapy with para-aminosalicylic acid (PAS), penicillin, mephenesin, imipramine and sulphonamides; it has even followed the application of a cream containing sulphonamide to the vagina (Klinghoffer, 1954). Lung biopsy in a patient with sulphonamide-induced pulmonary eosinophilia showed alveoli packed with eosinophils and histiocytes (Fiegenberg *et al.*, 1967).

DRUG-INDUCED LUPUS ERYTHEMATOSUS SYNDROME WITH PULMONARY COMPLICATIONS

The frequency with which treatment with some drugs has been accompanied by the development of a lupus erythematosus syndrome has suggested a causal relationship. In a series of cases of lupus erythematosus studied by Lee and Siegel (1968) 20 per cent of cases were considered to be drug-induced.

The respiratory component of the disease process in drug-induced lupus erythematosus is identical with that seen in systemic lupus erythematosus and the presenting factor is often pleurisy, with or without effusion. In some cases pleurisy may be associated with pericarditis; in other cases, the symptoms can be associated with a clinical illness which resembles pneumonia in some cases, and acute pulmonary oedema or pulmonary infarction in others. Another type of pulmonary manifestation of drug-induced lupus erythematosus results in shrinking lungs, in which the changes are due to widespread alveolar atelectasis without airway obstruction. The patient is dyspnoeic and X-rays show marked elevation of the diaphragm.

Drugs which have been incriminated as causative agents in lupus erythematosus are the penicillins and tetracyclines, gold salts, phenylbutazone, griseofulvin, hydrallazine, isoniazid, phenytoin, methoin (mephenytoin), streptomycin, procainamide, sulphonamides, para-aminosalylic acid (PAS), thiouracil, trimethadione and methyldopa.

DRUG-INDUCED POLYARTERITIS SYNDROME WITH PULMONARY COMPLICATIONS

Polyarteritis may present as a disorder of the respiratory system with asthma, transient lung shadows or destructive lung lesions resembling pneumonia, lung abscess or infarction. Drugs alleged to cause polyarteritis include iodides, organic arsenicals, mercurials, hydantoins, penicillins, gold salts, DDT, thiouracils, phenothiazines and sulphonamides (Rose and Spencer, 1957).

DRUG-INDUCED PULMONARY FIBROTIC SYNDROMES

The use of the ganglion-blocking hypotensive agents, hexamethonium, pentolinium, and mecamylamine, has been associated with intra-alveolar fibrinous oedema, which in some cases becomes converted into fibrous tissue. Whether these changes are directly due to the drugs or due to left ventricular failure is controversial (Doniach *et al.*, 1954). The clinical picture of the acute stage is that of pulmonary oedema; fibrosis may develop and become widespread, leading to honeycomb lung, bronchiolectasis, and bronchiectasis (Heard, 1962) [see PLATE 1]. Busulphan, a cytotoxic drug chemically related to hexamethonium, may also cause intra-alveolar fibrinous oedema converting to fibrous tissue (Heard and Cooke, 1968).

Prolonged ventilation with high concentrations of oxygen may result in lung disease, the microscopical features of which show two merging phases. An early exudative phase characterized by congestion, alveolar oedema, intra-alveolar haemorrhage, and fibrin exudate, with the formation of prominent hyaline membrane without an associated inflammatory component. A late proliferative phase of this condition shows alveolar and interlobular septal oedema and fibroblastic proliferation, with early fibrosis and prominent hyperplasia of the alveolar lining cells (Nash *et al.*, 1967). Oxygen should not be withheld from patients who need it for fear of possible toxic effect on the lungs, but the concentration should be reduced to 40 per cent or less as soon as measurements of arterial blood gas show that this can be done safely.

Pleuro-pulmonary fibrosis may also be related to methysergide therapy (Ballou, cited by Graham, 1968).

In reviewing the literature on methysergide-induced retroperitoneal fibrosis, Graham found numerous examples of pleuro-pulmonary episodes which had occurred in these patients but which had been overshadowed by the genito-urinary problem (Tubbs, 1946; Raper, 1955; Talbot and Mahoney, 1957; Hawk and Hazard, 1959; Reed and Stinley, 1959; Dineen *et al.*, 1960; Cameron *et al.*, 1961; Thompson *et al.*, 1961; Hoffman and Trippel, 1961; Partington, 1961; Benfield *et al.*, 1962; Olsson *et al.*, 1962; Viikari, 1963; Que and Mandema, 1964).

It is of interest that in Graham's review all 16 patients who presented the picture of pleuro-pulmonary fibrosis were male. Two female patients taking methysergide developed pulmonary complications which may or may not have been of the type previously described; in one, the symptoms were short-lived and the findings minimal and may have been related to infection. In the other, a diagnosis of repeated pulmonary infarction was made on clinical grounds and a vena cava ligation was performed. Three other patients either developed emphysema or suffered aggravation of existing emphysema during methysergide therapy; they were all males. Thus, it would seem that males are more prone than females to develop pulmonary problems under the influence of this drug.

Three of the above 16 male patients were known to have suffered from other fibrotic conditions, either currently or in the past; one had marked bilateral Dupuytren's contractures, one a keloid on the chest, and the third had a penile lesion biopsied 20 years previously, and diagnosed as balanitis xerotica obliterans, an inflammatory fibrosis.

The striking features of methysergide-induced pulmonary fibrosis has been the repeated episodes of pleuritic chest pain often accompanied by fever and pleural effusion, the presence of friction rubs being occasionally audible to the patient himself, and the chronic dense pleural thickening tending to cause gross limitation of motion of the chest. The X-ray findings show a large, often tumour-shaped, fibrotic lesion in the posterior chest which on biopsy shows inflammatory fibrosis encasing loculated fluid. There has been a tendency for these abnormalities to increase if methysergide therapy continues and for them slowly to improve when the drug is withdrawn.

Although in most instances the chief involvement seems to be pleural, the process in some patients definitely involves pulmonary parenchymal tissue and in one case was found to invade the chest wall as well. An acute fibrinous exudate was found in one patient, whereas, more commonly, a non-specific inflammatory process consisting of lymphocytes and plasma cells and marked fibrosis occurred. In two patients an increase in immunoglobulins was detected which disappeared some months after methysergide had been withdrawn. Although the process may start on one side, bilateral involvement before many months have passed seems to be the rule.

PULMONARY INFECTION AS A COMPLICATION OF DRUG THERAPY

Bacterial pneumonias and pulmonary tuberculosis are well recognized as complications of corticosteroid therapy, and, with increasing use of immunosuppressive agents, opportunistic infections of the lung with fungi (such as *Aspergillus*), actinomycetes (such as *Nocardia*), protozoa (such as *Pneumocystis carinii*), and viruses (such as cytomegalovirus) are now being seen (Symmers, 1965). Suppurative pneumonia and the formation of lung abscess are also common in 'main-line' drug addicts (Briggs *et al.*, 1967).

DRUG-INDUCED PULMONARY EMBOLISM

The association of pulmonary thrombo-embolism with the taking of oral contraceptive pills has been established beyond any shadow of doubt, following the investigation of Vessey and Doll (1969). The problem of thrombo-embolic disease caused by oral contraceptives is discussed fully in the chapter on drug-induced disorders of the clotting mechanism [see CHAPTER 6].

The lipoid granulomas which complicate the use of oily contrast media for bronchography have been known for many years. More recently, oil embolism has been described as a sequel to their use in lymphangiography (Gough *et al.*, 1964; Bron *et al.*, 1963; Hamilton *et al.*, 1964; Fraimow *et al.*, 1965).

DRUG-INDUCED PULMONARY HYPERTENSION

The possibility has been raised of an association between certain appetite suppressants and the development of pulmonary hypertension; a number of drugs of this type have been withdrawn from clinical use in many European countries and doctors in the United Kingdom have been asked to notify cases of this kind to the Committee on Safety of Drugs (Cahal, 1969).

New drug-induced respiratory syndromes are constantly appearing, but the mechanisms of most of them are still poorly understood; iodism is one of the longest known of these conditions and even with this agent mechanisms are still obscure. Any iodine-containing compound, however administered, can result in iodism. Symptoms may be immediate or delayed for several days. The respiratory tract may be involved diffusely with tracheobronchitis, asthma, pneumonia, or focally by angioneurotic oedema or haemorrhage.

In reviewing the contents of this chapter, it is apparent that no matter how drugs are given, they will reach the lung by the venous return and adverse respiratory reactions to drugs may follow administration by the most unlikely routes, e.g. severe iodism affecting the whole respiratory tract has occurred after the instillation of iodized talc into the pleural space to produce pleurodesis; oil embolism of the lungs has been recorded following myelography using a radio-opaque oil; and eosinophilic infiltration of the lung has been observed after the application of a sulphonamide-containing cream into the vagina.

In the majority of cases pulmonary reactions to drugs are due to the idiosyncrasies of the patients receiving them and since idiosyncrasies to these drugs are comparatively rare, little opportunity has arisen to study the mechanisms of these reactions. Only in rare cases are the pulmonary complications predictable, but there is one notable exception to this which is, of course, pulmonary embolism due to oral contraceptive medication.

RECOMMENDED FURTHER READING

DAVIES, P. D. B. (1969) Drug-induced lung disease, *Brit. J. Dis. Chest*, **63**, 57–70.

REFERENCES

BALLOU, J. B. (1968) cited by Graham, J. R. (1968).

BAYER, W. L., DAWSON, R. B., JR., and KOTIN, M. D. (1965) Allergic tracheobronchitis due to nitrofurantoin sensitivity. Report of a case, *Dis. Chest*, **48**, 429–30.

BENFIELD, J. R., HARRISON, R. W., MOULDER, P. V., LYON, E. S., and GRAFF, P. W. (1962) Bilateral nodular pulmonary granulomas and retroperitoneal fibrosis: Simulated metastatic malignant neoplasm and spontaneous remission of ureteral obstruction, *J. Amer. med. Ass.*, **182**, 579–81.

BRIGGS, J. H., MCKERRON, C. G., SOUHAMI, R. L., TAYLOR, D. J. E., and ANDREWS, H. (1967) Severe systemic infections complicating 'mainline' heroin addiction, *Lancet*, **ii**, 1227–31.

BRITISH MEDICAL JOURNAL (1969a) Asthma from aspirin, leading article, *Brit. med. J.*, **1**, 6.

BRITISH MEDICAL JOURNAL (1969b) Lung disease caused by drugs, leading article, *Brit. med. J.*, **3**, 729–30.

BRON, K. M., BAUM, S., and ABRAMS, H. L. (1963) Oil embolism in lymphangiography. Incidence, manifestations, and mechanism, *Radiology*, **80**, 194–202.

CAHAL, D. A. (1969) Appetite suppressants and pulmonary hypertension, *Lancet*, **i**, 947.

CAMERON, D. G., ING, S. T., BOYLE, M., and MATTHEWS, W. H. (1961) Idiopathic mediastinal and retroperitoneal fibrosis, *Canad. med. Ass. J.*, **85**, 227–32.

DAVIES, P. D. B. (1969) Drug-induced lung disease, *Brit. J. Dis. Chest*, **63**, 57–70.

DINEEN, J., ASCH, T., and PEARCE, J. M. (1960) Retroperitoneal fibrosis. An anatomic and radiologic review with a report of four new cases and an explanation of pathogenesis, *Radiology*, **75**, 380–90.

DONIACH, I., MORRISON, B., and STEINER, R. E. (1954) Lung changes during hexamethonium therapy for hypertension, *Brit. Heart J.*, **16**, 101–8.

FIEGENBERG, D. S., WEISS, H., and KIRSHMAN, H. (1967) Migratory pneumonia with eosinophilia associated with sulfonamide administration, *Arch. intern. Med.*, **120**, 85–9.

FRAIMOW, W., WALLACE, S., LEWIS, P., GREENING, R. R,. and CATHCART, R. T. (1965) Changes in pulmonary function due to lymphangiography, *Radiology*, **85**, 231–41.

GOUGH, J. H., GOUGH, M. H., and THOMAS, M. L. (1964) Pulmonary complications following lymphangiography; with a note on technique, *Brit. J. Radiol.*, **37**, 416–21.

GRAHAM, J. R. (1968) Fibrosis associated with methysergide therapy, in *Drug-Induced Diseases*, Vol. 3, eds. Meyler, L., and Peck, H. M., Excerpta Medica Foundation, Amsterdam, pp. 249–69.

HAMILTON, R. W., JR., HUSTEAD, R. F., PELTIER, L. F., KUENZIG, M. C., STRADINARK, J. F., and ROSENBAUM, S. M. (1964) Fat embolism: The effect of a particulate embolism on lung surfactant, *Surgery*, **56**, 53–6.

HAWK, W. A., and HAZARD, J. B. (1959) Sclerosing retroperitonitis and sclerosing mediastinitis, *Amer. J. clin. Path.*, **32**, 321–4.

HEARD, B. E. (1962) Fibrous healing of old iatrogenic pulmonary edema ('hexamethonium lung'), *J. Path. Bact.*, **83**, 159–64.

HEARD, B. E., and COOKE, R. A. (1968) Busulphan lung, *Thorax*, **23**, 187–93.

HOFFMAN, W. W., and TRIPPEL, O. H. (1961) Retroperitoneal fibrosis: Etiologic considerations, *J. Urol. (Baltimore)*, **86**, 222–31.

ISRAEL, H. L., and DIAMOND, P. (1962) Recurrent pulmonary infiltration and pleural effusion due to nitrofurantoin sensitivity, *New Engl. J. Med.*, **266**, 1024–6.

KEIGHLEY, J. F. (1966) Iatrogenic asthma associated with adrenergic aerosols, *Ann. intern. Med.*, **65**, 985–95.

KENNEDY, M. C. S. (1965) 'Bronchodilator' action of detropine citrate with and without isoprenaline by inhalation, *Brit. med. J.*, **2**, 916–17.

KLINGHOFFER, J. F. (1954) Löffler's syndrome following use of vaginal cream, *Ann. intern. Med.*, **40**, 343–50.

LEE, S. L., and SIEGEL, M. (1968) Drug-induced systemic lupus erythematosus, in *Drug-Induced Diseases*, Vol. 3, eds. Meyler, L., and Peck, H. M., Excerpta Medica Foundation, Amsterdam, pp. 239–48.

LANCET (1969) Drug-induced lung disease, annotation, *Lancet*, **ii**, 628–9.

LUEBBERS, P. (1962) Allergic reaction to Furadantin, *Dtsch. med. Wschr.*, **87**, 2209–11.

MUIR, D. C. F., and STANTON, J. A. (1963) Allergic pulmonary infiltration due to nitrofurantoin, *Brit. med. J.*, **1**, 1072.

MURRAY, M. J. (1968) Pulmonary reactions to nitrofurantoin, in *Drug-Induced Diseases*, Vol. 3, eds. Meyler, L., and Peck, H. M., Excerpta Medica Foundation, Amsterdam, pp. 157–60.

MURRAY, M. J., and KRONENBERG, R. (1965) Pulmonary reactions simulating cardiac pulmonary edema caused by nitrofurantoin, *New Engl. J. Med.*, **273**, 1185–7.

NASH, G., BLENNERHASSETT, J. B., and PONTOPPIDAN, H. (1967) Pulmonary lesions associated with oxygen therapy and artificial ventilation, *New Engl. J. Med.*, **276**, 368–74.

OLSSON, S., SJOBERG, J. E., WAHLQVIST, L., and ZEDERFELDT, B. (1962) Idiopathic retroperitoneal fibrosis, *Acta. chir. scand.*, **113**, 427–38.

PARTINGTON, P. F. (1961) Diffuse idiopathic fibrosis, *Amer. J. Surg.*, **10**, 239–44.

PEPYS, J. (1969) *Hypersensitivity Diseases of the Lungs due to Fungi and Organic Dusts*, Basel.

QUE, G. S., and MANDEMA, E. (1964) A case of idiopathic retroperitoneal fibrosis presenting as a systemic collagen disease, *Amer. J. Med.*, **36**, 320–9.

RAPER, F. P. (1955) Bilateral, symmetrical peri-ureteric fibrosis, *Proc. roy. Soc. Med.*, **48**, 736–40.

REED, W. G., and STINLEY, R. W. (1959) Massive periaortic and periarterial fibrosis: Report of a case, *New Engl. J. Med.*, **261**, 320–3.

ROSE, G. A., and SPENCER, H. (1957) Polyarteritis nodosa, *Quart. J. Med.*, **26**, 43–81.

SAMTER, M., and BEERS, R. F., JR. (1967) Concerning the nature of intolerance to aspirin, *J. Allergy*, **40**, 281–93.

SAMTER, M., and BEERS, R. F., JR. (1968) Intolerance to aspirin. Clinical studies and consideration of its pathogenesis, *Ann. intern. Med.*, **68**, 975–83.

SYMMERS, W. ST. C. (1965) Opportunistic infections, *Proc. roy. Soc. Med.*, **58**, 341–6.

TALBOT, H. S., and MAHONEY, E. M. (1957) Obstruction of both ureters by retroperitoneal inflammation, *J. Urol. (Baltimore)*, **78**, 738–47.

THOMPSON, R. J., JR., CARTER, R., GIBSON, L. D., REISWIG, O. K., and HINSHAW, D. B. (1961) Acute idiopathic retroperitoneal fibrosis, *Ann. Surg.*, **153**, 399–406.

TUBBS, O. S. (1946) Superior vena cava obstruction due to chronic mediastinitis, *Thorax*, **1**, 247–56.

VESSEY, M. P., and DOLL, R. (1969) Investigation of relation between use of oral contraceptives and thromboembolic disease. A further report, *Brit. med. J.*, **2**, 651–7.

VIIKARI, S. (1963) Idiopathic retroperitoneal fibrosis: Report of a case, *Ann. Chir. Gynaec. Fenn.*, **52**, 132–8.

8

DISORDERS OF GASTRO-INTESTINAL FUNCTION

DRUG-INDUCED MALABSORPTION SYNDROME

The primary function of the gastro-intestinal tract is the absorption of fat, protein, carbohydrate, vitamins and minerals from the lumen into the blood or lymphatic systems. There is evidence that specific drug therapy may cause malabsorption of many of the essential components of the diet.

DRUG-INDUCED MALABSORPTION OF FAT

Studies by Tygstrup and co-workers (1959, 1961) on tuberculous patients indicated that p-aminosalicylic acid lowered the plasma cholesterol and caused malabsorption of radioactive triolein from the gut. Levine (1968) investigated the effect of PAS on fat absorption in seven healthy, young adult male volunteers who were fed a measured 100 gram fat, gluten-free diet. The gluten-free diet was used in these studies to prevent possible gluten sensitivity or enteropathy developing. During the four-week study period, acid PAS, recrystallized in the presence of ascorbic acid (PAS-C), was given in a dosage of 6 grams per day, and subsequently, after a 10-day recovery period, the dosage was increased to 12 grams per day. PAS-C was used to minimize gastro-intestinal symptoms and also to achieve higher PAS blood levels. This improved patient tolerance and the initial absorption.

The oral administration of 12 grams per day of PAS-C for 4 weeks induced moderate steatorrhoea, without diarrhoea, in all seven subjects, although 6 grams per day of PAS-C failed to produce malabsorption of fats. The salicylate exhibited no direct toxic effect on intestinal epithelium, as determined by light microscopy. Jejunal mucosal biopsies performed before, during and after PAS-C administration, at either the 6 gram/day or 12 gram/day dosage, did not show any alterations in the normal histology pattern. The degree of steatorrhoea did not appear to account entirely for the diminished serum cholesterol concentrations observed during this regime.

DRUG-INDUCED MALABSORPTION OF FOLIC ACID

The megaloblastic anaemia that is a well-recognized but infrequent complication of anticonvulsant therapy (Badenoch, 1954; Hawkins and Meynell, 1958) is associated with low serum-folate levels (Klipstein, 1964) and responds well to conventional doses of folic acid by mouth (Chanarin et al., 1958). The mechanism for this defect of folate metabolism is uncertain, but suggestions include interference with folate-coenzyme formation or function (Hawkins and Meynell, 1954; Girdwood and Lenman, 1956), interference with folic absorption (Meynell, 1966; Dahlke and Mertens-Roesler, 1967), displacement of folic acid from its carrier plasma protein (Klipstein, 1964) and inhibition of gastro-intestinal folate conjugase (Druskin et al., 1962). Although it has been suggested as a mechanism (Druskin et al., 1962; Kiorboe and Plum, 1966; Dahlke and Mertens-Roesler, 1967), little attention has been given to the possible adverse effect of anticonvulsant drugs on the absorption of conjugated folate, which constitutes 80 per cent of the dietary folate (Butterworth et al., 1958).

Hoffbrand and Necheles (1968) showed that phenytoin (diphenylhydantoin) inhibited folate absorption from folate polyglutamates, which are major components of food folate. Phenytoin was also shown to inhibit the activity of folate conjugase from human jejunal mucosa at a pharmacological concentration in in vitro studies. Folate conjugase is thought to split dietary folate polyglutamates into the simpler folate monoglutamate form before absorption and it is therefore likely that phenytoin reduces absorption of folate polyglutamates by inhibiting this enzyme.

It was concluded by these workers that folate deficiency in patients receiving phenytoin medication was at least partly due to reduced absorption of food folate polyglutamates.

Rosenberg and associates (1968) also showed that oral administration of phenytoin impaired intestinal absorption of conjugated folate in some healthy volunteers although it did not significantly affect the absorption of free folate. These investigators also confirmed that phenytoin inhibited the in vitro deconjugation of polyglutamate folate by homogenates of human intestinal mucosa. These observations would suggest that the mechanism for the folate deficiency and megaloblastic anaemia, which may accompany chronic anticonvulsant therapy with phenytoin, may be due to inhibition of an enzyme system responsible for the intestinal deconjugation of folate sources in the diet.

DRUG-INDUCED MALABSORPTION OF VITAMIN B_{12}

A specific type of PAS-induced malabsorption related only to the vitamin B_{12} absorption process has been suggested by Scandinavian investigators, while others have been unable to confirm a relationship between PAS therapy and diminished vitamin B_{12} concentrations. Determination of faecal fat, d-xylose tolerance, and intestinal biopsies usually gave normal findings, although steatorrhoea and diminished urinary d-xylose excretion were each found in one patient.

Malabsorption of vitamin B_{12} was found by Lindenbaum (1968) in six of 11 patients receiving 12 grams of acid PAS daily, and two patients had concomitant malabsorption of d-xylose and folic acid. It would appear therefore that the selectivity of PAS-induced malabsorption of vitamin B_{12} is relative, probably representing another manifestation of the occult mild malabsorption found in some subjects receiving this drug.

MULTIFACTORIAL MALABSORPTION DUE TO DRUG-INDUCED PANCREATIC NECROSIS

Pancreatic dysfunction manifests itself in terms of pain, steatorrhoea, protein malabsorption and raised serum amylase levels.

Pancreatic necrosis may occur in children on corticosteroid therapy; Labram (1963) mentioned observations on 25 children treated with corticoids for lipoid nephrosis. Severe pancreatic complications were observed in 10 children: there were three of these cases with necrosis of the entire pancreas, and seven with focal lesions. Of these, three children died due to pancreatic complications. In a comparable group of 27 children not on steroid therapy, focal pancreatic lesions were only found in four cases and these were not fatal.

Pancreatic necrosis is not exclusively restricted to lipoid nephrosis; it has also been described in the course of steroid therapy for asthma, polymyositis, and other conditions requiring such treatment (Baar and Wolff, 1957; Marczynska-Robowska, 1957).

One definite conclusion that may be drawn from these observations is that it is always advisable to consider the possibility of a pancreatic lesion in children who present with an acute abdomen while on corticosteroid therapy. Amylase determinations in blood and urine should be performed routinely in these cases.

DRUGS CAUSING GASTRO-INTESTINAL ULCERATION AND HAEMORRHAGE

ANTI-INFLAMMATORY AGENTS

It is of considerable pharmacological interest to note that the whole spectrum of anti-inflammatory agents in clinical use will cause dyspepsia, and that the corticosteroids and non-steroidal anti-inflammatory agents (phenylbutazone, oxyphenbutazone, indomethacin and salicylates) cause gastric ulceration in a high

proportion of cases. These same drugs are also implicated in a large proportion of cases of gastro-intestinal haemorrhage.

Nearly all the available anti-inflammatory agents have been shown to cause erosion of mucous membranes in animal tests, and it is not unduly pessimistic to predict that all future anti-inflammatory agents will also, to a greater or lesser degree, cause gastric erosion, since, by the very nature of their anti-inflammatory activity, they damp down the essential regenerative processes in the gastro-intestinal tract.

Corticosteroids

Corticosteroid-induced ulcers can develop rapidly although sometimes they occur only after prolonged treatment. Low dosage, for example less than 15 mg of prednisolone daily, seems to entail slightly less risk of gastric complications than do higher doses. No difference in frequency of gastric complications has been demonstrated between the different synthetic corticosteroids when they are used in comparable therapeutic dosage.

Steroid ulcers show no male or female predominance; their localization is the opposite to the 'natural' ulcer distribution, and about 60 per cent are found in the stomach. They rarely cause subjective complaints so that their presence remains unnoticed until a haemorrhage or perforation occurs. Steroid ulcers generally respond well to conventional ulcer treatment (bed-rest, diet, antacids), even when steroid medication has to be continued, although healing is somewhat slower than with the classical peptic ulcer. Therefore abrupt stoppage of corticosteroid treatment because of a complicating ulcer is not necessary, and indeed could be dangerous. The fact that a patient has a history of peptic ulcer is not an absolute contraindication for steroid treatment; in such cases it is advisable to prescribe an appropriate diet and antacids prophylactically.

It has been considered that a relationship exists between the frequency of the development of a steroid ulcer and its complications on one hand, and the nature of the pre-existing disease for which the steroid treatment has been instituted on the other. Spiro and Milles (1960) found an increase in the frequency of gastric ulcers in patients with rheumatoid arthritis who were on corticosteroids, but Duprez and Simons (1963) mentioned only sporadic and slight gastro-intestinal disturbances in 1,094 patients with bronchial asthma who were treated with corticoids.

The steroid ulcers of the stomach may present in many ways, differing from a slight tenderness in the upper abdomen to an abdominal catastrophe. Some characteristics of these ulcers are:

1. The complications (bleeding and perforation) are often the first symptoms. These are often obscured by the lowered level of visceral sensitivity, and the severity of the complication is frequently masked by

the absence of fever, shock, muscular irritability or abnormal white blood cell count.

2. A steroid-induced ulcer may complicate any disease for which the steroid therapy has been instituted.

3. The duration of the steroid therapy does not determine the onset of an induced ulcer. Severe, and even lethal, complications have been reported only a few days after corticosteroid treatment had started.

4. There is a direct correlation between high dosage of steroids and development of ulcers and their complications.

Acetylsalicylic Acid

Dyspepsia and heart-burn are experienced by 7 per cent of all users of acetylsalicylic acid (aspirin). This percentage is much larger, about 30 per cent, among patients who suffer from peptic ulcer and take aspirin. Occult blood in the faeces is unfortunately all too frequently encountered during aspirin medication, even if the drug is used in conventional doses (1·5 to 3 grams per day). Stubbé (1962) found occult blood loss in 62·5 per cent of 461 rheumatic patients taking aspirin. The same frequency of occult blood loss was also found in normal controls during aspirin administration; indeed anaemia due to aspirin-induced chronic blood loss is now well recognized. Enteric coating of aspirin, while not affecting adequate salicylate levels in the blood, does greatly reduce the frequency of occult blood loss. This constitutes an argument in favour of the stomach as the source of blood and of the insensitivity of the intestinal mucosa to local salicylate inflammation.

Acute upper haemorrhage also can be caused by aspirin; of 166 patients with haematemesis, 33 per cent had taken aspirin less than 6 hours previously, as against 5 per cent of unselected controls. Jones and associates (1959) estimated that 40 per cent of all X-ray negative upper gastro-intestinal bleeding was caused by acetylsalicylic acid. Studies after oral challenge have demonstrated that effervescent aspirin (which contains $NaHCO_3$ in excess), or good enteric coating, ensures a relatively low frequency of gastro-intestinal bleeding. If required the drug can also be administered in suppositories, or alternatively sodium salicylate can be prescribed by mouth, although this is less effective as an analgesic.

When confronted with major gastric haemorrhage after aspirin medication, one should not be hasty in resorting to an emergency gastrectomy, particularly when gastric X-rays disclose no lesion; in that case the surgeon sometimes finds a diffuse haemorrhagic gastritis, and total gastrectomy is a rather drastic intervention for a condition which, as a rule, heals spontaneously within a few days of the aspirin being stopped. However, there is a special warning regarding patients on anticoagulant therapy; they are at special risk from aspirin-induced haematemesis.

The mechanism of aspirin-induced bleeding is multifactorial; it causes focal necrosis, erosions, capillary thrombosis and haemorrhages. The traumatic influence acting from the lumen is chiefly of a chemical nature, and radically changes the ionic fluxes through the mucosa. However, another factor also involved is prolongation of the bleeding time, as has been clearly demonstrated by Stubbé (1962). This makes it understandable why bleeding is so prominent with aspirin, and why even intravenous administration of the drug can lead to blood loss.

Indomethacin

Lövgren and Allander (1964) reported a series of 18 patients receiving 200–300 mg of indomethacin daily; five of these patients developed gastro-duodenal ulcers, of whom two died, one after massive haemorrhage and one after resection for multiple gastric ulcers. Three of these five patients had a previous history of gastric or duodenal ulcers but barium meal examinations were negative at the onset of treatment.

Lockie and Norcross (1966) noted the development of 14 peptic ulcers in their series of 180 patients on indomethacin; eight of these patients had ulcers previously and 11 had also been on corticosteroids or salicylates. There were five perforations and seven haemorrhages in this series.

Boardman and Hart (1967) reviewed the side-effects of indomethacin and recorded dyspepsia in 7·8 per cent of 228 patients. However, the most conclusive evidence of gastric ulceration caused by indomethacin has been provided by Taylor and co-workers (1968) who described 10 cases of gastric ulceration, mainly prepyloric. Due to their radiological appearance, malignancy was suspected in seven of these cases. Other drugs known to cause gastric ulceration (e.g. phenylbutazone, oxyphenbutazone, corticosteroids) were absent from treatment although one patient received aspirin, and one patient corticotrophin. Only one of these patients had a previous history suggestive of gastric ulceration. In five of the patients in this series healing of the ulcer occurred with no other treatment than antacids and withdrawal of indomethacin; two patients showed ulcer healing with carbenoxolone treatment, and one patient showed healing of the pre-pyloric lesion while continuing with indomethacin at a reduced dosage. However, in two cases the ulcers did not heal and one of these required a gastrectomy; the other patient died of a massive haemorrhage and melaena. In the latter, necroscopy showed a benign ulcer 1 cm in diameter on the posterior wall of the stomach.

In three of these patients gastric ulceration occurred when the patients were receiving indomethacin suppositories alone, thus a direct irritant effect of the agent can be excluded in these cases.

Phenylbutazone

Phenylbutazone medication is often associated with gastric complications regardless of the route of administration; these complications can be expected not only after ingestion of tablets, but also following intra-muscular or rectal administration. Phenylbutazone-induced ulcers are frequently localized in the duodenum. Sometimes they occur within a few days of treatment, but more usually they occur when the period of treatment exceeds 2 weeks. A brief course of treatment with this drug, therefore, raises fewer objections than maintenance therapy, especially when large doses are involved; a low daily dosage (not exceeding 400 mg) and administration every other day can reduce the frequency of gastric complications.

Mefenamic Acid

Mefenamic acid has been reported as causing gastric irritation and diarrhoea, although there are other reports of constipation following treatment. There has been no report of gastric ulceration being caused by mefenamic acid alone although Prescott (1968) has cited one case of acute gastric ulcer in which mefenamic acid was taken together with corticosteroids, and another case where haematemesis without radiological evidence of gastric ulcer occurred during mefenamic acid treatment. A further warning of importance in this aspect of gastric irritation is that mefenamic acid has been linked with a possible potentiation of the effects of the coumarin anticoagulants.

MODE OF ACTION OF ULCEROGENIC DRUGS

Reserpine treatment has been implicated in peptic ulceration and perforation in a few cases (West, 1958), and its ulcerogenic action would appear to be due to increased vagal activity causing increased acid secretion. Other drugs which affect acid secretion such as the xanthines (caffeine and theophylline), phenylbutazone and the corticosteroids appear to do so by their direct stimulant action on parietal cells.

Corticosteroids do not seem to affect the basal overnight acid secretion in man (Kirsner and Ford, 1956; Carbone and Liebowitz, 1958; Beck et al., 1960; Strickland et al., 1969). Strickland and co-workers (1969) showed that prednisolone in a total daily dose of 20 mg given for 1 month caused no change in basal acid secretion in a group of 14 healthy male subjects, although it did cause a significant increase in histamine stimulated gastric acid secretion. In contrast, a group not taking corticosteroids showed no significant change in stimulated acid secretion when tested on two occasions 1 month apart. These investigators pointed out that the stimulated secretory volume was not significantly altered by prednisolone but that the increase was one of acid concentration. Experiments in dogs (Reid et al., 1961) and in rats (Foley and Glick, 1962) have shown that continuous steroid administration causes an increase in total parietal cell mass.

Other ulcerogenic drugs such as cinchophen and aspirin have no influence in promoting gastric acid secretion, and Winkelman and Summerskill (1960) showed that there was no correlation between gastric secretion and aspirin-induced bleeding. Nevertheless, it is a wise precaution to avoid giving aspirin to patients with known peptic ulceration, since the mode of action of aspirin on gastro-intestinal bleeding is multifactorial.

Aspirin destroys the protective mucus layer over the gastric epithelium and causes focal necrosis and superficial erosions of the epithelium together with capillary thrombosis and haemorrhage. In addition, apart from the damage caused by aspirin itself, the gastric mucosa is left exposed to the enzymatic action of the gastric secretions.

Apart from the actions already described, the anti-inflammatory group of drugs slow down the natural repair processes which would otherwise tend to correct their erosive tendencies. If the action of anti-inflammatory agents on the gastro-intestinal mucosa was to delay or prevent the repair of wear and tear injuries to the bowel, then similar lesions could reasonably be expected to occur elsewhere in the alimentary canal. In fact, such lesions have been described during treatment with both steroids and phenylbutazone. Parker and Thomas (1959) reported several cases of fatal intestinal perforations occurring during the course of steroid therapy for rheumatoid arthritis. These perforations occurred in the duodenum, the caecum or the sigmoid colon. The severe arteritis with fibrinoid necrosis present in the intestinal wall in these cases has been partly ascribed to the steroid therapy. Duprez and Simons (1963) reported four cases of intestinal necrosis in patients on corticosteroid therapy in whom no arteritis was found; in these cases, the intestinal necrosis was localized in the duodenum in one patient and affected larger parts of the colon or even the entire large bowel in the other three patients.

Bravo and Lowman (1968) recorded an illustrative case of a 70-year-old man, who received prolonged treatment with phenylbutazone for severe arthritis, and who presented with severe rectal bleeding and diarrhoea. The rectal bleeding ceased when drug treatment was stopped. However, acute flare-ups of the arthritis necessitated re-institution of the phenylbutazone and again there was severe rectal bleeding. A barium enema examination followed the final episode and showed a conical narrowing of the sigmoid colon with evidence of ulceration. This lesion simulated a carcinoma from clinical and radiological aspects. Operation disclosed an induration of the sigmoid and descending colon and the indurated segment was resected. Grossly, it contained two large ulcers with sharply demarcated edges. Microscopically, these lesions consisted of dense chronic inflammatory infiltrate. Infectious and malignant disease were therefore excluded and, in view of the clinical history, it was concluded that these ulcers were caused by the phenylbutazone treatment.

Debenham (1966) described a case of ulceration and perforation of the caecum during oxyphenbutazone therapy; histologically, the ulcer showed a chronic inflammatory infiltrate with a granulomatous base.

GASTRO-INTESTINAL HAEMORRHAGE DUE TO ANTICOAGULANTS

Gastro-intestinal haemorrhage caused by anticoagulants usually originates as haematomas in the wall of the stomach or intestine. These haematomas are frequently found in the submucosa in the small bowel especially the jejunum, and they may vary in width from several centimetres up to 20 centimetres or longer. Occasionally a large number may be found along the entire digestive tract; however, this is uncommon and more usually the lesion is limited to one or two large haematomas, accompanied by several punctate haemorrhages. Frequently the mesentery is also filled with blood. A notable feature is that the more peripheral mesenteric arterioles continue to pulsate normally. At laparotomy blood has frequently been found in the abdominal cavity, and the amount may vary from a few millilitres to several hundred millilitres (Perez-Mesa, 1960).

The haematoma in the intestinal wall makes the affected piece of gut firmer in consistency, and as a result offers some degree of obstruction to all oncoming peristaltic waves. Therefore the obstruction may give rise to an initial phase of increased peristaltic activity coupled with colicky abdominal pains and diarrhoea which may be blood-stained. This is frequently followed by a phase of peristaltic hypoactivity and ultimately ileus. Whether this ileus is of the paralytic or obstructive type depends on the size of the haematomas. A large solitary haematoma is likely to cause an ileus of the mechanical type, whereas diffusely scattered haematomas in the intestinal wall and extravasation into the mesentery and peritoneum probably cause an ileus of the paralytic type.

X-ray changes in a patient with these intra-mural haematomas show luminal narrowing with spiculated and thickened transverse folds (Felson and Levin, 1954; Senturia et al., 1961; Wiot et al., 1961; Kramer and Hill, 1964) and if there is obstruction, a few dilated loops may be seen proximal to this; occasionally fluid levels may be seen in them (Kramer and Hill, 1964).

Accurate recognition of the cause of the obstruction or ileus is necessary and the anticoagulants should be discontinued. Conservative treatment or resection of the affected bowel should be dictated by the clinical condition of the patient also bearing in mind the level of anticoagulation.

GASTRO-INTESTINAL BLEEDING CAUSED BY ETHACRYNIC ACID

The American National Institutes of Health have recently issued a preliminary warning concerning gastro-intestinal bleeding caused by ethacrynic acid. Their evidence was drawn from a study carried out at Tufts University, Massachusetts, at the request of the National Institute of General Medical Sciences, and involved 1,602 patients. Amongst these, 157 patients received ethacrynic acid intravenously, 67 received frusemide, and 189 received other diuretics. The remaining 1,189 patients served as controls. It was found that 20 per cent of patients having ethacrynic acid intravenously developed gastro-intestinal bleeding compared with about 5 per cent in each of the other three groups.

RECTAL BLEEDING DUE TO VASCULAR OCCLUSION ASSOCIATED WITH ORAL CONTRACEPTIVE MEDICATION

Vascular occlusion of the colon in young women has been reported by several investigators in association with oral contraception (Reed and Coon, 1963; Brennan et al., 1968; Kilpatrick et al., 1968; Ward and Stevenson, 1968; Brindle and Henderson, 1969). For example, the case reported by Brindle and Henderson was that of a 24-year-old woman, para 2, who had been on *Enavid E* for 15 months, and developed a severe cramp-like abdominal pain of acute onset followed by nausea and watery diarrhoea. Within 6 hours of onset she was passing bright red blood per rectum. Stool culture was negative, Widal test was negative and sigmoidoscopy showed bright red blood to 20 cm. Radiological findings showed gross scalloping in the colon, together with picket-fence appearance in the distal ileum. These conformed to the criteria laid down for a diagnosis of reversible vascular occlusion. It was difficult to determine whether the occlusion was arterial or venous but the distribution of the disease, together with the timing of the onset of melaena in relation to pain suggested venous thrombosis.

DRUG-INDUCED ILEUS

Ganglion-blocking drugs, hexamethonium, pentamethonium, pentolium tartrate, mecamylamine, and pempidine may all cause constipation. It is essential to control the constipation due to these drugs since it can develop into paralytic ileus which persists even when the drug is stopped, and can be fatal. Munster and Milton (1961) described a series of 12 cases of paralytic ileus caused by ganglion-blocking drugs.

Goldstone (1952) described a case of ileus which developed in a middle-aged hypertensive man treated with pentamethonium. Although it was realized that the drug could cause vomiting, distension and constipation there had been no previous report of abdominal pain or X-ray findings characteristic of the obstruction that occurred. At laparotomy the whole of the small-gut was grossly distended, although the caecum and large bowel were of normal calibre. The gut was emptied of gas by puncture and the investigators commented that it was remarkable that after deflation the gut did not contract but merely became flaccid. The patient died 48 hours after operation.

If ileus does occur, routine intestinal suction, intravenous fluids and subcutaneous neostigmine injections should be given hourly.

DRUG-INDUCED PAROTITIS

PHENYLBUTAZONE AND OXYPHENBUTAZONE

The clinical picture of phenylbutazone-induced parotitis appears to be slightly variable in different cases described in the literature. For example, Cohen and Banks (1966) described a 44-year-old man who presented with a fever and symmetrical enlargement of the parotid glands. The symptoms suggested mumps, but the complement fixation tests for mumps S and V antibodies excluded this diagnosis. The patient made a spontaneous recovery. A year later the man suffered a similar short febrile illness with bilateral enlargement of the parotid glands. On each of the two occasions, his illness had started 2 days after starting phenylbutazone therapy, which had been prescribed for tennis elbow; the salivary-gland swelling began to subside when the phenylbutazone was discontinued.

Murray-Bruce (1966) described a case where phenylbutazone was given by intramuscular injection to a merchant seaman for gout; the patient developed parotid swelling and this lasted for 1 month while he continued on the phenylbutazone treatment. The swelling subsided when the patient was changed to sulphinpyrazone. A similar attack occurred about 3 years later when the patient again received phenylbutazone for his gout, but on this occasion his parotid glands remained enlarged but pain free.

Rogers (1966) described a case where phenylbutazone was given to a 71-year-old man on two occasions; at each time, 48 hours after commencing treatment, he developed a pyrexial illness and swelling of all his salivary glands. In this patient, the salivary gland swelling took 7 days to subside after the first episode, even though the treatment was immediately stopped.

Simpson (1966) described a case of a woman aged 74 years in whom phenylbutazone caused submaxillary swelling on two occasions, and Gross (1969) described a case of febrile parotitis caused by oxyphenbutazone in a 57-year-old woman. On the third day of oxyphenbutazone treatment, the patient developed a temperature of 40°C (104°F) and painless parotid swelling; serological tests for mumps were negative. The association between parotitis and drug therapy was then suspected. Similar cases have also been reported by Cardoe (1964) and Stahl (1966) following oxyphenbutazone therapy.

Patients with phenylbutazone or oxyphenbutazone parotitis respond to corticosteroid treatment or withdrawal of drug by a dramatic drop in fever with prompt recovery; this suggests an allergic basis for the parotitis. It is also important to note that in many of the reported cases, the second episode of parotitis has been worse than the first; this too would be in keeping with an allergic mechanism.

ISOPRENALINE (ISOPROTERENOL)

Borsanyi and Blanchard (1961 and 1962) described symptomatic swelling of the parotid glands due to isoprenaline. These cases differed from those caused by phenylbutazone or oxyphenbutazone in that there was no febrile episode or feeling of malaise.

HYPOTENSIVE DRUGS

Bretylium tosylate and guanethidine sulphate have also been reported as causing parotid pain and swelling. With bretylium, parotid pain is a fairly frequent side-effect; its cause is unknown, and although it usually improves when the drug is stopped it may persist for a long time.

RECOMMENDED FURTHER READING

BRUMMELKAMP, W. H. (1965) The 'acute abdomen' caused by steroids and anticoagulants, in *Drug-Induced Diseases*, Vol. 2, eds. Meyler, L., and Peck, H. M., Excerpta Medica Foundation, Amsterdam, pp. 35–46.

COOKE, A. R. (1967) The role of adrenocortical steroids in the regulation of gastric secretion, *Gastroenterology*, **52**, 272–81.

TEN THIJE, O. J. (1965) Peptic ulcer due to drugs, in *Drug-Induced Diseases*, Vol. 2, eds. Meyler, L., and Peck, H. M., Excerpta Medica Foundation, Amsterdam, pp. 30–4.

REFERENCES

BAAR, H. S., and WOLFF, O. H. (1957) Pancreatic necrosis in cortisone-treated children, *Lancet*, **i**, 812–15.

BADENOCH, J. (1954) The use of labelled vitamin B_{12} and gastric biopsy in the investigation of anaemia, *Proc. roy. Soc. Med.*, **47**, 426–7.

BECK, I. T., FLETCHER, H. W., McKENNA, R. D., and GRIFF, H. (1960) Effect of small and massive doses of prednisone on gastric secretory activity, *Gastroenterology*, **38**, 740–9.

BOARDMAN, P. L., and HART, F. D. (1967) Side-effects of indomethacin, *Ann. rheum. Dis.*, **26**, 127–32.

BORSANYI, S. J., and BLANCHARD, C. L. (1961) Asymptomatic enlargement of the parotid glands due to the use of isoproterenol, *Maryland med. J.*, **10**, 572–3.

BORSANYI, S. J., and BLANCHARD, C. L. (1962) Asymptomatic parotid swelling and isoproterenol, *Laryngoscope (St Louis)*, **72**, 1777–83.

BRAVO, A. J., and LOWMAN, R. M. (1968) Benign ulcer of the sigmoid colon. An unusual lesion that can simulate carcinoma, *Radiology*, **90**, 113–15.

BRENNAN, M. F., CLARKE, A. M., and MACBETH, W. A. A. G. (1968) Infarction of the midgut associated with oral contraceptives, *New Engl. J. Med.*, **279**, 1213–14.

BRINDLE, M. J., and HENDERSON, I. N. (1969) Vascular occlusion of the colon associated with oral contraception *Canad. med. Ass. J.*, **100**, 681–2.

BUTTERWORTH, C. E., JR., SANTINI, R., JR., and PÉREZ-SANTIAGO, E. (1958) The absorption of glycine and its conversion to serine in patients with sprue, *J. clin. Invest.*, **37**, 20–7.

CARBONE, J. V., and LIEBOWITZ, D. (1958) The effect of adrenal corticoids on gastric secretion and the suppression of corticoid-induced hypersecretion of anticholinergics, *Metabolism*, **7**, 70–7.

CARDOE, N. (1964) The place of oxyphenbutazone in the treatment of rheumatoid arthritis and allied conditions, *Med. J. Aust.*, **2**, 986–8.

CHANARIN, I., MOLLIN, D. L., and ANDERSON, B. B. (1958) Folic acid deficiency and the megaloblastic anaemias, *Proc. roy. Soc. Med.*, **51**, 757–63.

COHEN, L., and BANKS, P. (1966) Salivary gland enlargement and phenylbutazone, *Brit. med. J.*, **1**, 1420.

DAHLKE, M. B., and MERTENS-ROESLER, E. (1967) Malabsorption of folic acid due to diphenylhydantoin, *Blood*, **30**, 341–51.

DEBENHAM, G. P. (1966) Ulcer of the cecum during oxyphenbutazone (Tandearil) therapy, *Canad. med. Ass. J.*, **94**, 1182–4.

DRUSKIN, M. S., WALLEN, M. H., and BONAGURA, L. (1962) Anticonvulsant-associated megaloblastic anemia. Response to 25 Microgm. of folic acid administered by mouth daily, *New Engl. J. Med.*, **267**, 483–5.

DUPREZ, A., and SIMONS, M. (1963) A propos de quelques drames abdominaux au cours de traitements à la cortisone, *Acta gastro-ent. belg.*, **26**, 609–20.

FELSON, B., and LEVIN, E. J. (1954) Intramural hematoma of the duodenum: Diagnostic roentgen sign, *Radiology*, **63**, 823–31.

FOLEY, W. A., and GLICK, D. (1962) Studies in histochemistry, LXVI. Histamine, mast and parietal cells in stomach of rats and effects of cortisone treatment, *Gastroenterology*, **43**, 425–9.

GIRDWOOD, R. H., and LENMAN, J. A. R. (1956) Megaloblastic anaemia occurring during primidone therapy, *Brit. med. J.*, **1**, 146–7.

GOLDSTONE, B. (1952) Death associated with methonium treatment, *S. Afr. med. J.*, **26**, 552–4.

GROSS, L. (1969) Oxyphenylbutazone-induced parotitis, *Ann. intern. Med.*, **70**, 1229–30.

HAWKINS, C. F., and MEYNELL, M. J. (1954) Megaloblastic anaemia due to phenytoin sodium, *Lancet*, **ii**, 737–8.

HAWKINS, C. F., and MEYNELL, M. J. (1958) Macrocytosis and macrocytic anaemia caused by anticonvulsant drugs, *Quart. J. Med.*, **27**, 45–63.

HOFFBRAND, A. V., and NECHELES, T. F. (1968) Mechanism of folate deficiency in patients receiving phenytoin, *Lancet*, **ii**, 528–30.

JONES, F. A., READ, A. E., and STUBBE, J. L. (1959) Alimentary bleeding of obscure origin. A follow-up study and commentary, *Brit. med. J.*, **1**, 1138–42.

KILPATRICK, Z. M., SILVERMAN, J. F., BETANCOURT, E., FARMAN, J., and LAWSON, J. P. (1968) Vascular occlusion of the colon and oral contraceptives. Possible relation, *New Engl. J. Med.*, **278**, 438–40.

KIORBOE, E., and PLUM, C. M. (1966) Megaloblastic anaemia developing during treatment of epilepsy, *Acta med. scand.*, **179**, Suppl. 445, 349.

KIRSNER, J. B., and FORD, H. (1956) Gastric secretory stimulation: Effects of phenylbutazone, histalog, ACTH, adrenal steroids and reserpine in man, *J. Lab. clin. Med.*, **48**, 824–5.

KLIPSTEIN, F. A. (1964) Subnormal serum folate and macrocytosis associated with anticonvulsant drug therapy, *Blood*, **23**, 68–86.

KRAMER, R. A., and HILL, R. L. (1964) Intramural small bowel bleeding during anticoagulant therapy, *Arch. intern. Med.*, **113**, 213–17.

LABRAM, C. (1963) Accidents de la corticothérapie particuliers ou récemment décrits, *Concours med.*, **85**, 5375–8, 6189–92.

LEVINE, R. A. (1968) Steatorrhea induced by para-aminosalicylic acid, *Ann. intern. Med.*, **68**, 1265–70.

LINDENBAUM, J. (1968) personal communication cited by Levine, R. A. (1968)

LOCKIE, L. M., and NORCROSS, B. M. (1966) in *Arthritis and Allied Conditions*, 7th ed., ed. Hollander, J. L., London, p. 345.

LÖVGREN, O., and ALLANDER, E. (1964) Side-effects of indomethacin, *Brit. med. J.*, **1**, 118.

MARCZYNSKA-ROBOWSKA, M. (1957) Pancreatic necrosis in a case of Still's disease, *Lancet*, **i**, 815–16.

MEYNELL, M. J. (1966) Megaloblastic anaemia in anticonvulsant therapy, *Lancet*, **i**, 487.

MUNSTER, A., and MILTON, G. W. (1961) Paralytic ileus due to ganglion blocking agents, *Med. J. Aust.*, **48**, 210–13.

MURRAY-BRUCE, D. J. (1966) Salivary gland enlargement and phenylbutazone, *Brit. med. J.*, **1**, 1599–600.

PARKER, R. A., and THOMAS, P. M. (1959) Intestinal perforation and widespread arteritis in rheumatoid arthritis during treatment with cortisone, *Brit. med. J.*, **1**, 540–2.

PEREZ-MESA, C. (1960) Paralytic ileus associated with prolonged bishydroxycoumarin (dicumarol) therapy, *Surgery*, **48**, 351–6.

PRESCOTT, L. F. (1968) Antipyretic analgesic drugs, in *Side Effects of Drugs*, Vol. VI, eds. Meyler, L., and Herxheimer, A., Excerpta Medica Foundation, Amsterdam, p. 132.

REED, D. L., and COON, W. W. (1963) Thromboembolism in patients receiving progestational drugs, *New Engl. J. Med.*, **269**, 622–4.

REID, N. C. R. W., HACKETT, R. M., and WELBOURN, R. D. (1961) The influence of cortisone on the parietal cell population of the stomach in the dog, *Gut*, **2**, 119–22.

ROGERS, R. D. (1966) Salivary gland enlargement and phenylbutazone, *Brit. med. J.*, **2**, 113.

ROSENBERG, I. H., GODWIN, H. A., STREIFF, R. R., and CASTLE, W. B. (1968) Impairment of intestinal deconjugation of dietary folate: A possible explanation of megaloblastic anaemia associated with phenytoin therapy, *Lancet*, **ii**, 530–2.

SENTURIA, H. R., SUSMAN, N, and SHYKEN, H. (1961) The roentgen appearance of spontaneous intramural hemorrhage of the small intestine associated with anticoagulant therapy, *Amer J. Roentgenol.*, **86**, 62–9.

SIMPSON, R. W. (1966) Salivary gland enlargement and phenylbutazone, *Brit. med. J.*, **2**, 113.

SPIRO, H. M., and MILLES, S. S. (1960) Clinical and physiologic implications of the steroid-induced peptic ulcer, *New Engl. J. Med.*, **263**, 286–94.

STAHL, R. (1966) Parotitis in Tandearil treatments, *Nord. méd.*, **75**, 170.

STRICKLAND, R. G., FISHER, J. M., and TAYLOR, K. B. (1969) Effect of prednisolone on gastric function and structure in man, *Gastroenterology*, **56**, 675–86.

STUBBÉ, L. TH. F. L. (1962) The noxious effect of acetylsalicylic acid preparations on the gastro-intestinal tract, in *Drug-Induced Diseases*, eds. Meyler, L., and Peck, H. M., Assen, Netherlands, pp. 145–55.

TAYLOR, R. T., HUSKISSON, E. C., WHITEHOUSE, G. H., DUDLEY HART, F., and TRAPNELL, D. H. (1968) Gastric ulceration during indomethacin therapy, *Brit. med. J.*, **4**, 734–7.

TRAPNELL, D. H. (1968) Gastric ulceration during indomethacin therapy, *Brit. med. J.*, **4**, 734–7.

TYGSTRUP, N., WINKLER, K., and WARBURG, E. (1959) Effect of p-aminosalicylic acid on serum-cholesterol, *Lancet*, **i**, 503.

TYGSTRUP, N., WINKLER, K., and JORGENSEN, K. (1961) Treatment of hypercholesterolaemia with para-aminosalicylic acid, *Ugeskr. Laeg.*, **123**, 255.

WARD, G. W., and STEVENSEN, J. R. (1968) Colonic disorder and oral contraceptives, *New Engl. J. Med.*, **278**, 910.

WEST, W. O. (1958) Perforation and hemorrhage from duodenal ulcer during the administration of Rauwolfia serpentina: Report of five cases, *Ann. intern. Med.*, **48**, 1033–9.

WINKELMAN, E. I., and SUMMERSKILL, W. H. (1960) Gastric secretion in relation to gastrointestinal bleeding from salicylate compounds, *Gastroenterology*, **40**, 56–63.

WIOT, J. F., WEINSTEIN, A. S., and FELSON, B. (1961) Duodenal hematomata induced by coumarin, *Amer. J. Roentgenol.*, **86**, 70–5.

9

DISORDERS OF HEPATIC FUNCTION

DRUG DETOXICATION BY THE LIVER

Many drugs are metabolized by the liver and there they are made more water soluble for subsequent extraction into the bile. This process is achieved by a variety of enzymes (oxidizing, reducing, hydrolyzing or conjugating) located largely in the hepatic microsomes, part of the smooth endoplasmic reticulum of the liver cell.

Metabolism of the drug in the liver may increase potency, e.g. phenylbutazone, reduce potency, e.g. pethidine, or even produce a toxic derivative, e.g. chloramphenicol. Sometimes also metabolism by the liver is necessary to make the drug clinically effective, e.g. cyclophosphamide (Sherlock, 1968a).

There has been much discussion about the effects of specific drugs in patients with underlying liver disease; it is common knowledge, for example, that morphine may precipitate coma in patients with cirrhosis, and that paraldehyde causes profound sleep in some patients with liver disease. It is difficult to show that the half-life of these and other drugs is increased in patients with cirrhosis, although recent investigations have shown that this is probably so; chloramphenicol has been demonstrated to have an increased serum half-life in patients with cirrhosis due to a slower rate of glucuronide conjugation (Kunin et al., 1959) and similar results have been reported in patients with liver disease given a salicylamide load (Barniville and Misk, 1959). Any

drug should be given with caution to these patients; if a sedative is required then only half the normal dose of, for example, butobarbitone or promethazine should be given (Sherlock, 1968a).

The rate at which a drug is metabolized by the liver may be increased by the process of enzyme induction. A great many drugs activate the microsomal enzymes of the endoplasmic reticulum, which can actually be shown to hypertrophy after their use. This may explain why certain drugs, particularly barbiturates and meprobamate, become less effective and have a shorter duration of action with repeated use. Even patients with underlying liver disease are able to improve their hepatic metabolism in this way to some extent and it is also probable that this is the process by which the alcoholic becomes increasingly tolerant of alcohol. Indeed, in the latter stages of alcoholism when the liver is damaged, the alcohol tolerance is diminished; this is probably due to a reduction of hepatic detoxicating enzymes, particularly alcohol dehydrogenase, in the cirrhotic liver (Sherlock, 1968a).

Enzyme induction is non-specific and is not confined to the enzymes actually concerned in the metabolism of the drug being administered. This principle of non-specific enzyme induction has been applied therapeutically; a patient with deep, unconjugated hyperbilirubinaemia was given phenobarbitone in order to induce the enzymes which metabolize bilirubin and did indeed show a marked reduction in icterus (Whelton et al., 1968).

FIG. 9.1. *Sites at which drugs interfere with bilirubin metabolism*

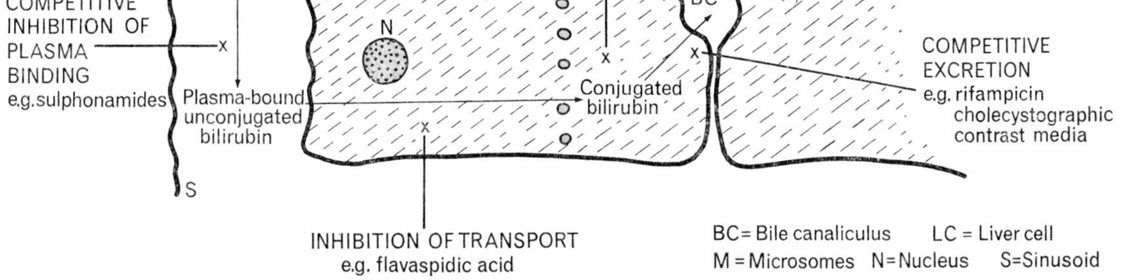

DRUG INTERFERENCE WITH BILIRUBIN METABOLISM

The metabolism and excretion of bilirubin can be interfered with at a number of points [FIG. 9.1]; these have been documented by Sherlock (1968a).

1. Drugs causing haemolysis increase the load of unconjugated bilirubin on the liver cell.
2. Drugs such as sulphonamides and salicylates compete with serum albumin for binding with bilirubin.
3. Drugs like flavaspidic acid, the active principle of male fern extract, interfere with the transport of bilirubin through the hepatic cell.
4. Drugs like novobiocin can inhibit conjugation of the bilirubin as a glucuronide.
5. Cholecystographic contrast media and the antibiotic rifampicin compete with conjugated bilirubin for excretion into the biliary canaliculus.

The inhibition of bilirubin conjugation by the antibiotic novobiocin is well documented and is worthy of specific mention in this context due to its association with severe neonatal jaundice.

Finland and Nichols (1957) reported yellow pigmentation of the skin and sclera after administration of novobiocin; this was ascribed to accumulation of a metabolic product of the antibiotic. In 1961, Sutherland and Keller investigated a three-fold increase in the incidence of severe neonatal jaundice in infants treated with novobiocin. It was suggested that the interference with metabolism must occur at or before the conversion of unconjugated bilirubin to bilirubin glucuronide.

Hargreaves and Holton (1962) showed that the addition of novobiocin to rat liver slices lowered the rates of conjugation of bilirubin and o-aminophenol, because the conjugating system of intact liver cells is complex, involving, amongst other steps, both the enzymic production of uridine diphosphoglucuronic acid and the utilization of this glucuronyl donor substance by a specific transferase; an attempt was made to define the point of inhibition more precisely. Diphosphoglucuronic acid was added to the broken liver cell preparation and the transferase stage of conjugation examined. Inhibition of the glucuronyl transferase system was considerable at concentrations of novobiocin within the range obtained in the serum of adults after therapeutic doses (Simon et al., 1956).

There are low levels of glucuronyl transferase in the livers of new born infants (Lathe and Walker, 1958); this is considered to be the main reason for accumulation of bilirubin in the neonatal period and presumably accounts for the greater susceptibility of the newborn to become jaundiced when treated with novobiocin. In view of the danger of kernicterus, novobiocin should be used with caution in the newborn.

The antibiotic rifampicin has shown considerable promise as an antitubercular agent either alone or in combination with ethambutol, especially against tuberculosis resistant to 'main-line' agents. However, jaundice has been reported following its use. Lesobre and co-workers (1969) reported 12 cases in a series of 50 patients; four of these cases died; three of these were alcoholics. Lees and others (1970) reported four cases in 50 patients; all were elderly with impaired liver function.

Keberle et al. (1968) have described the metabolic fate of rifampicin; it would appear to compete with conjugated bilirubin for excretion into the biliary canaliculi. Treatment with this antibiotic has also been associated with two severe cases of thrombocytopenia [see CHAPTER 4].

DIRECT HEPATOXICITY CAUSED BY DRUGS

In general permanent liver damage due to therapeutic agents is rare and progression to cirrhosis is most unusual (Sherlock, 1968a).

Tetracyclines depress liver metabolism but in the usual therapeutic dosage they are quite safe. Their use in the last trimester of pregnancy has, however, been associated with acute fatty liver, a particularly serious complication of pregnancy. Intravenous tetracycline should be avoided in large doses (greater than 3 grams per day), especially when protein synthesis is stressed or deficient as in pregnancy or malnutrition (Kunelis et al., 1965).

Cytotoxic drugs such as 6-mercaptopurine, methotrexate, and 5-fluoro-2-deoxyuridine can give a picture similar to hepatitis. In addition, these agents can cause damage to the vascular epithelium and injury to the central hepatic veins within the liver lobule; a Budd-Chiari (hepatic venous occlusion) syndrome can thus be produced (Reed and Cox, 1966). It is perhaps a measure of the potential hepatoxicity of agents of this type that it may be difficult to separate the hepatic changes induced by disease for which the cytotoxic drug is being given from the drug effects themselves.

Aubrey (1970) has reported massive hepatic necrosis after cyclophosphamide; this is the first report of such an effect. The patient had received cyclophosphamide after mastectomy for an anaplastic cirrhous carcinoma; a total dose of 2,800 mg was administered. The condition was fatal and at necropsy the liver was shrunken (weight 430 grams); its cut surface was pale and granular, and the normal lobular pattern was totally destroyed. Microscopically there was a complete absence of normal hepatic tissue, with only the reticulin framework of the hepatic cords and sinusoids remaining. There was a mild diffuse infiltration by mononuclears and lymphocytes, with occasional polymorphs. The only visible tissue was represented by clusters of small bile ducts around the sites of the portal tracts. There was no evidence of biliary obstruction, metastatic carcinoma, or any other lesions. The only recognized hepatotoxic agent which the patient received was halothane, and this only on one occasion.

DRUG-INDUCED HEPATITIS

HYDRAZINE-TYPE MAO INHIBITORS AND OTHER AGENTS

The hepatitis-like drug reactions cannot be clinically distinguished from ordinary acute viral hepatitis. Since there is no specific test for this common viral infection, the possibility of a coincident and unrelated viral hepatitis can never be completely excluded despite negative tests for SH or Australia antigen. The reaction is usually unrelated to duration or dose of therapy, but may be more frequent after multiple exposures to the drug; it may develop up to three weeks after stopping the drug. The incidence of these drug-induced hepatic reactions is small but they have a very high mortality of 20–25 per cent (Sherlock, 1968a).

Several drugs have been incriminated in this type of reaction; the most important are the hydrazine-type monoamine oxidase inhibitors. This group includes iproniazid, pheniprazine, phenoxypropazine, phenelzine, and isocarboxazid. Liver damage has not been reported with the MAO inhibitor tranylcypromine which is not a hydrazine derivative. The mortality of hydrazine-induced hepatitis is 25 per cent or more, and the major cause of this hepatitis was iproniazid, which has now been withdrawn. Hepatotoxicity occurred in 1 in 5,000 patients treated with iproniazid (Randolph and Joseph, 1953; Gellis and Murphy, 1955).

This rather heavy indictment of the hydrazine-base MAO inhibitors in hepatocellular damage is by no means the whole story and, indeed, may present but one side of the evidence for their sole committal. Using iproniazid as an example Griffith and Oblath (1962) carried out a careful analysis of the results of prior published investigations and of questionnaires answered by the physicians attending the first 100 reported cases of jaundice among the approximately 500,000 iproniazid-treated patients during 1957 and 1958. Their objective was to determine the validity or otherwise of the evidence pointing to the sole implication of these MAO inhibitors in liver damage. The findings of this analysis were somewhat startling. They found a multiple duplication of cases reported on; confusion and diagnostic unreliability of laboratory test results; a high incidence of jaundice in patients with no hepatic damage; the possibility of unreported cardiac involvement; the near impossibility of determining whether hepatitis is drug-caused because of listing in the histories of such potentially hepatotoxic or contributing factors as malnutrition, multiple inoculations, pre-existing jaundice or hepatitis, or exposure to these and other diseases, and the previous ingestion of a number of drugs reported as having been hepatotoxic.

One might well assume, with some justification, that these factors although not clearing iproniazid in hepatic dysfunction, certainly lessen the probability that this drug was the sole and immediate cause of all the jaundice attributed to its administration.

Ibufenac, an anti-arthritic agent, was also withdrawn from clinical use because of its high tendency to cause hepatitis (Thompson et al., 1964); it is not a hydrazine. Isoniazid, a hydrazide, also causes this complication although documented cases are exceedingly rare; the patients in most cases reported have also been receiving another antitubercular drug such as para-aminosalicylic acid which is well known as a potential hepatotoxin (Simpson and Walker, 1960; Reynolds, 1962). However, recently Martin and Arthaud (1970) described a patient in whom hepatitis developed shortly after he began taking isoniazid for a recent tuberculin skin test (PPD) conversion. Challenge with isoniazid was followed by a recurrence of hepatitis that was confirmed by a histological study. Although the course of this particular case was benign, fatal cases have been recorded (Reynolds, 1962), one of these in a patient who received no other anti-tubercular drugs (Cohen et al., 1961).

Cinchophen, although rarely used today, can cause a hepatitis reaction; indeed it was the first drug to be associated with this condition and has become obsolete as a uricosuric agent because of the high incidence of serious and sometimes fatal liver damage that accompanied its use.

HALOTHANE

There is considerable controversy whether hepatic injury in the form of a fulminating hepatitis is induced by exposure to halothane. In view of its exceedingly wide usage and its undoubted value as a safe anaesthetic the pertinent details of this controversy are included here.

Over 400 cases of liver damage after halothane anaesthesia were reported in the literature by 1967. Among these the most clear cut associations are those described by Belfrage et al., 1966; Klein and Jeffries, 1966 and Lischner et al., 1967. In general, the reaction was severe with a fatal outcome in about one-third of cases. Concern was such that in the United States, the National Halothane study was set up and published its findings in 1966 on a possible association between halothane anaesthesia and post-operative hepatic necrosis. This study, based on a review of 856,000 patients, and other retrospective studies, encompassing an additional 300,000 patients, provided the major evidence against a cause-and-effect relationship between halothane and post-operative liver damage. These studies indicated that massive hepatic necrosis is uncommon after surgical anaesthesia and that massive necrosis is no more frequent after exposure to halothane than to other anaesthetic agents. When, in addition, one considers that millions of halothane anaesthetics are administered each year, and compares this number with the relatively few reported cases of liver damage, it is not surprising that many have concluded that halothane-induced hepatic necrosis does not exist. Support was given to this view by Lorhan (1969) who estimated that of the 20–24 million anaesthetics given each year, 12–15 million were halothane. He computed that the risk of liver complication was 1 in 333,000.

Some investigators have therefore directed their attention to other factors that might account for liver damage in the post-operative period, with coincidental viral hepatitis one of the more popular considerations.

Trey and colleagues (1968) reported the findings from 150 patients collected over a two-year period from 73 centres. Thirty-six of these 150 cases of fulminant hepatic necrosis had developed this condition within 21 days of exposure to halothane, and of these 36 patients, 32 had fatal outcome.

Klatskin and Kimburg (1969) reported an interesting case of an anaesthetist who had previously suffered from hay fever and asthma who developed an attack of hepatitis after a period of exposure to halothane. The hepatitis was accompanied by enlargement of the liver, the tip of the spleen was palpable and the patient was icteric. At this time, a diagnosis of viral hepatitis was made.

Over the next 5 years, the patient experienced six relapses which coincided with his return to work and re-exposure to halothane. In each relapse the illness was of acute onset heralded by fever, rigor, myalgia, headache and nausea. During the course of his illness, serial liver biopsies were taken which gave a continuous record of the change in liver histology.

The first biopsies were taken 3 years and 9 months after the initial episode and during the patient's fourth relapse:

Needle biopsy of the liver revealed obliteration of the normal lobular architecture by smooth-contoured, slender connective-tissue septums containing a moderate number of lymphocytes, monocytes and ductules. In some areas, the septums outlined nodules of parenchyma, but in others, they radiated into the lobules from intact but enlarged portal triads. Only an occasional eccentric central vein could be identified. The parenchyma had a normal plate pattern and gave no evidence of inflammation, degeneration, necrosis or bile stasis. These findings were interpreted as evidence of an early, inactive posthepatic cirrhosis.

The second biopsy was taken after the patient's sixth relapse, which occurred 5 years and 4 months after the initial illness:

On needle biopsy, the liver showed the same type of cirrhosis seen 19 months previously. However, there were several notable differences: the fibrosis and nodule formation were more extensive; the septums were broader, and contained many more ductules, lymphocytes and monocytes; there were numerous zones of recent collapse bridging adjacent triads and central veins; in these zones, a loose meshwork of reticulin, containing sinusoids, collections of lymphocytes, monocytes, proliferating reticuloendothelial cells, and numerous degenerating hepatocytes and acidophilic bodies, replaced normal parenchyma; and the parenchymal plates adjacent to the zones of collapse were irregular in contour, thickened and occasionally arranged in the form of rosettes.

These features were interpreted as evidence of an advancing posthepatic cirrhosis with superimposed subacute hepatic necrosis. Since both recurrent viral hepatitis and drug sensitization can produce lesions of this type, it was not possible to distinguish between these two possibilities on histologic grounds alone. However, considering the sequence of events in this case, it appeared highly probable that both the initial attack of hepatitis and the subsequent relapses were attributable to halothane hypersensitivity. Consistent with the histologic evidence of progression of the cirrhosis was the reappearance of splenomegaly, which had not been noted since the initial attack of hepatitis 5 years previously, and the apparent development of mild hypersplenism, as evidenced by leucopenia and thrombocytopenia.

At this stage it was thought worth while to make a definite diagnosis of halothane sensitivity and prior to this a further liver biopsy was made:

Needle biopsy of the liver on December 1st revealed a further increase in the degree of fibrosis, diminution in the number of septal inflammatory cells and disappearance of the zones of collapse, parenchymal inflammation and necrosis noted two months earlier. The septums were much broader and more densely collagenized than previously, but the remaining parenchyma appeared normal. Although there were many circumscribed nodules, several small areas showed a normal lobular architecture. The histological picture was considered typical of moderately advanced, but inactive posthepatitic cirrhosis. It was evident that the acute hepatitis seen two months earlier had healed completely, and that collagenization of the zones of collapse had added to the fibrosis first demonstrated 21 months previously.

One week after the liver biopsy a subanaesthetic dose of halothane was given as follows:

After an overnight fast and without premedication, 0·1 to 0·2 per cent halothane in oxygen was given for a period of exactly five minutes. The halothane was administered via an air-tight face mask connected to a non-rebreathing system in a temperature compensated apparatus. Fifty ml of 5 per cent glucose solution in water was administered intravenously. The patients remained alert throughout, but experienced mild giddiness toward the end of the inhalation procedure. The blood pressure and pulse rate remained stable.

At 2 p.m. four hours after exposure to halothane, the patient began to experience severe aching in the legs, a symptom that he had previously noted at the onset of his hepatitis relapses, and half an hour later, he had a shaking chill that lasted for $1\frac{1}{2}$ hours. Soon thereafter, the temperature rose abruptly, reaching 102·2°F at 4 p.m. and 102·8°F at 8 p.m. and there was a concomitant increase in the pulse rate from 80 to 108. The temperature dropped to a normal level at midnight, and did not rise again. However, tachycardia and malaise persisted for an additional 24 hours. No notable changes in hepatic function or blood count were noted six hours after halothane challenge. However, by the next morning, serum glutamic oxalacetic transaminase activity had risen considerably, with a slight increase in serum bilirubin. There was no tenderness over the liver or any change in its size. However, the spleen, which had not been palpable on admission, could now be felt on fingerbreadth below the left costal margin. No rash or lymphadenopathy was noted. The serum glutamic oxalacetic transaminase level continued to rise for 48 hours after halothane challenge, and then fell slowly. The serum bilirubin concentration rose no further and returned to its base-line level within a few days. There was an increase in eosinophils.

Needle biopsy of the liver was carried out four days after halothane challenge. In addition to cirrhosis found 10 days previously during the control period, the liver showed acute hepatitis, manifested by an intense mononuclear inflammatory reaction in the septums and the presence within the parenchyma, especially adjacent to the septums, of many small zones of recent collapse containing numerous acidophilic bodies, proliferating reticuloendothelial cells, and monocytes. The serum glutamic acid dehydrogenase did not return to normal for a period of six weeks after halothane challenge.

Klatskin and Kimberg (1969) concluded that the attacks in this case were attributable to hypersensitivity reactions rather than to a direct hepatotoxic action of halothane. This view would agree with Sherlock (1964) that halothane is not a true hepatotoxic agent in the same way as are other halogenated hydrocarbons, notably carbon tetrachloride and chloroform.

DRUG-INDUCED INTRAHEPATIC CHOLESTASIS

PHENOTHIAZINES

Jaundice with the clinical and biochemical features of biliary obstruction occurs as a rare complication following the therapeutic use of some drugs, including a number of phenothiazines. The mechanism of this jaundice is stasis of bile in the canaliculi of the centrilobular zones of the liver lobules. Chlorpromazine jaundice will be considered as an example of this type of phenothiazine reaction. Other drugs producing a similar effect will then be referred to more briefly.

Many reports have appeared of jaundice occurring during treatment with chloropromazine. Probably about 1 per cent of the patients who take the drug for more than two weeks develop jaundice (Waitzkin, 1958). In most cases, jaundice occurred 7 to 36 days after treatment started, although occasionally it first appeared after administration of the drug had been discontinued for as long as 18 days. However, the appearance of

jaundice has been unrelated to total dose consumed, and it has been described after amounts as small as 75 mg. Jaundice has usually been preceded by a prodromal stage of fever, abdominal discomfort, vomiting or diarrhoea for a few days. An enlarged, tender liver has been recorded in some patients, and splenomegaly was occasionally found. The clinical and biochemical findings closely mimicked those of extrahepatic biliary obstruction. Stools were pale and urine contained bile pigment. Serum bilirubin and alkaline phosphatase levels were raised; cephalin flocculation and thymol turbidity have almost always been normal; the prothrombin time was normal and eosinophilia in the blood was sometimes found early in the course of the jaundice.

On withdrawal of chlorpromazine, the jaundice has usually subsided gradually during the succeeding 4 weeks, with ultimate complete recovery. There have been several cases, however, in which jaundice was very prolonged, even up to 3 years (Read *et al.*, 1961), and in 10 per cent of cases jaundice lasted for more than 3 months. On the other hand, in some patients, the jaundice faded even though the drug was still being taken regularly. In few cases, in spite of apparent clinical recovery, histological changes in the liver have persisted and the ultimate prognosis must await prolonged follow-up. Occasional cases of xanthomatous biliary cirrhosis following chlorpromazine administration have been reported.

It has been suggested that corticosteroids or corticotrophin hastened the disappearance of the jaundice, although it is doubtful whether this treatment greatly modified the progress of the disorder. Knowledge of a previous history of chlorpromazine ingestion should save many unnecessary laparotomies, but in cases in which the jaundice persists for a prolonged period after stopping the drug, the possibility of obstruction to the extrahepatic bile duct occurring in a patient who just happened to have had chlorpromazine must, of course, be considered (Bourke and Ritchie, 1967). Prolonged jaundice usually merits surgical exploration of the bile ducts with cholangiography performed at the time of operation to exclude obstruction to the main bile ducts (Read *et al.*, 1961).

Many liver biopsies have now been performed in this type of jaundice and there has been a general uniformity of findings; the most characteristic features were the biliary thrombi found within the distended canaliculi of the centrilobular zones, with little or no evidence of hepatic cell necrosis [see PLATE 3A].

The mechanism by which chlorpromazine produces canalicular stasis of bile is still obscure. It has been suggested, although without proof, that the bile stasis is the result of increased viscosity of the bile associated with excessive permeability of the bile canaliculi, or possibly with a defect in the normal process of hydration of bile. However, it has not been possible to reproduce this effect of chlorpromazine in animals. The lack of correlation with total dosage, and the time relationship between start of therapy and onset of jaundice, and the presence of eosinophilia have suggested that a sensitization phenomenon is more likely. This has been supported by reports of an acceleration reaction of the same type produced by a small dose of chlorpromazine in patients who have recovered from chlorpromazine jaundice (Hollister, 1957). On the other hand, the response to the 'challenging' dose has not always occurred, and the occasional disappearance of jaundice while the drug was continued is difficult to understand.

An unexplained pyrexia during chlorpromazine therapy should suggest the possibility of incipient obstructive jaundice. In some milder examples of this drug reaction, jaundice may not develop, and fever, increased serum alkaline phosphatase, and eosinophilia may be the only indications. Chlorpromazine should probably be avoided in patients with previous liver disease, in malnourished patients, or when other potentially hepatotoxic agents are being used. Clearly, the further administration of chlorpromazine to a patient who has previously become jaundiced following that drug would be most unwise.

Jaundice appears to occur less often following the use of some of the newer phenothiazine drugs than with chlorpromazine. There have been reports of occasional cases of jaundice after prochlorperazine, pecazine, trifluoperazine, and promazine, but it is not at present possible to estimate its frequency with these newer drugs.

There is no method of testing in which patients chlorpromazine jaundice is likely to develop, indeed cutaneous tests for sensitivity are thought to be valueless (Hollister, 1957). No cross-sensitivity with promazine has been demonstrated, so possibly other phenothiazine derivatives might be substituted for chlorpromazine after development of sensitivity.

C-17 SUBSTITUTED STEROIDS

Methyltestosterone

Jaundice of the intrahepatic obstruction type is a well recognized complication of therapy with oral methyltestosterone (Foss and Simpson, 1959), although it does not occur after the use of parenteral testosterone propionate. Usually methyltestosterone has to be taken for several months before jaundice occurs; the clinical and biochemical features of the jaundice are somewhat similar to those already described for chlorpromazine. After stopping the hormone, the condition clears rapidly without residual damage to the liver.

The histology of a biopsy specimen of liver showed biliary stasis in the canaliculi in the central zones of the lobules, with very little, if any, evidence of hepatic cellular damage. There are, however, some differences from the appearances in chlorpromazine jaundice (Werner *et al.*, 1950). The portal zones were normal in intrahepatic cholestasis due to methyltestosterone, whereas in the lesions following chlorpromazine or arsphenamine there was cellular infiltration of these zones. The jaundice following methyltestosterone also

differed from that of chlorpromazine in that retreatment with the drug after recovery from jaundice was not followed by a recurrence of the reaction (Werner *et al.*, 1950), and to some extent its occurrence was related to dosage and duration of treatment rather than to a sensitivity reaction. The jaundice of methyltestosterone does not have the features of a hypersensitivity reaction, as with chlorpromazine, but probably most patients given a high enough dosage for a sufficient period will develop some interference with biliary flow.

Norethandrolone

This anabolic steroid may give rise to jaundice similar to that following methyltestosterone (Schaffner *et al.*, 1959). It is interesting to note that both methyltestosterone and norethandrolone relieve the itching of obstructive jaundice, although liable themselves to cause a deepening of the jaundice. It has been suggested that these drugs produce this therapeutic effect by interfering with the excretion into the bile, not only of the bile pigments, but also the substance responsible for the itching (Sherlock, 1968b). When liver tests were performed at intervals during treatment with norethandrolone, impairment of bromsulphthalein excretion occurred in 35 of 47 patients. There was a clear relationship between the dose of norethandrolone and the degree of bromsulphthalein retention (Kory *et al.*, 1959). These changes in hepatic function reverted to normal when the drug was stopped.

Methyltestosterone and norethandrolone should be prescribed only when there are clear indications for their use, and it is probable that the occurrence of jaundice can be minimized by using the smallest dose capable of producing the required therapeutic benefit.

Oral Contraceptives

The 'pill' is composed of an oestrogen and a progestogen; either or both of these components is usually a C-17 substituted derivative of testosterone and as such can be regarded as having potential cholestatic properties.

The rarity of cases of jaundice among the many millions of women taking the pill has various possible explanations. In part, it is due to the very small dose of cholestatic drug consumed, and in part, it is related to the underlying susceptibility, possibly genetic, of the women being treated. It is interesting that the only large series of patients reported with jaundice complicating oral contraceptive therapy have come from Scandinavia and Chile (Orellana-Alcalde and Dominguez, 1966). It is from these countries that the largest series of patients with cholestatic jaundice of the last trimester of pregnancy have been described. Moreover, about half the number of patients who react to the pill by developing cholestasis have suffered from this condition during pregnancy. This suggests that the sufferers have a dual sensitivity to a steroid contained in the pill and to a steroid produced during pregnancy. The end-result in both cases is cholestasis of variable severity; therefore it is recommended that oral contraceptives should not be given to patients who have experienced jaundice or itching in the last trimester of pregnancy (Sherlock, 1968a).

Patients with underlying liver disease may also react abnormally, and the 'pill' should not be prescribed for patients with underlying liver disease or within 6 months of recovery from viral hepatitis. Most instances of jaundice associated with the oral contraceptives are seen in the first three cycles of administration. If jaundice is seen after this it is probably unrelated to the 'pill' (Sherlock, 1968a).

MISCELLANEOUS AGENTS
Organo-arsenicals
Intrahepatic cholestasis as a drug-induced reaction was first described following the use of arsphenamine. Today, however, this reaction is only of historical interest since this organo-arsenical, once widely used in the treatment of syphilis, is no longer used. After arsphenamine, the histological appearance of the liver resembled that following the use of chlorpromazine. In most cases jaundice developed after the second or third intravenous injection of the first course of treatment, and persisted for weeks or months with eventual recovery. Neoarsphenamine replaced arsphenamine in the treatment of syphilitic infections owing to the ease with which injection solutions could be prepared, and to the fact that it was less toxic. Unfortunately, however, it proved to be less toxic to the spirochaetes as well, and has now been replaced by the penicillins. As with arsphenamine, it was also toxic to the liver.

As a group the organic arsenicals are all toxic to the liver to a greater or lesser extent; their degree of toxicity is almost certainly directly related to the amount of arsenic incorporated into their molecular configuration. Another member of this group is the pentavalent arsenical, tryparsamide which is still used in the treatment of early cases of African trypanosomiasis (sleeping sickness).

Phenindione
Jaundice from intrahepatic cholestasis has been described in patients receiving treatment with the anticoagulant phenindione (Sherlock et al., 1961; Perkins, 1962a, 1962b; British Medical Journal, 1963). The mechanism of the jaundice is obscure and although damage to hepatic parenchymal cells may occur the hepatitis was mainly cholestatic in type (Portal and Emanuel, 1961). Combined disturbance of liver and renal function has been reported in a hypersensitivity reaction to phenindione (Wallace, 1964) and in several cases of jaundice during therapy there has been other evidence of a general reaction, particularly skin lesions.

Triacetyloleandomycin and Other Antibiotics
Hepatic dysfunction, with or without jaundice, due to antibiotics has been rarely reported. There are several reported instances in which jaundice has been caused by chloramphenicol (Salm, 1953) and by triacetyloleandomycin (Koch and Assay, 1958). Robinson (1961, 1962) has presented evidence of hepatic abnormality resulting from the propionyl ester of erythromycin and from the triacetyl salt of oleandomycin in a substantial percentage of all patients treated with these antibiotics for 14 days or longer; their aetiological role was further substantiated by properly controlled challenge with these agents after all signs of previously existing dysfunction had subsided. This hepatotoxic effect would seem to be confined to the use of the ester since it has not been reported with erythromycin base (McKenzie and Doyle, 1966).

Some impairment of hepatic function has been reported following very large intravenous doses of chlortetracycline and oxytetracycline; however, in normal clinical doses hepatic damage does not occur.

Chlorpropamide and Tolbutamide
Chlorpropamide, a sulphonylurea hypoglycaemic agent, has also been reported to cause cholestatic jaundice especially when doses greater than 250 mg per day have been used. Cases have occurred within 2 to 5 weeks from start of therapy and have been characterized by an elevation of the serum alkaline phosphatase level, a positive cephalin flocculation test and the presence of intracanalicular biliary stasis (Camerini-Dávalos et al., 1962; Haunz et al., 1964). When chlorpropamide has been stopped the jaundice has disappeared and the liver returned to normal.

Similar reports have been received concerning the closely related compound tolbutamide, although the incidence of jaundice is a little less than with chlorpropamide; with both drugs cholestatic jaundice can, however, be regarded as a rare complication of therapy (Arnold and Lauener, 1964; Popper et al., 1965).

With both drugs, jaundice is probably a manifestation of hypersensitivity; it does not appear to be related entirely to dose and it may be accompanied by skin rashes and eosinophilia (Friedman, 1962).

Other Drugs
Other drugs reported to cause intrahepatic cholestasis on rare occasions are thiouracil and propylthiouracil, two members of the thiourea group of antithyroid agents, methimazole, a member of the imidazole group of antithyroid drugs, the diuretic chlorothiazide, the antitubercular agent p-aminosalicylic acid (PAS) and sulphadiazine, a short-acting sulphonamide. In addition a complex hepatic-cholestatic reaction can follow treatment with some of the newer antitubercular agents including cycloserine, ethionamide, and pyrazinamide (Sherlock, 1968a).

DRUG-INDUCED HEPATIC NEOPLASIA
THORIUM DIOXIDE
Very few drugs have been even tentatively incriminated as a cause of neoplasia at any site. One of these few is

Thorotrast, a colloidal suspension of 232-thorium dioxide. This agent has been used extensively since 1928 as a radiographic contrast medium, either to outline body cavities such as the renal pelvis, or the cerebral ventricles or for visualization of blood vessels.

In 1961 Suckow and co-workers drew attention to the association between *Thorotrast* administration and haemangioendothelioma of the liver. Sherlock (1968*b*) described this tumour as very rare and also described its association with *Thorotrast*. The clinical course of hepatic haemangioendothelioma is a rapid deterioration with cachexia, blood-stained ascites; bruit may be heard over the liver.

In Portugal, Da Silva Horta *et al.* (1965) checked records of 2,377 individuals who had received injections of *Thorotrast* between 1930 and 1952. A total of 1,107 cases were traced; of these 699 had died and 408 were still living; certified cause of death was obtained for the former group.

Twenty-two cases of haemangioendothelioma had occurred; this tumour is virtually thorium-dioxide specific in the liver. The latent period between *Thorotrast* injection and onset of this fatal condition was, with a single exception, 20 years or more. In this investigation, liver cirrhosis was recorded in 42 cases, and 17 of these were fatal, the incidence of cirrhosis was significantly higher than in the general population. There were also 16 cases of fatal blood dyscrasia: six acute and two

chronic myeloid leukaemia, six aplastic anaemia (pancytopenia) and two were recorded as fatal purpuras. Eighty-one local granulomas occurred and eight of these caused death. Blood dyscrasias and leukaemias were significantly higher than in the general population.

As a result of this earlier survey Boyd *et al.* (1968) undertook a survey on 137 patients who had received *Thorotrast* by intra-arterial injection between the years 1933–1955. Although mortality amongst the patients reflected the diseases (mainly cerebrovascular) that brought them to original investigation, it was noted that there were 12 deaths from neoplasia among 109 patients who survived more than one year after the *Thorotrast* administration. Four cases of primary liver tumours were found in this group, three were tumours of the intrahepatic bile ducts and one case was a haemangioendothelioma. A further case with oat-cell carcinoma also showed, at laprotomy, liver changes suggestive of haemangioendothelioma.

Other cases of carcinoma of other organs and tissue have been described in association with the use of thorium dioxide many years previously. The literature on these cases has been reviewed by Meyler (1966).

Thorium dioxide (*Thorotrast*) is no longer used; however, tumours caused by its use in the past are still presenting themselves and the possibility of prior use of this agent in cases of primary liver tumour should be investigated.

RECOMMENDED FURTHER READING

GREENE, N. M., ed. (1968) *Halothane*, Clinical Anesthesia Series 1/1968, Philadelphia.

HARGREAVES, T. (1970) Oral contraceptives and liver function, *J. clin. Path.*, **23**, Suppl. (Ass. Clin. Path.), **3**, 1–10.

OCKNER, R. K., and DAVIDSON, C. S. (1968) Hepatic effects of oral contraceptives, in *Drug-Induced Diseases*, Vol. 3, eds. Meyler, L., and Peck, H. M., Excerpta Medica Foundation, Amsterdam, pp. 229–33.

SHERLOCK, S. (1968) *Diseases of the Liver and Biliary System*, 4th ed., Oxford.

REFERENCES

ARNOLD, C. R., and LAUENER, R. W. (1964) Oral hypoglycaemic drugs, *Canad. med. Ass. J.*, **91**, 395–6.

AUBREY, D. A. (1970) Massive hepatic necrosis after cyclophosphamide, *Brit. med. J.*, **3**, 588.

BARNIVILLE, H. T. F., and MISK, R. (1959) Urinary glucuronic acid excretion in liver disease and the effect of a salicylamide load, *Brit. med. J.*, **1**, 337.

BELFRAGE, S., AHLGREN, I., and AXELSON, S. (1966) Halothane hepatitis in an anaesthetist, *Lancet*, **ii**, 1466–7.

BOURKE, J. B., and RITCHIE, H. D. (1967) Laparotomy for jaundice, *Lancet*, **ii**, 521–3.

BOYD, J. T., LANGLANDS, A. O., and MACCABE, J. J. (1968) Long-term hazards of Thorotrast, *Brit. med. J.*, **2**, 517–21.

BRITISH MEDICAL JOURNAL (1963) Anticoagulants in Today's Drugs, *Brit. med. J.*, **1**, 801–3.

CAMERINI-DÁVALOS, R., LOZANO-CASTANEDA, O., and MARBLE, A. (1962) Five years' experience with tolbutamide, *Diabetes*, **11**, 74–80.

COHEN, R., KALSER, M. H., and THOMPSON, R. V. (1961) Fatal hepatic necrosis secondary to isoniazid therapy, *J. Amer. med. Ass.*, **176**, 877–9.

DA SILVA HORTA, J., DA MOTTA, L. C., ABBATT, J. D., and RORIZ, M. L. (1965) Malignancy and other latent effects following administration of Thorotrast, *Lancet*, **ii**, 201–5.

FINLAND, M., and NICHOLS, R. (1957) Current therapeutics CXIV. Novobiocin, *Practitioner*, **179**, 84–92.

FOSS, G. L., and SIMPSON, S. L. (1959) Oral methyl testosterone and jaundice, *Brit. med. J.*, **1**, 259–63.

FRIEDMAN, A. (1962) Hepatic function of diabetic patients on chlorpropamide, *Med. Ann. D.C.*, **31**, 447–51.

GELLIS, S. N., and MURPHY, R. V. (1955) Hepatitis following isoniazid, *Dis. Chest*, **28**, 462–4.

GRIFFITH, G. C., and OBLATH, R. W. (1962) Jaundice and hepatitis in patients who have received hydrazine-base monoamine oxidase inhibitors, *Amer. J. med. Sci.*, **244**, 593–604.

HARGREAVES, T., and HOLTON, J. B. (1962) Jaundice of the newborn due to novobiocin, *Lancet*, **i**, 839.

HAUNZ, E. A., CORNATZER, W. E., and LUPER, G. (1964) Liver function in chlorpropamide therapy. Five-year clinical study of 181 patients, *J. Amer. med. Ass.*, **188**, 237–40.

HOLLISTER, L. E. (1957) Allergy to chlorpromazine manifested by jaundice, *Amer. J. Med.*, **23**, 870–9.

KEBERLE, H., SCHMID, K., and MEYER-BRUNOT, H. G. (1968) *The Metabolic Fate of Rifampicin*, A Symposium, Ciba Foundation, Basel.

KLATSKIN, G., and KIMBERG, D. V. (1969) Recurrent hepatitis attributable to halothane sensitization in an anesthetist, *New Engl. J. Med.*, **280**, 515–22.

KLEIN, N. C., and JEFFRIES, G. H. (1966) Hepatotoxicity after methoxyflurane administration, *J. Amer. med. Ass.*, **197**, 1037–9.

KOCH, R., and ASSAY, L. D. (1958) Oleandomycin, a laboratory and clinical evaluation, *J. Pediat.*, **53**, 676–82.

KORY, R. C., BRADLEY, M. H., WATSON, R. N., CALLAHAN, R., and PETERS, B. J. (1959) A six month evaluation of an anabolic drug norethandrolone in underweight persons, II. Bromsulphthalein (BSP) retention and liver function, *Amer. J. Med.*, **26**, 243–8.

KUNELIS, C. T., PETERS, J. L., and EDMONDSON, H. A. (1965) Fatty liver of pregnancy and its relationship to tetracycline therapy, *Amer. J. Med.*, **38**, 359–77.

KUNIN, C. M., GLAZKO, A. J., and FINLAND, M. (1959) Persistence of antibiotics in blood of patients with acute renal failure, II. Chloramphenicol and its metabolic products in the blood of patients with severe renal disease or hepatic cirrhosis, *J. clin. Invest.*, **38**, 1498–508.

LATHE, G. H., and WALKER, M. (1958) Inhibition of bilirubin conjugation in rat liver slices by human pregnancy and neonatal serum and steroids, *Quart. J. exp. Physiol.*, **43**, 257–65.

LEES, A. W., ASCHER, B., HASHEM, M. A., and SINA, B. M. (1970) Jaundice after rifampicin, *Brit. J. Dis. Chest*, **64**, 90–5.

LESOBRE, O., RUFFINO, J., TEYSSIER, L., ACHARD, F., and BREFORT, G. (1969) Jaundice occurring during treatment with rifampicin, *Rev. Tuberc. (Paris)*, **33**, 393–403.

LISCHNER, M. W., MACNABB, G. M., and GALAMBOS, J. T. (1967) Fatal hepatic necrosis following surgery: Possible relation to methoxyflurane anesthesia, *Arch. intern. Med.*, **120**, 725–8.

LORHAN, P. H. (1969) Halothane and liver damage, *New Engl. J. Med.*, **280**, 562.

MARTIN, C. E., and ARTHAUD, J. B. (1970) Hepatitis after isoniazid administration, *New Engl. J. Med.*, **282**, 433–4.

MCKENZIE, I., and DOYLE, A. (1966) Two cases of jaundice following ilosone, *Med. J. Aust.*, **1**, 349–51.

MEYLER, L. (1966) Radioactive isotopes, in *Side Effects of Drugs*, Vol. V, eds. Meyler, L., *et al.*, Excerpta Medica Foundation, Amsterdam, pp. 466–71.

NATIONAL HALOTHANE STUDY (1966) Possible association between halothane anesthesia and postoperative hepatic necrosis, Cooperative Study, Summary of National Halothane Study, Sub-committee on National Halothane Study of Committee on Anesthesia, National Academy of Sciences and National Research Council, *J. Amer. med. Ass.*, **197**, 775–8.

ORELLANA-ALCALDE, J. M., and DOMINGUEZ, J. P. (1966) Jaundice and oral contraceptive drugs, *Lancet*, **ii**, 1278–80.

PERKINS, J. (1962a) Phenindione jaundice, *Lancet*, **i**, 125–7.

PERKINS, J. (1962b) Phenindione sensitivity, *Lancet*, **i**, 127.

POPPER, H., RUBIN, E., GARDIOL, D., SCHAFFNER, F., and PARONETTO, F. (1965) Drug induced liver disease: A penalty for progress, *Arch. intern. Med.*, **115**, 128–36.

PORTAL, R. W., and EMANUEL, R. W. (1961) Phenindione hepatitis complicating anticoagulant therapy, *Brit. med. J.*, **2**, 1318–19.

RANDOLPH, H., and JOSEPH, S. (1953) Toxic hepatitis with jaundice occurring in a patient treated with isoniazid, *J. Amer. med. Ass.*, **152**, 38–40.

READ, A. E., HARRISON, C. V., and SHERLOCK, S. (1961) Chronic chlorpromazine jaundice: With particular reference to its relationship to primary biliary cirrhosis, *Amer. J. Med.*, **31**, 249–58.

REED, G. B., and COX, A. J. (1966) The human liver after radiation injury, *Amer. J. Path.*, **48**, 597–611.

REYNOLDS, E. (1962) Isoniazid jaundice and its relationship to iproniazid jaundice, *Tubercle (Edinb.)*, **43**, 375–81.

ROBINSON, M. M. (1961) Hepatotoxic side effects of propionyl erythromycin ester lauryl sulfate and triacetyloleandomycin, in *Antimicrobial Agents and Chemotherapy*, American Society for Microbiology, Detroit, pp. 394–400.

ROBINSON, M. M. (1962) Hepatic dysfunction associated with triacetyloleandomycin and propionyl erythromycin ester lauryl sulfate, *Amer. J. med. Sci.*, **243**, 502–9.

SALM, R. (1953) Acute necrosis of liver following chloramphenicol therapy, *Edinb. Med. J.*, **60**, 334–6.

SCHAFFNER, F., POPPER, H., and CHESROW, E. (1959) Cholestasis produced by the administration of norethandrolone, *Amer. J. Med.*, **26**, 249–54.

SHERLOCK, S. (1964) The hepatotoxic effects of anaesthetic drugs, *Proc. roy. Soc. Med.*, **57**, 305–7.

SHERLOCK, S. (1968a) Drugs and the liver, *Brit. med. J.*, **1**, 227–9.

SHERLOCK, S. (1968b) *Diseases of the Liver and Biliary System*, 4th ed., Oxford, pp. 298, 371–3, 657–8.

SHERLOCK, S., BARBER, K. M., BELL, J. L., and WATT, P. J. (1961) Anticoagulants and the liver, in *Symposium on Anticoagulant Therapy*, ed. Pickering, G. W., London, p. 14.

SIMON, H. J., McCUNE, R. M., DINEEN, P. A. P., and ROGERS, D. E. (1956) Studies on novobiocin, new antimicrobial agent, *Antibiot. Med.*, **2**, 205–18.

SIMPSON, D. G., and WALKER, J. H. (1960) Hypersensitivity to para-aminosalicylic acid, *Amer. J. Med.*, **29**, 297–306.

SUCKOW, E. E., HENEGAR, G. C., and BASERGA, R. (1961) Tumours of the liver following administration of Thorotrast, *Amer. J. Path.*, **38**, 663–77.

SUTHERLAND, J. M., and KELLER, W. H. (1961) Novobiocin and neonatal hyperbilirubinemia. An investigation of the relationship in an epidemic of neonatal hyperbilirubinemia, *Amer. J. Dis. Child*, **101**, 447–53.

THOMPSON, M., STEPHENSON, P., and PERCY, J. S. (1964) Ibufenac in the treatment of arthritis, *Ann. rheum. Dis.*, **23**, 397–404.

TREY, C., LIPWORTH, L., CHALMER, T. C., DAVIDSON, C. S., GOTTLIEB, L. S., POPPER, H., and SAUNDERS, S. J. (1968) Fulminant hepatic failure. Presumable contribution of halothane, *New Engl. J. Med.*, **279**, 798–801.

WAITZKIN, G. (1958) Hepatic dysfunction due to chlorpromazine hypersensitivity, *Ann. intern. Med.*, **49**, 607–19.

WALLACE, D. C. (1964) Cerebral vascular disease in relation to long-term anticoagulant therapy, *J. chron. Dis.*, **17**, 527–37.

WERNER, S. C., HANGER, F. M., and KRITZLER, R. A. (1950) Jaundice during methyl testosterone therapy, *Amer. J. Med.*, **8**, 325–31.

WHELTON, M. J., KRUSTEV, L. P., and BILLING, B. H. (1968) Reduction in serum bilirubin by phenobarbital in adult unconjugated hyperbilirubinemia, *Amer. J. med.*, **45**, 160–4.

10

DISTURBANCES OF PORPHYRIN METABOLISM

The porphyrins are highly coloured red pigment substances which are related to the synthetic pathways used in the production of haem and hence of haemoglobin, myoglobin and the cytochromes. The steps in this pathway are shown in FIGURE 10.1. This synthesis can probably occur in cells generally, but the most important organs in which it takes place are the bone marrow and liver.

It has been known for a long time that certain drugs, especially barbiturates, can derange liver porphyrin metabolism in man. A drug may, for example, cause increased porphyrin excretion in a person with no previous abnormality of porphyrin metabolism and no genetic disposition to porphyria, or it may precipitate an overt episode of hepatic porphyria in a patient who is a carrier of the genetic defect in the latent state.

This is different from the disturbance of porphyrin metabolism caused by lead, which concerns primarily, if not entirely, the erythropoietic system (Gajdos and Gajdos-Török, 1964; Goldberg and Rimington, 1962) and will not be discussed here.

INCREASED PORPHYRIN EXCRETION CAUSED BY DRUGS IN NORMAL PERSONS

This metabolic disturbance is like the experimental porphyrias induced by drugs in animals, and when the increased porphyrin formation is accompanied by clinical symptoms of photosensitivity it should be considered among the toxic varieties of the symptomatic hepatic porphyrias.

There is some divergence of opinion as to whether barbiturates and other drugs, known to precipitate attacks in patients with acute intermittent porphyria, can derange the liver porphyrin metabolism of normal individuals. However, several cases have been described in which a marked increase in porphyrin excretion and appearance of clinical symptoms of photosensitivity have been linked with the administration of certain drugs, cases in which there was no obvious evidence of a genetic background of porphyria. Drugs that have been implicated in this disorder are: sulphonal (Harris, 1898), phenobarbitone (Haxthausen, 1927) and, more recently, tolbutamide (Rook and Champion, 1960), chlorpropamide (Zarowitz and Newhouse, 1965), and oestrogens (Becker, 1965; Copeman et al., 1966; Felsher and Redecker, 1966).

Most of these drugs can produce a condition of hepatic porphyria in animals or in tissue culture of liver cells; this provides some support for the belief that they may also produce a porphyria-like syndrome in normal persons with the appearance of cutaneous symptoms in the most severe cases. However, it is a fact that out of the very large number of patients receiving these drugs, only a very small proportion develop the porphyria-like syndrome; therefore the existence of some concurrent factor might be suspected, and the presence of a genetic disposition to porphyria in these patients obviously cannot be excluded. Indeed, there is no evidence that an acute attack of porphyria can be precipitated by drugs in the absence of a genetic disposition. In general, clinical experience indicates very strongly that symptoms of acute porphyria appear in those patients who are carriers of the genetic defect in a latent state.

A moderate increase in the excretion of porphyrins, or of their precursors, without clinical symptoms is probably not uncommon among normal persons receiving certain drugs. For example, a small but significant increase in faecal and blood porphyrin levels has been observed by Rimington et al. (1963) and by Ziprkowski et al. (1966), in persons receiving the anti-fungal, griseofulvin, in the usual therapeutic doses, and a significantly increased excretion of urinary delta-aminolaevulinic acid has been reported in a group of healthy females receiving oral contraceptives (Koskelo et al., 1966). Van Der Grient (1968) has reviewed the recent literature on griseofulvin and porphyrin metabolism in man and in animal studies, and concludes by recommending that griseofulvin be withheld from patients with a familial history of porphyria. With regard to oral contraceptives, it is interesting to note that Perlroth and co-workers (1965) showed that, in established acute intermittent porphyria, the administration of an oral contraceptive resulted in amelioration of the disease; obviously at present there is inadequate evidence to determine the true role of oral contraceptives in porphyrin metabolism.

ADVERSE EFFECT OF SOME DRUGS ON THE CLINICAL AND BIOCHEMICAL PICTURE OF HEPATIC PORPHYRIA

Non-barbiturate and Barbiturate Hypnotics

Hepatic porphyrias are inherited as Mendelian dominants and are characterized by excess production of

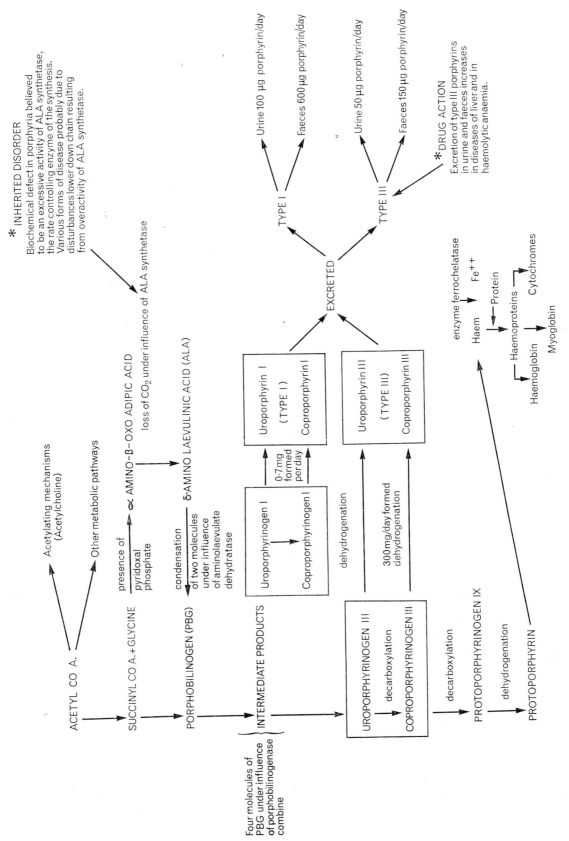

FIG. 10.1. *Overall scheme of porphyrin synthesis*

porphyrin and related compounds by the liver. Acute intermittent porphyria is the most frequent, and the clinical features include a combination of abdominal colic, vomiting, and severe constipation, often with peripheral neuritis and psychological disturbance. Photosensitivity is absent. The urine darkens on standing and gives a positive Erhlich test; it contains coproporphyrin and uroporphyrin in large quantities. The liver synthesizes excess of the porphyrin precursors delta-aminolaevulinic acid and porphobilinogen (Sherlock, 1968).

It is now widely accepted that the administration of some drugs to patients with genetic hepatic porphyria of the acute intermittent or mixed types can worsen the course of the disease and also precipitate attacks in persons with latent porphyria. The worsening action involves not only the metabolic picture and excretion of pyrrole compounds, but also the clinical symptoms especially the nervous symptoms. This is a far more serious complication of the therapeutic use of barbiturates and several other drugs than in the induction of porphyria in normal persons. Patients with the genetic trait can be very sensitive to these drugs, and in a relatively small number of them, a single dose at times may be sufficient to change an asymptomatic abnormality of metabolism to a very serious clinical syndrome menacing life. Although an acute attack of the disease can be triggered by several other factors such as the ingestion of alcohol, dietary indiscretions (see Mac-Alpine et al., 1968) an acute infection, pregnancy or menstruation, drug administration is probably the most important precipitating factor.

The causal relationship between some drugs and this disease has been known for many years. In 1889, Stockvis described the case of an elderly woman who, after taking the hypnotic sulphonal, passed dark red urine containing a pigment similar to haematoporphyrin and who subsequently died. One year later, Harley (1890) reported the case of a patient, who, after ingestion of sulphonal exhibited many of the neurological features of what is now known as acute intermittent porphyria. Several other cases of acute porphyria were described in the following years and in some of these sulphonal or the related drugs tetronal and trional had been taken before the onset of symptoms.

The importance of barbiturates in relation to acute porphyria was also suspected fairly soon after the introduction of these agents in clinical therapy. Dobrschansky (1906) described a typical case of acute porphyria in a patient who had received prolonged treatment with barbitone, and in the following years several other groups reported deterioration in the clinical and metabolic state of porphyric patients after administration of barbiturates (Denny-Brown and Sciarra, 1945; Eliaser and Kondo, 1942; Prunty, 1946; Whittaker and Whitehead, 1956). From the study of a large number of patients in Sweden and Great Britain respectively, Waldenström (1937) and Goldberg (1959) were both convinced that barbiturates could precipitate

attacks in persons with latent porphyria of the acute intermittent variety and that they seriously affected the prognosis of the disease. In South Africa, patients with mixed porphyria are extremely sensitive to barbiturates, and in these patients most, if not all, acute attacks appear to be precipitated by administration of either barbiturates or other drugs (Dean, 1963). In patients with hereditary coproporphyria, acute attacks can also be precipitated by barbiturates and other drugs (Goldberg et al., 1967).

The onset of an acute attack, however, does not necessarily follow the administration of barbiturates, and Waldenström (1937, 1939), Schmid (1966), Eales (1966) and With (1965) have experience of patients with latent genetic porphyria of all three varieties, who were given barbiturates without ill effect. From a survey of all porphyric patients hospitalized in Seattle over an 11-year period and given barbiturates for general anaesthesia, Ward (1965) concluded that the precipitation of an acute attack was a very rare complication of barbiturate anaesthesia; some other authors (Discombe and D'Silva, 1945; Günther, 1922; Turner, 1938) even failed to find any relation between barbiturates and acute porphyria. Several likely explanations can be offered for this discrepancy in findings. Firstly, some of these studies, in which an adverse effect of barbiturates was not noted or occurred only rarely, may have included patients with hepatic porphyrias of the acquired varieties, who are not expected to show any abnormal sensitivity to barbiturates. This is likely to be the case, as suggested by Eales (1966), for the survey conducted by Ward in which no discrimination appears to have been made between different types of hepatic porphyrias. A second very important reason is that there seems to be a considerable difference in sensitivity to barbiturates between different patients with latent porphyria: some develop very serious symptoms and even fatal paralysis after a single dose, others require prolonged administration of relatively large doses before showing symptoms (Goldberg, 1959). Therefore, the absence of symptoms of an acute attack after administration of single isolated doses of barbiturates to a patient, as was the case for the members of the family described by With (1965), does not necessarily mean that a patient can go on taking barbiturates with impunity. Finally, the study of the literature suggests that there may also be a difference in sensitivity to barbiturates between the various genetic varieties of hepatic porphyria: South African mixed porphyria is probably the most sensitive, the acute intermittent variety less so, and hereditary coproporphyria possibly even less.

More recently other drugs have been implicated in the precipitation of attacks of acute porphyria in patients who possess the genetic trait. Such drugs include sulphonamides, non-barbiturate sedatives, hypoglycaemics, anticonvulsants, tranquillizers and griseofulvin. A list of these drugs, which all resemble barbiturates in the production of acute porphyria, is given in TABLE 10.1. In addition, sex hormones and chloroquine have been reported to affect the condition of porphyric patients.

TABLE 10.1

DRUGS THAT INDUCE ACUTE PORPHYRIA (A) OR CUTANEOUS PORPHYRIA (C) IN MAN
(based on De Matteis, 1967)

Sulphonal	A & C
Trional	A
Tetronal	A
Sulphonamides	A
Amidopyrine	A
Barbiturates	A & C
Chlordiazepoxide	A
Dichloralphenazone	A
Meprobamate	A
Phenytoin	A
Tolbutamide	A & C
Chlorpropamide	A & C
Griseofulvin	A
Oestrogens, progestogens and androgens including oral contraceptives	A & C
Chloroquine	C

SEX HORMONES (OESTROGENS, PROGESTOGENS AND ANDROGENS)

The relationship of sex hormones to porphyria is a diverse one; they can precipitate acute attacks of porphyria on the one hand, and on the other they can prevent the appearance of acute attacks in those patients in whom exacerbation of clinical symptoms occur regularly with menstruation.

Watson and associates (1962) described a female patient with a latent mixed hepatic porphyria who was being treated with stilboestrol for carcinoma. Her urinary porphobilinogen and uroporphyrin increased above their previous high levels and cutaneous manifestations developed, but no abdominal or nervous symptoms ensued.

There have been several reports of impaired liver function and jaundice after oral contraceptive therapy (Cohen et al., 1964); this could cause diversion of the porphyrins from the enteric route of excretion to the blood and urine and result in photosensitivity. In mixed porphyria photosensitivity is often associated with impairment of liver excretory function. It is not surprising therefore that oestrogens and progestogens administered separately or together, in oral contraceptives, have been reported to affect the biochemical picture and clinical state of patients with acute intermittent porphyria. Increased excretion of porphyrin precursors and, less frequently, appearance of symptoms indicative of clinical exacerbation have been observed in patients of both sexes (Levit et al., 1957; Redeker, 1963; Welland et al., 1964; Wetterberg, 1964). An acute attack with peripheral paralysis in a patient with porphyria of the mixed type has been reported by Nayrac and co-workers (1964). Dean (1963) reported increased blood and urinary porphyrin levels with the appearance of jaundice and photosensitivity in a patient with mixed porphyria who had been taking an oral

contraceptive containing lynoestrenol and mestranol (e.g. Lyndiol).

In clear contrast to these findings, Haeger-Aronsen (1963) has described one case, and Perlroth and associates (1965) have described two cases, where the exacerbation of acute intermittent porphyria occurring in association with menstruation was prevented by combined oestrogen and progestogen therapy. The fact that these hormones can exacerbate acute intermittent porphyria in some patients and ameliorate the condition in others, together with the fact that menstruation and pregnancy can adversely affect the course of the disease, would indicate most strongly that the hormonal balance of the patient is a prime factor in the pathogenesis of attacks of this disease.

It is not known, however, in what way the hormonal state is implicated or which hormone or endocrine system is primarily involved. In one of the patients described by Perlroth et al. (1965), complete control of the porphyric symptoms was also obtained by treatment with either an androgen or an oestrogen alone, as well as by administration of a combination of an oestrogen with a progestogen. Androgenic therapy was similarly effective in another patient described by Schmid (1966). These observations suggest that a physiological response common to all three hormonal treatments may prevent acute attacks in these patients. Perlroth et al. (1965) have suggested that inhibition of the secretion of pituitary gonadotrophins, with stabilization of endogenous steroid production at a low level, may be the effective mechanism. This interpretation pre-supposes that a high level of endogenous sex hormones may be conducive to an attack of acute porphyria, whereas a high level of exogenous synthetic hormones may not; but this concept is not borne out by the finding by Redecker (1963) and Wetterberg (1964) of acute episodes after administration of synthetic sex hormones. Another possibility is that the recurring hormonal imbalance responsible for the periodic exacerbation of the clinical symptoms in these patients lies outside the gonodotrophins-ovary system and that large doses of sex hormones may affect other functions of the pituitary in addition to the secretion of gonadotrophin.

SYMPTOMATIC CUTANEOUS PORPHYRIA AND CHLOROQUINE

In the last 10 years or so there have been a number of reports on the effect of the administration of the antimalarial chloroquine to porphyric patients (Linden et al., 1954; Marsden, 1959; Cripps and Curtis, 1962; Gertler, 1962; Rimington, 1964; Sweeney et al., 1965). Unlike the barbiturates and the other agents so far considered in relation to porphyria, chloroquine affects hepatic porphyria of the symptomatic variety (porphyria cutanea tarda) in which cutaneous symptoms are present without abdominal or neurological disturbances.

This purely cutaneous form of the disease is hereditary and appears in middle age; it may occur secondary to hepatocellular disease. There is a well established relationship between this condition and alcoholism and usually there is evidence of hepatic dysfunction and raised serum bilirubin levels. Liver biopsy sections show subacute hepatitis or cirrhosis. Uroporphyrin is increased in the liver. Exacerbation of symptoms has been connected with deterioration of liver function. At this time porphyrins which would be normally excreted into the bile may be directed via the kidneys to the urine. The tendency to porphyria is made manifest by coincident liver disease. In the healthy liver the porphyrin is excreted harmlessly into the bile; in the diseased or damaged liver it is retained in the blood. The porphyria itself may be hepatotoxic (Sherlock, 1968).

Chloroquine is concentrated to a remarkable degree in the liver, indeed this is the advantage for its use as a tissue amoebicide in the treatment of liver amoebiasis. It exerts no effective action on amoebae elsewhere and is quite valueless, for example, in the treatment of intestinal amoebiasis. It is not surprising therefore that with this specific concentration in the liver, chloroquine in the presence of porphyria cutanea tarda causes a hepatic reaction with transient fever, general malaise, tachycardia, a rise in serum transaminases and hepatic necrosis. Hepatic uroporphyrin decreases and urinary excretion increases (Kofman et al., 1955). This effect does not recur and on regiving the chloroquine when the uroporphyrin excretion has considerably decreased, further administration of chloroquine does not cause any new increase in urinary uroporphyrin (Sweeney et al., 1965). Sweeney and co-workers (1965) were not able to state how long this refractory period to chloroquine effects lasted; however, since then Sherlock (1968) has commented that this period may last for up to five months.

The nine cases reported by Sweeney et al. (1965) all had alcoholism in common as a pre-disposing factor of their symptomatic cutaneous porphyria and although these patients had a severe reaction lasting 3 days following a 2 to 8 day latent period after chloroquine administration they subsequently showed clinical improvement of their cutaneous porphyria. It is doubtful, however, whether the improvement could be related to the use of chloroquine and the authors were more of the opinion that a good diet, absence of alcohol and sunlight and attention to their skin lesions were the causes of this. They considered that evidence of liver dysfunction contra-indicated the use of chloroquine in symptomatic porphyria.

The massive uroporphyrinuria reported by Sweeney et al. (1965) was not accompanied by a significantly increased excretion of porphyrin precursors, and they suggested, for this reason, that the liver was the probable source of the urinary uroporphyrin and it was from that site that it was released during the reaction to chloroquine. A very careful study of the effects of chloroquine on liver porphyrin metabolism has been made by Felsher and Redeker (1966) in five patients with symptomatic porphyria. A marked increase in

urinary porphyrin excretion was observed after chloroquine administration and was accompanied by a 50 per cent reduction of uroporphyrin in the liver. This supported the view that chloroquine causes a release of uroporphyrin from the liver rather than an increased synthesis at that site. No effect on porphyrin and porphobilinogen excretion was observed when chloroquine was given to two patients with acute intermittent porphyria; chloroquine did not induce porphyria in liver cells cultured in vitro as do most of the agents responsible for precipitating attacks in patients with porphyria of the acute and mixed types.

Chloroquine is known to form complexes with ferrihaemic acid and protoporphyrin in vitro, and Felsher and Redeker (1966) suggested that the formation of a similar complex might occur between chloroquine and liver uroporphyrin, leading to a large concentration of chloroquine in the liver cells, to liver damage, and, finally to leakage of the accumulated uroporphyrin. These investigators also reported a marked clinical and biochemical improvement in their patients once the initial transient reaction to chloroquine had subsided. No further symptoms of porphyria were seen in these patients for several months.

FIG. 10.2. *Structural relationship within the 4-aminoquinolines*

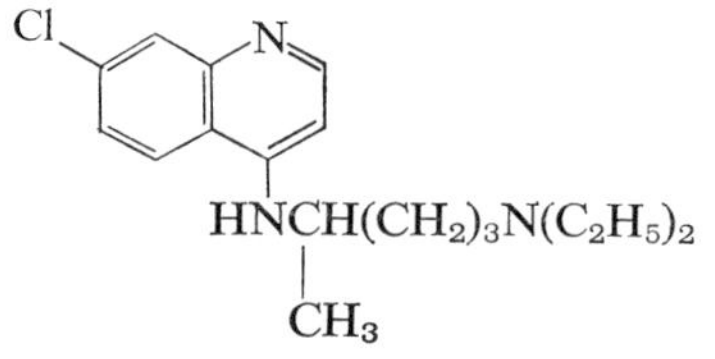

Chloroquine

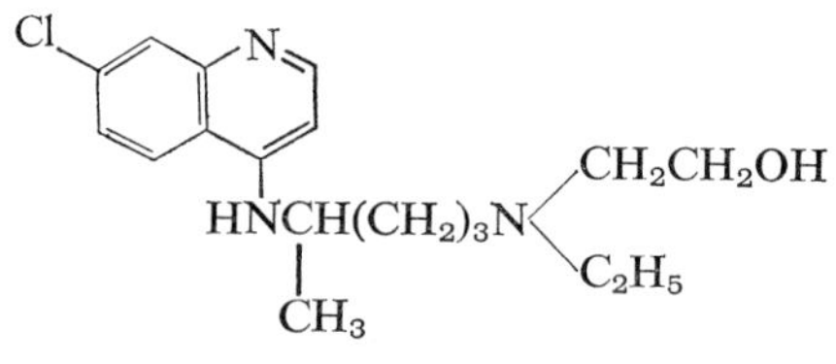

Hydroxychloroquine

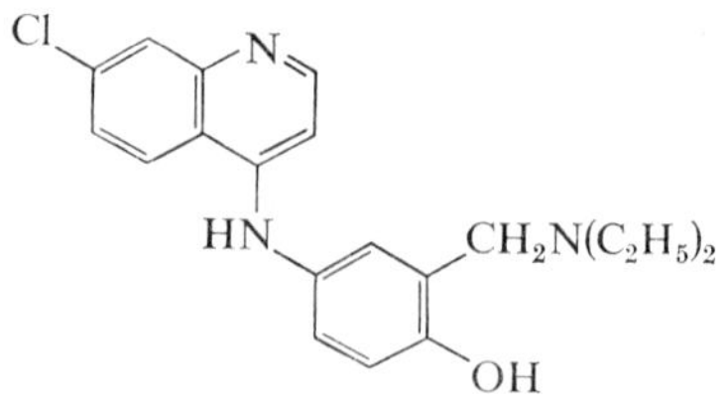

Amodiaquine

Apart from its use in the chemotherapy of malaria and amoebiasis, chloroquine is effective in relatively large doses in the treatment of discoid and systemic lupus erythematosus and in rheumatoid arthritis. This 'anti-inflammatory' use of chloroquine has become widespread in recent years and obviously the chance of chloroquine reaction in symptomatic cutaneous porphyria has also increased correspondingly especially when coincident with alcoholism. Evidence of liver dysfunction must contra-indicate the use of chloroquine with the possible exception of tissue amoebiasis of the liver for which the drug is specifically indicated. There is a very close structural relationship between chloroquine and other members of the 4-aminoquinoline series of antimalarials [FIG. 10.2], and it is to be expected that with the latter, amodiaquine and hydroxychloroquine, similar effects might occur on porphyrin metabolism.

ERYTHROPOIETIC PROTO-PORPHYRIA AND PHOTO-SENSITIZING DRUGS

A further type of abnormality of porphyrin metabolism, erythropoietic protoporphyria, has not so far been linked with drug administration. This may well be due to its rare occurrence. This condition is characterized by excess of erythrocyte protoporphyrin and the cardinal symptom is photosensitivity with erythematous papules and vesicles on face, ears and extremities after exposure to sunlight. The urine is pink or reddish and liver biopsies show characteristic focal, intrahepatic deposits of pigment containing protoporphyrin (Cripps and Scheuer, 1965).

Although there have been no reports of drug precipitation or exacerbation of this condition, it is interesting to learn that when certain farm animals, notably sheep and pigs, feed on buckwheat (*Fagopyrum esculentum*), which contains phytoporphyrin, they may develop hypersensitivity and if bare or slightly covered areas of their skin are then exposed to sunlight, vesiculation, ulceration or even pyrexia and constitutional symptoms may ensue (Thorne, 1966). This would suggest that dietary factors and drugs might possibly influence the course of erythropoietic protoporphyria; certainly it is within the realms of possibility. Any drug that produces photosensitivity would be expected to have an adverse effect on this condition. Unfortunately there is a large number of drugs implicated in photosensitivity reactions, including certain tetracyclines, sulphonamides, sulphonylurea derivatives, phenothiazines, and thiazide diuretics. In addition, methoxasalen (8-methoxypsoralen), trioxsalen (trimethylpsoralen), and other psoralens used in the treatment of vitiligo (leucoderma), produce intolerance to sunlight when taken orally or applied topically (D'Arcy, 1965, 1966). The psoralens also might well be expected to have a deleterious effect on the course of erythropoietic protoporphyria; indeed trioxsalen is specifically contra-indicated in porphyria (Council on Drugs, 1966).

RECOMMENDED FURTHER READING

BRITISH MEDICAL ASSOCIATION (1968) *Porphyria a Royal Malady*, London.
DE MATTEIS, F. (1967) Disturbances of liver porphyrin metabolism caused by drugs, *Pharmacol. Rev.*, **19**, 523–59.
GOLDBERG, A. (1968) The porphyrias, in *Porphyria a Royal Malady*, British Medical Association, London, pp. 66–8.
SCHMID, R. (1966) The porphyrias, in *The Metabolic Basis of Inherited Disease*, eds. Stanbury, J. B., Wyngaarden, J. B., and Frederickson, D. S., New York, pp. 813–70.

REFERENCES

BECKER, F. T. (1965) Porphyria cutanea tarda induced by estrogens, *Arch. Dermat.*, **92**, 252–6.
COHEN, S. N., PHIFER, K. O., and YIELDING, K. L. (1964) Complex formation between chloroquine and ferrihaemic acid *in vitro*, and its effect on the antimalarial action of chloroquine, *Nature (Lond.)*, **202**, 805–6.
COPEMAN, P. W. M., CRIPPS, D. J., and SUMMERLY, R. (1966) Cutaneous hepatic porphyria and oestrogens, *Brit. med. J.*, **1**, 461–3.
COUNCIL ON DRUGS (1966) An agent for stimulating pigmentation or tolerance to sunlight: Trioxsalen (Trisoralen), *J. Amer. med. Ass.*, **197**, 43.
CRIPPS, D. J., and CURTIS, A. C. (1962) Toxic effect of chloroquine on porphyria hepatica, *Arch. Derm.*, **86**, 575–81.
CRIPPS, D.J., and SCHEUER, P.J. (1965) Hepatobiliary changes in erythropoietic protoporphyria, *Arch. Path.*, **80**, 500–8.
D'ARCY, P. F. (1965) The pharmacological basis of drug treatment in dermatology, *Pharm. J.*, **194**, 637–43.
D'ARCY, P. F. (1966) The sun and the skin, *Pharm. J.*, **196**, 477–81.
DEAN, G. (1963) *The Porphyrias. A Story of Inheritance and Environment*, London.

DEAN, G. (1965) Oral contraceptives in porphyria variegata, *S. Afr. Med. J.*, **39**, 278–80.
DENNY-BROWN, D., and SCIARRA, D. (1945) Changes in nervous system in acute porphyria, *Brain*, **68**, 1–16.
DISCOMBE, G., and D'SILVA, J. L. (1945) Acute idiopathic porphyria, *Brit. med. J.*, **2**, 491–3.
DOBRSCHANSKY, M. (1906) Einiges über Malonal, *Wien. Med. Presse*, **47**, 2145–51.
EALES, L. (1966) Porphyria and thiopentone, *Anesthesiology*, **27**, 703–4.
ELIASER, M., and KONDO, B. O. (1942) Electrocardiographic changes associated with acute porphyria, *Amer. Heart J.*, **24**, 696–702.
FELSHER, B. F., and REDEKER, A. G. (1966) Effect of chloroquine on hepatic uroporphyrin metabolism in patients with porphyria cutanea tarda, *Medicine (Baltimore)*, **45**, 575–83.
GAJDOS, A., and GAJDOS-TÖRÖK, M. (1964) Études de l'activité de l'acide δ-aminolévulinique-synthétase dans les mitochondries des hépatocytes de lapin et de rat blanc intoxiqués par l'acetate de plomb, *Rev. franç. Étud. clin., biol.*, **9**, 629–32.

GERTLER, W. (1962) Latente Porphyria cutanea tarda. manifestiert durch Resochintherapie bei Vitiligo, *Derm. Wschr.*, **146**, 376–7.

GOLDBERG, A. (1959) Acute intermittent porphyria. A study of 50 cases, *Quart. J. Med.*, **28**, 183–209.

GOLDBERG, A., and RIMINGTON, C. (1962) *Diseases of Porphyrin Metabolism*, Springfield, Ill.

GOLDBERG, A., RIMINGTON, C., and LOCHHEAD, A. C. (1967) Hereditary coproporphyria, *Lancet*, **i**, 632–6.

GÜNTHER, H. (1922) Die Bedeutung der Hämatoporphyrine in Physiologie und Pathologie, *Ergebn. allg. Path. Anat.*, **20**, 608–764.

HAEGER-ARONSEN, B. (1963) Various types of porphyria in Sweden, *S. Afr. J. Lab. clin. Med.*, **9**, 288–95.

HARLEY, V. (1890) Two fatal cases of an unusual form of nerve disturbance associated with dark-red urine, probably due to defective tissue oxidation, *Brit. med. J.*, **2**, 1169–70.

HARRIS, D. F. (1898) On the red ally of urohaematoporphyrin: A retrospect of twelve cases, *Brit. med. J.*, **1**, 361–2.

HAXTHAUSEN, H. (1927) Ein Fall von Hydroa aestivale ähnehndem Lichtausschlag bei einem Patienten mit Hämatoporphyrinurie, hervorgerufen durch Luminal, *Derm. Wschr.*, **84**, 827–9.

KOFMAN, S., JOHNSON, G. C., and ZIMMERMAN, H. J. (1955) Apparent hepatic dysfunction in lupus erythematosus, *Arch. intern. Med.*, **95**, 669–76.

KOSKELO, P., EISALO, A., and TOIVONEN, I. (1966) Urinary excretion of porphyria precursors and coproporphyrin in healthy females on oral contraceptives, *Brit. med. J.*, **1**, 652–4.

LEVIT, E. J., NODINE, J. H., and PERLOFF, W. H. (1957) Progesterone-induced porphyria, *Amer. J. Med.*, **22**, 831–3.

LINDEN, I. H., STEFFEN, C. G., NEWCOMER, V. D., and CHAPMAN, M. (1954) Development of porphyria during chloroquine therapy for chronic discoid lupus erythematosus, *Calif. Med.*, **81**, 235–8.

MACALPINE, I., HUNTER, R., and RIMINGTON, C. (1968) Porphyria in the Royal Houses of Stuart, Hanover and Prussia, in *Porphyria a Royal Malady*, British Medical Association, London, pp. 17–57.

MARSDEN, C. W. (1959) Porphyria during chloroquine therapy, *Brit. J. Derm.*, **71**, 219–22.

NAYRAC, P., GRAUX, P., FOURLINNIE, J. C., and PETIT, H. (1964) A propos de deux cas de porphyries (dont une forme mixte déclenchée par l'association oestradiol-progestérone), *Lille méd.*, **9**, 704–11.

PERLROTH, M. G., MARVER, H. S., and TSCHUNDY, D. P. (1965) Oral contraceptive agents and the management of acute intermittent porphyria, *J. Amer. med. Ass.*, **194**, 1037–42.

PRUNTY, F. T. G. (1946) Acute porphyria: Investigations on pathology of porphyrins and identifications of excretion of uroporphyrin, I, *Arch. intern. Med.*, **77**, 623–42.

REDEKER, A. (1963) Conference discussion, *S. Afr. J. Lab. clin. Med.*, **9**, 302–3.

RIMINGTON, C. (1964) Drug and enzyme interactions in the porphyrias, *Proc. roy. soc. Med.*, **57**, 511–14.

RIMINGTON, C., MORGAN, P. N., NICHOLLS, K., EVERALL, J. D., and DAVIES, R. R. (1963) Griseofulvin administration and porphyrin metabolism. A survey, *Lancet*, **ii**, 315–22.

ROOK, A., and CHAMPION, R. H. (1960) Porphyria cutanea tarda and diabetes, *Brit. med. J.*, **1**, 860–1.

SCHMID, R. (1966) The porphyrias, in *The Metabolic Basis of Inherited Disease*, eds. Stanbury, J. B., Wyngaarden, J. B., and Fredrickson, D. S., New York, pp. 813–70.

SHERLOCK, S. (1968) The liver in the porphyrias, in *Diseases of the Liver and Biliary System*, 4th ed., Oxford, pp. 514–16.

STOCKVIS, B. J. (1889) Over twee Zeldzame Kleurstoffen in urine van zieken, *Ned. T. Geneesk.*, **25**, 409–17.

SWEENEY, G. D., SAUNDERS, S. J., DOWDLE, E. B., and EALES, L. (1965) Effects of chloroquine on patients with cutaneous porphyria of the 'symptomatic' type, *Brit. med. J.*, **1**, 1281–5.

THORNE, N. (1966) Cosmetics and the dermatologist. The lucites and sunscreening preparations, *Brit. J. clin. Pract.*, **20**, 443–4, 447.

TURNER, W. J. (1938) Studies on porphyria, III. Acute idiopathic porphyria, *Arch. intern. Med.*, **61**, 762–73.

VAN DER GRIENT, A. J. (1968) Antifungal drugs, in *Side Effects of Drugs*, Vol. VI, eds. Meyler, L., and Herxheimer, A., Excerpta Medica Foundation, Amsterdam, pp. 315–19.

WALDENSTRÖM, J. (1937) Studien über die Porphyrie, *Acta med. scand., Suppl.*, **82**, 254.

WALDENSTRÖM, J. (1939) Neurological symptoms caused by so called acute porphyria, *Acta psychiat. scand.*, **14**, 375–9.

WARD, R. J. (1965) Porphyria and its relation to anesthesia, *Anesthesiology*, **26**, 212–15.

WATSON, C. J., RUNGE, W., and BOSSENMAIER, I. (1962). Increased urinary porphobilinogen and uroporphyrin after administration of stilboestrol in a case of latent porphyria, *Metabolism*, **11**, 1129–33.

WELLAND, F. H., HELLMAN, E. S., GADDIS, E. M., COLLINS, A., HUNTER, G. W., JR., and TSCHUDY, D. P. (1964). Factors affecting the excretion of porphyrin precursors by patients with acute intermittent porphyria, I. The effect of diet, *Metabolism*, **13**, 232–50.

WETTERBERG, L. (1964) Oral contraceptives and acute intermittent porphyria, *Lancet*, **ii**, 1178–9.

WHITTAKER, S. R. F., and WHITEHEAD, T. P. (1956) Acute and latent porphyria, *Lancet*, **i**, 547–51.

WITH, T. K. (1965) Porphyria, *Lancet*, **i**, 916–17.

ZAROWITZ, H., and NEWHOUSE, S. (1965) Coproporphyrinuria with cutaneous reaction induced by chlorpropamide, *N.Y. Med. J.*, **65**, 2385–7.

ZIPRKOWSKI, L., SVEINBERG, A., CRISPIN, M., KRAKOWSKI, A., and SAIDMAN, J. (1966) The effect of griseofulvin in hereditary porphyria cutanea tarda, *Arch. Derm.*, **93**, 21–7.

11

DISORDERS OF CARBOHYDRATE AND FAT METABOLISM

DIABETOGENIC EFFECT OF DRUGS

DIURETICS

Thiazides (Benzothiadiazines)

Many of the diuretics are most certainly implicated in diabetogenic effects. Of this group of agents the thiazide diuretics are worthy of particular mention.

Chlorothiazide was the first member of this group to be used extensively in the clinic and this was rapidly followed by hydrochlorothiazide and many related compounds of increased diuretic potency.

Thiazide diuretics can induce hyperglycaemia in normal animals (Wolff and Parmley, 1963); however, clinical results are not so clear cut, nor are they so convincing, since most patients reported showed either some diabetic symptoms before thiazide treatment commenced or were suffering from hypertension, a condition which can be associated with impaired carbohydrate tolerance.

Generally clinical studies have shown that the thiazides are potentially diabetogenic in high dosage to early diabetics, to those who have a familial history of diabetes, to those patients with some form of hypertension, and during pregnancy.

The possibility that thiazide diuretics can induce a diabetes-like state was first noted by Finnerty (1959) and Wilkins (1959), who reported that hyperglycaemia and glycosuria developed in patients taking such drugs. Other reports soon appeared relating the aggravation of known diabetes, or the uncovering of 'latent diabetes' to the administration of thiazide compounds. Zatuchni and Kordasz (1961) reported the effects of a single dose of chlorothiazide (1 gram) or trichlormethiazide (8–16 mg) on the two-hour post-prandial blood sugar level in 25 patients hospitalized for reasons other than diabetes. Fourteen (56 per cent) of the 25 patients had abnormal (above 120 mg/100 ml) two-hour blood glucose levels after the thiazide dosage. However, it must be noted that 10 (40 per cent) had abnormally high levels even prior to administration of the diuretic, and that six of these worsened after the single dosage treatment. Only four out of the 25 patients showed an apparent alteration from normal to abnormal blood glucose levels.

In earlier studies Dinon et al. (1958) reported that there was no evidence of altered carbohydrate metabolism in 121 oedematous and hypertensive patients treated with chlorothiazide at dose levels of 0·5–2 grams daily.

Further investigations on this effect were carried out by Goldner and colleagues (1960), who also studied a group of hospitalized patients, 20 of whom were diabetic and 20 of whom were non-diabetic with no family history of the disease. The drugs administered in this study were chlorothiazide (500–1,000 mg/day), hydrochlorothiazide (100–300 mg/day) and dihydroflumethiazide (20 mg/day). Each drug was given for at least 5 days. None of the non-diabetic patients, and only six of the diabetic patients showed an increase in fasting blood sugar level following treatment, and such effects were only seen at the higher levels of dosage.

In a similar study, Runyan (1962) found that benzthiazide in large doses (50 mg t.i.d.) for 1 week resulted in a 45 per cent increase in fasting blood sugar level of patients with mild uncomplicated diabetes. When dosage was reduced to 50 mg daily the increase in fasting blood sugar level was only 14 per cent. Shapire and colleagues (1961) studied the effects of thiazides on carbohydrate metabolism in middle-aged and elderly hypertensive patients and showed that chlorothiazide (1 gram/day) for 2 weeks raised the fasting blood sugar level in patients who were judged as 'potential diabetics', due to family history of diabetes or to previous abnormal glucose tolerance tests, but did not affect non-diabetic control subjects.

The effect of long-term administration of thiazide diuretics on carbohydrate metabolism has also been studied by a number of clinicians. Roediger and associates (1964) compared the effects of 3 months chlorothiazide therapy (1gram/day) with 3 months bendroflumethiazide treatment (10mg/day) in 35 patients under treatment for hypertension and diabetes mellitus. Fasting blood sugar levels were raised to comparable levels (147–160 mg/100 ml.) with either thiazide. Wolff et al. (1963) focused attention on the long-term effects of benzothiadiazine on hypertensive patients. They reported a mean fasting blood glucose level of 88·4 mg/100 ml in patients receiving placebo dosage and a value of 97 mg/100 ml in those patients on the thiazide diuretic. Five patients developed frank diabetes mellitus whilst on thiazide therapy, and, in two of these patients, a return to normal glucose levels followed after treatment was discontinued. The remaining three patients were not obese, had no family history of diabetes, and, prior to the thiazide treatment, had normal carbohydrate tolerance. Apparently these patients suffered permanent damage in their ability to handle carbohydrate.

Brown and Brown (1967) studied 11 normal men with negative family histories of diabetes who received 50 mg hydrochlorothiazide daily for 5 months. At the end of that time one man showed diminished ability to utilize carbohydrates. That individual, plus four others, continued taking the drug for a total of 14 months, at which time three of the five displayed an abnormal oral glucose tolerance test. Thus it would appear that thiazide-induced carbohydrate intolerance is not limited to persons with other disease states or with a family history of diabetes but can occur in normal individuals.

The effect of thiazide compounds on glucose tolerance in pregnancy has been investigated by Sugar (1961) who reported aggravation of known diabetes during pregnancy by thiazide diuretics. Ketoacidosis occurred in two pregnant patients, one receiving chlorothiazide (50 mg/day) and the other benzhydroflumethiazide (5 mg/day). In contrast to this finding Esbenshade and Smith (1965) did not observe any increase in the two-hour post-prandial blood glucose level of 23 third trimester patients on hydrochlorothiazide (50 mg twice daily) for 7 days in spite of the fact that four of these patients had a familial history of diabetes.

The mechanism of the diabetogenic action of the thiazides has been studied, but there is little clear evidence of the precise mechanisms involved. It has been suggested that thiazides may act as stressing agents on carbohydrate metabolism, and that this effect, mediated by hypokalaemia, reduced insulin secretion; a further hypothesis is that those patients who exhibit hyperglycaemia on thiazide treatment have an inborn error of carbohydrate metabolism which is uncovered by the drug treatment. In view of these theories, the work of Wales *et al.* (1967) is of particular interest. Normal subjects undergoing metabolic stress due to high fat diet during two-week periods did not show hyperglycaemia or decreased glucose tolerance after hydrochlorothiazide treatment at normal therapeutic dosage. Nor was there any change in plasma levels, serum FFA or serum pyruvate levels. The thiazide dosage did, however, produce other metabolic changes, notably hyperuricaemia and hypokalaemia.

It is difficult to draw hard and fast conclusions from these studies, except that patients taking thiazides are at potential diabetogenic risk, especially if there is a tendency to or a latent possibility of diabetes mellitus. Certainly such patients should be periodically evaluated during treatment for the potency of their carbohydrate handling ability. Knowledge of carbohydrate tolerance prior to commencement of thiazide therapy would be a wise precaution.

Frusemide and Ethacrynic Acid

Impairment of glucose tolerance is also reported after frusemide, another oral diuretic which is structurally dissimilar to the benzothiadiazines (thiazides). Frusemide is a member of a group of monosulphamyl diuretics, which also includes quinethazone, chlorthalidone, and clorexolone, while ethacrynic acid is a related desulphamyl compound.

Konigstein (1965) showed that five of eleven non-diabetic obese subjects showed deterioration of glucose tolerance following an oral dosage of 75 mg frusemide daily for 5 days, although two diabetic subjects who showed deterioration of glucose tolerance on thiazide therapy showed no impairment while taking frusemide 20–25 mg daily for many months. Toivonen and Mustala (1966) described deterioration of glucose tolerance in one patient treated with frusemide 80 mg daily for 4 weeks; the glucose tolerance reverted to normal after cessation of therapy.

Ethacrynic acid is a related desulphamyl compound, and although ethacrynic acid has been implicated in impaired glucose tolerance the evidence for this is somewhat controversial and there are conflicting opinions as to whether or not this diuretic is diabetogenic.

Jones and Pickens (1967) described a single case of a non-diabetic woman whose glucose tolerance had become impaired after thiazide therapy, but had returned to normal after treatment ceased. Diuretic treatment was then recommended with ethacrynic acid and her glucose tolerance again became impaired, and diuretic treatment was again discontinued with a return to a normal glucose tolerance curve. Jones and Pickens (1967) suggested that any patient, who has shown glycosuria and diminished glucose tolerance on thiazide diuretics, should be carefully monitored when placed on an ethacrynic acid diuretic regime.

Feldman and Diamond (1967) studied 15 patients, some of whom had normal glucose tolerance and others who had mild or severe diabetes. Glucose tolerance curves were done prior to initiation of ethacrynic acid therapy and were repeated after 1 month and 3 months of continuous medication. Only one patient, a non-diabetic, showed a decrease in glucose tolerance. Glucose tolerance reverted to normal in this patient after withdrawal of the diuretic.

Lebacq and Marcq (1967) studied 24 normal subjects and 15 diabetics; carbohydrate intolerance was induced or increased by the diuretic in eight of the 24 normals and in eight of the 15 diabetics. Serum amylase levels were unchanged during treatment. Ethacrynic acid resulted in lower insulin levels in the fasting state and lessened the increase in insulin levels following glucose ingestion.

A further report suggesting that ethacrynic acid does not cause abnormalities of carbohydrate metabolism was published by Dige-Petersen (1966), but the balance of evidence suggests that it does. No direct comparison has yet been made between the diabetogenic effect of ethacrynic acid and the thiazides.

Diazoxide

Diazoxide was the outcome of research to separate the

antihypertensive and diuretic properties of chloro-thiazide, to which it has a close structural resemblance. There are, however, important differences in the pharmacology of chlorothiazide and diazoxide. Diazoxide has no diuretic properties and produces a sharp and immediate fall in blood pressure when given intravenously, which chlorothiazide does not.

Diazoxide causes a predictable hyperglycaemia when administered to animals or man and it has therefore proved easier to study the mechanism of the diabetogenic effect with it than with the thiazide diuretics. It may be unwise to assume that the diabetogenic action of diazoxide and the thiazide diuretics are the same because their pharmacological actions are different.

Diazoxide is a potent diabetogenic agent in man and its effect is increased by combining it with a thiazide diuretic. Dollery et al. (1962) reported two patients who were treated with diazoxide 400 mg daily for hypertension. As the patients became oedematous, hydrochlorothiazide was added to treatment in a dose of 50 mg daily. In each case after about 4 weeks' treatment the patients became diabetic with high fasting blood sugar levels. One of these patients was known to have a normal glucose tolerance test before diazoxide was given and the glucose tolerance test returned to normal 17 days after stopping the drugs. The plasma insulin-like activity, assayed by the rat epididymal-fat-pad technique, was reduced during the diabetic period.

Okun et al. (1963) used diazoxide and trichlormethiazide together to treat hypertension and found that approximately half the patients developed hyperglycaemia. Subsequently, it was shown that this effect could be reproduced in animals. Kvam and Stanton (1964) gave diazoxide, 100–400 mg/kg to fasting rats. A rise in blood glucose followed, which could be antagonized by administration of tolbutamide. Serum insulin-like activity in rats receiving diazoxide was not significantly lower than in control rats, though a marked hyperglycaemia had been produced. A beta adrenergic blocking drug (MJ 1999) was capable of modifying the hyperglycaemia produced by diazoxide. Potassium deficiency in the rats strikingly exaggerated the hyperglycaemic action of diazoxide, while potassium supplements (KCl 750 mg/kg) reduced it. Tabachnick et al. (1964) carried out an extensive investigation into the pharmacological basis of the hyperglycaemia produced by diazoxide. They produced hyperglycaemia in de-pancreatized dogs, alloxan-treated mice, propylthiouracil-treated mice and nephrectomized mice. These observations suggested that the main locus of action was not in the pancreas, thyroid or kidneys. Diazoxide hyperglycaemia was partly suppressed by adrenalectomy, hypophysectomy or administration of isopropyl-methoxamine, a specific inhibitor of the metabolic effects of adrenaline. However, some doubt is cast upon the importance of the participation of the sympathetic nervous system in this effect, since reserpine-treated mice respond to diazoxide with hyperglycaemia. These previous observations suggest that diazoxide diabetes is produced by an extra-pancreatic action.

Seltzer and Allen (1965) studied eight normal subjects given 600 mg of diazoxide and 8 mg of trichlormethiazide daily for 5 days. Blood glucose and plasma insulin (immuno-assay) were determined after oral and intravenous glucose loads at the end of the 5-day period on the drugs and again 2 weeks later. Diazoxide raised the fasting, 60 and 120 minute blood sugars and reduced the rise in plasma insulin produced by the glucose load. The ratios of total insulin response to total glycaemia stimulus were 1·81 in controls and 0·4 during diazoxide. In the intravenous glucose tolerance tests plasma insulin was maximal at 5 minutes in controls and then paralleled the falling blood sugar. Diazoxide almost completely inhibited insulin release under these circumstances. Seltzer and Allen (1965) concluded that diazoxide diabetes stems from the same functional defects which typify spontaneous diabetes. There is initially a sluggish response to acute stimulus and proportionately less insulin production per unit of secretory stimulus. Since the abnormalities produced in normal controls could rapidly be reversed by withdrawal of the drugs they suggested that this might prove a useful experimental model for further study of human diabetes.

Diazoxide has been used to treat children with leucine-sensitive hypoglycaemia and patients with insulin-producing tumours (Unger, 1966). Drash and Wolff (1964) found that diazoxide in doses of 12 mg/kg per day elevated the blood glucose response to oral glucose in a four-year-old boy with leucine-sensitive hypoglycaemia. Samols and Marks (1966) reported similar observations in two children with leucine-sensitive hypoglycaemia. It is of interest that this unwanted and potentially dangerous hyperglycaemic effect of diazoxide should have been put to good use in treating patients with intractable hypoglycaemic attacks.

There is very strong evidence that diazoxide has both a peripheral and pancreatic action. Its ability to produce hyperglycaemia in de-pancreatized or alloxan diabetic animals proves the peripheral action, while the alterations in plasma insulin produced in intact animals, or slices of pancreas, suggests an effect on insulin formation or release. Howell and Taylor (1966) showed that diazoxide inhibits insulin secretion from the rabbit pancreas in vitro in response to glucose.

All the widely used thiazide diuretics have been reported to cause hyperglycaemia (benzthiazide, chlorothiazide, hydrochlorothiazide, hydroflumethiazide, trichlormethiazide). What comparative evidence there is suggests that they are equally likely to cause hyperglycaemia. Abnormalities of glucose tolerance brought about by short-term administration of diuretics or diazoxide are reversible. It is uncertain what proportion of the abnormalities found in patients treated with diuretics for long periods are due to drugs. Some of these are not reversible.

The practical outcome of the clinical observations of

the diabetogenic action of thiazides, frusemide and possibly ethacrynic acid is that care should be taken in prescribing any of these drugs to diabetics since the control of diabetes may be severely interfered with and adjustment of oral hypoglycaemia therapy or insulin requirements may be necessary.

CORTICOSTEROIDS

Most patients who develop steroid diabetes have a predisposition to diabetes mellitus as shown by a positive family history of the disease. It is rare for a steroid-induced diabetic to develop ketosis, but this has been described by Blereau and Weingarten (1964). In this case, a 29-year-old man was given corticosteroid therapy for pulmonary sarcoidosis; his glucose tolerance test before steroid therapy was normal. He developed severe hyperglycaemia (520 mg/100 ml) acidosis and ketosis. After withdrawal of steroids his glucose tolerance test returned to normal. Schubert and Schulte (1963) reported a series of 214 patients treated with corticosteroids for periods in excess of 3 days; 14 per cent developed steroid diabetes. Disturbances of carbohydrate metabolism were observed earlier in patients on high doses of steroids or who had liver disease which retarded the elimination of the steroid as a glucuronide. Matsunaga et al. (1963) found that of 235 patients treated on steroid therapy 5·5 per cent developed diabetes. No patients on corticotrophin or cortisone developed steroid diabetes although 7 per cent of those patients treated with prednisolone, 23 per cent of those treated with paramethasone, and 20 per cent of those treated with betamethasone developed diabetes.

Systemic administration or topical application of corticosteroids to a diabetic under good control may disturb carbohydrate balance and the requirements for insulin or oral hypoglycaemic agents may increase. Kershbaum (1963) reported four cases of diabetes treated with topical fluocinolone acetonide for skin conditions, who experienced an increase in insulin or tolbutamide requirements after commencing this therapy.

A further complication of steroid therapy in diabetic patients is the development of ketonuria without accompanying glycosuria. This has been reported by Madison (1964) who observed this in four diabetic patients who were treated with topical triamcinolone acetonide for necrobiosis lipoidica. No explanation for this phenomenon is known.

ORAL CONTRACEPTIVES

Impairment of glucose tolerance in women taking oral contraceptives has been recognized since the drugs were introduced (Waine et al., 1963) and has been confirmed by some (Petersen et al., 1966; Wynn and Doar, 1966) but debated by others (Taylor and Kass, 1968; Clinch et al., 1969). Descriptions of the severity of the impairment and its frequency have varied in the reports and evidence has been presented that the impairment was transient and that it reverted to pretreatment levels while contraceptives were continued or when they were discontinued.

For the purpose of this review it is convenient to classify reports on impairment of carbohydrate metabolism due to oral contraceptive agents into three categories: studies in diabetic women, studies in women with potential diabetes, and studies in normal subjects.

There are many early reports suggesting that oral contraceptives adversely affected carbohydrate tolerance and caused a change in diabetic control. Usually there was an increased insulin demand and the previously stable diabetic became unstable. An illustrative case is one that has been described by Paros (1964). A patient with previously stable diabetes was given norethynodrel with ethinyloestradiol; after the third day of medication, glycosuria, polyuria and polydipsia reappeared and insulin demand increased. Even after discontinuation of the contraceptive it was nearly 2 months before the diabetes was stable again.

With regard to the second category, Paros (1964) reported on 12 patients who had a positive family history of diabetes, of whom seven showed increased blood sugar levels after using oral contraceptives.

In a recent study, Szabo et al. (1970) have drawn attention to the unwise complacency surrounding the use of these agents in women with potential diabetes. The inserts packaged with oral contraceptive agents advise caution when taken by women with manifest diabetes, but give no guidance regarding their use in those with potential diabetes. In their study Szabo et al. (1970) performed oral glucose tolerance tests periodically on 15 women who had shown abnormal tolerance to glucose in the third trimester, but who had normal tolerance after delivery. Subsequently five of these women received a combination of norethindrone (1 mg) and mestranol (0·05 mg) as an oral contraceptive cyclically. The other 10 women practised other methods of contraception and served as controls to the study.

Abnormal glucose tolerance recurred in all five women while they were taking the contraceptive agent. When therapy ceased the glucose tolerance test remained diabetic in three cases; it temporarily improved but became abnormal again in the fourth woman. The fifth woman was lost to follow-up observation after discontinuing contraceptive pills. Three of the 10 controls showed deterioration of the glucose tolerance test.

The authors concluded that screening tests for diabetes should be performed early during contraceptive treatment, and that women with latent diabetes should be excluded from hormonal birth control.

It is, however, in the third category that the full effect of the contraceptive agent on an otherwise normal carbohydrate tolerance is shown and in this respect the studies of Gershberg et al. (1964), Clinch et al. (1969) and Wynn and Doar (1969) are illustrative of the problems created.

Gershberg and colleagues (1964) investigated 59 patients of whom 51 had used norethynodrel with mestranol for 2 years or longer. Blood sugar levels were measured fasting, and 1 and 2 hours after administration of glucose. The fasting level was outside normal limits in 6 of these patients, and the two-hour blood sugar level was raised above normal limits in 27 of these women.

Clinch et al. (1969) studied the effect of oral contraceptive medication in 42 women. An intravenous glucose tolerance test was used in preference to the oral test. Blood glucose levels were higher than normal in 32 of the 42 women when they were on contraceptive medication.

Wynn and Doar (1969) made longitudinal studies of plasma glucose, non-esterified fatty acids (NEFA), insulin and blood pyruvate levels during oral and intravenous glucose tolerance tests in women treated with combined oral contraceptive preparations.

Group A consisted of 91 women tested before and during oral contraceptive medication. In terms of total area between the plasma curve and the abscissa, oral and intravenous glucose tolerance deteriorated during therapy in respectively 78 per cent and 70 per cent of these women. Thirteen per cent of women in this group developed chemical diabetes mellitus as a result of medication.

Group B consisted of 39 women tested during contraceptive therapy and again after discontinuing medication. An improvement occurred in the oral glucose tolerance in 90 per cent and in the intravenous glucose tolerance in 85 per cent after medication was discontinued.

Group C consisted of 22 women whose glucose tolerance tests were similar to those measured in group B, while on oral contraceptives. These women were re-tested while continuing on contraceptives and there was no change in the oral or intravenous glucose tolerance.

Plasma-NEFA levels were unchanged before and after oral or intravenous glucose tolerance tests in Groups A and B. As a result of medication, the fasting blood pyruvate rose in Group A. The mean fasting insulin levels were unchanged in Groups A and B on or off therapy.

The conclusion drawn from these studies by Wynn and Doar (1969) was that the impaired glucose tolerance was steroid diabetes caused by elevated plasma cortisol levels secondary to the oestrogen component of the oral contraceptive.

Oestrogen-progestogen oral contraceptives, especially of the combined type, offer almost complete protection against pregnancy. All other methods are substantially less effective and in assessing the significance of the iatrogenic risks of oral contraception due consideration must be given to the dangers of unwanted pregnancy, especially since pregnancy itself can worsen a diabetic or potential diabetic state.

It is understandable, although somewhat disappointing, that medical opinion, whilst headlining the association between the use of oral contraceptives and thrombo-embolic disorders (e.g. Vessey, 1970), has not also given some authoritative warning to doctors that some of their patients may also be at risk from a breakdown of carbohydrate homeostasis, especially if they are controlled diabetics or, perhaps more important, if they are undiagnosed potential diabetics. Certainly a routine investigation of carbohydrate metabolism status would be a wise and sensible precaution, if not in all patients, then certainly in those who might be suspected through familial history or 'avoirdupois' to have an impaired or a 'strained' carbohydrate tolerance. The danger of precipitating permanent diabetes has, we believe, not been properly appreciated, and it is perhaps towards gaining informative data on this aspect that long-term studies should be initiated.

CYCLOPHOSPHAMIDE

Development of diabetes mellitus has been described by Pengelly (1965) in three women who were being treated with cyclophosphamide for carcinoma of the breast.

ISONIAZID

Reports of glycosuria and hyperglycaemia have been reported during treatment with isoniazid (Dickson, 1962). In a group of 50 patients receiving isoniazid, three developed glycosuria and two of these presented all the classical characteristics of true diabetes. The urine of the third reverted to normal on the cessation of isoniazid therapy. There was no pre-existent diabetes in any of these cases.

PHENYTOIN (DIPHENYLHYDANTOIN)-INDUCED HYPERGLYCAEMIA

Millichap (1965) first showed that diphenylhydantoin and other anticonvulsants could cause hyperglycaemia. Belton et al. (1965) confirmed, in rabbit experiments, that diphenylhydantoin and phenobarbitone at anticonvulsant doses caused a significant rise in blood sugar.

Millichap (1969) records that, in view of the hyperglycaemic action of diphenylhydantoin, this drug could be used to control the hypoglycaemic seizures seen in leucine-sensitive hypoglycaemia. Over a 12-month period, diphenylhydantoin successfully maintained a normal fasting blood sugar level in a child with leucine-sensitive hypoglycaemia and controlled the child's convulsions. The abnormal hypoglycaemic response to leucine was not prevented in a subsequent sensitivity test, but the child did not convulse.

The mechanism of the hyperglycaemic action of diphenylhydantoin has been variously suggested as being due to a direct action of diphenylhydantoin on the hypothalamus (Belton et al., 1965), to stimulation of the pituitary and the adrenal cortex (Woodbury, 1952) and, more recently, it has been suggested that the hyperglycaemia is due to an impairment of the insulin response to carbohydrate, i.e. causing a relative hypo-insulinaemia (Peters and Samaan, 1969).

HYPOGLYCAEMIC EFFECT OF DRUGS

PROPRANOLOL

Kotler *et al.* (1966) noted that propranolol precipitated hypoglycaemia in an insulin-dependent diabetic, but did not change his total insulin requirement. Abramson *et al.* (1966) have suggested that propranolol increases sensitivity to insulin in normal subjects by damping down the rebound of blood glucose level after its initial fall, while Sussman *et al.* (1967) suggested that propranolol could be a potent stimulator of insulin secretion and that the observed hypoglycaemia could have been due to raised circulating insulin levels.

Divitiss *et al.* (1968) showed that blockade of beta-adrenergic receptors by propranolol inhibited, within certain limits, the usual response of blood glucose to tolbutamide during the tolbutamide load test. They thought that the antagonistic effect of β-receptor blockade took place at the level of insulin release from the granules in the β-cells of the islets of Langerhans, and that insulin was released from β-cell granules only in the presence of β-adrenergic activity. An alternative hypothesis was that decreased splanchnic blood flow due to blockade of β-adrenergic receptors reduced access to the pancreas of the injected tolbutamide.

Whatever the mechanism of action of propranolol, Reveno and Rosenbaum (1968) thought that its effect might be of value in the management of the labile diabetic. The object of their studies was to flatten the unpredictable hyperglycaemic peaks and, if possible, to reduce the variable insulin requirement. Oral propranolol in varying dosage and timing was tried in four patients treated with calorie diet restriction, isophane (NPH) insulin and supplementary crystalline insulin, treatment which had either failed to achieve good control of persistent hyperglycaemia, or had poorly controlled glycosuria and hyperglycaemic attacks.

The combined propranolol, diet and insulin regime produced a severe hypoglycaemic reaction in one patient which persisted even though the dosage of insulin and propranolol was reduced. In a second patient, a severe hypoglycaemic reaction also occurred and this ceased when propranolol dosage was reduced, although persistent glycosuria and raised morning blood sugar levels remained. In the third patient, an improved status resulted from the combined treatment which continued for over 6 months although heavy proteinuria continued and fresh retinal haemorrhages recurred at intervals. In the final case, the insulin requirement was reduced by the combined treatment, although fasting blood sugar levels remained high and glycosuria was unaltered. The previous episodes of hypoglycaemia which occurred on diet and insulin alone did not recur.

It may be assumed that in the labile diabetic the β-adrenergic blockade of propranolol, by opposing catecholamine action, might enhance hypoglycaemia in sufficient degrees to overcome the hyperglycaemia resulting from the multiple factors at play in this disease. This assumption, as stated by Reveno and Rosenbaum (1968) would necessarily ascribe a dominant role to the catecholamines and a weak compensatory or defensive reaction to these multiple factors. It is more likely, however, that there is already a trend towards hypoglycaemia when propranolol is effective and that the induced hypoglycaemia is the result of β-blockade interfering with the attainment of normoglycaemia.

The authors (Reveno and Rosenbaum, 1968) concluded that propranolol has no practical value in the management of the brittle diabetic.

THALIDOMIDE

Meade and Rosalki (1961) found a flat glucose tolerance after a 100 gram load in a woman who had been receiving 50 mg thalidomide for 18 months. The drug was then stopped and a week later a normal rise in blood glucose after a 50 gram glucose load was observed. The patient agreed to restart thalidomide and again the blood sugar levels failed to rise after oral glucose. Oral *d*-xylose and intravenous glucose tests were normal. In this patient, therefore, thalidomide interfered with active absorption of glucose.

DRUG-INDUCED DISORDERS OF FAT METABOLISM

DRUG-INDUCED INCREASES IN PLASMA TRIGLYCERIDE LEVEL WITH ORAL CONTRACEPTIVES

Wide acceptance of oral contraceptive therapy has been associated with an increasing recognition of diverse metabolic side-effects. However, particular concern has arisen following reports of increased levels of plasma triglycerides in women receiving this form of contraception (Aurell *et al.*, 1966 and Wynn and others, 1966, 1969). The increase in triglyceride levels in these women was such that sex differential between men and women of similar ages was reduced. These observations have raised the possibility that the relative immunity from atherosclerotic vascular disease enjoyed by premenopausal women may be severely jeopardized.

A detailed investigation of this problem was carried out by Hazzard *et al.* (1969) using 10 young women of 20–33 years in good health, with normal menses, and who were non-obese, within the 95 percentile of the ideal Metropolitan Life Assurance standards. Identical studies were performed before and after 14 days' treatment with ethinyloestradiol 0·05 mg and medroxy-progesterone acetate 10 mg daily. During this treatment, none of the 10 subjects showed a net gain in weight, and the mean plasma triglyceride level rose from 45 mg/100 ml to 64 mg/100 ml (p < 0·005); the post-hepatic lipolytic activity fell from 0·373 μEq FFA/ml/min to 0·199 μEq FFA/ml/min (p < 0·001); the mean basal immunoreactive insulin levels increased in eight of 10 subjects, the mean increase for the group was from 10·5 μV/ml before treatment to 14·5 μV/ml during treatment ($p < 0.05$). The one subject, who showed no increase in plasma triglyceride during the initial 14-day period, and, who was subsequently followed up for three complete cycles, showed a rise in plasma triglyceride level of nearly 100 per cent during the second cycle.

It would appear that the rise in plasma triglyceride level might be due to increased endogenous (hepatic) triglyceride synthesis which would be supported by the increase in immunoreactive insulin levels and/or decreased triglyceride removal as suggested by the fall in post-hepatic lipolytic activity.

Wynn *et al.* (1969) made a longitudinal study of the effects of oral contraceptives on fasting serum lipid and low-density lipoprotein levels in two groups of women. Group A consisted of 116 women tested before and during contraceptive therapy. Group B consisted of 48 women initially tested during therapy and tested again after this had been discontinued. In both groups, while on contraceptive therapy, there was a higher mean serum triglyceride and cholesterol level. Elevated mean fasting $S_f 0$–12, $S_f 20$–100 and $S_f 100$–400 serum lipoprotein levels were found during therapy, but $S_f 12$–20 lipoprotein and chylomicron triglyceride levels were unchanged. Serum triglyceride levels increased in 95 per cent of Group A women during therapy and decreased in 88 per cent of Group B women after therapy was discontinued. No relationship was found between the nature of the oestrogen-progesterone combination, day of treatment cycle, duration of therapy, degree of obesity, parity, or family history of diabetes or of oral glucose tolerance abnormality.

'The clinical significance of these findings is unknown, but they cannot be ignored, since they raise the possibility of irreversible structural changes such as atherosclerosis after 10 or 20 years on oral contraceptives. Both raised serum lipid levels and chemical diabetes are associated with an increased incidence of occlusive vascular disease. The risks of venous thrombosis, pulmonary embolism and cerebral thrombosis have already been shown to be raised in women taking oral contraceptives. . . .

'In view of these doubts, the wisdom of administering such compounds to *healthy* women for many years must be seriously considered.' (*Lancet*, leading article, 1969.)

RECOMMENDED FURTHER READING

DOLLERY, C. T. (1968) Changes in carbohydrate metabolism after the use of diuretics, in *Drug-Induced Diseases*, Vol. 3, eds. Meyler, L., and Peck, H. M., Excerpta Medica Foundation, Amsterdam, pp. 95–102.

DOLLERY, C. T. (1968) Diuretic drugs, in *Side Effects of Drugs*, Vol. VI, eds. Meyler, L., and Herxheimer, A., Excerpta Medica Foundation, Amsterdam, pp. 212–22.

DE LANGE, W. E., and DOORENBOS, H. (1968) Hormones and synthetic substitutes, in *Side Effects of Drugs*, Vol. VI, eds. Meyler, L., and Herxheimer, A., Excerpta Medica Foundation, Amsterdam, pp. 383–421.

MEYLER, L., DALDERUP, C., VAN DIJL, W., and BOUMA, H. G. D., in *Side Effects of Drugs*, Vol. V, eds. Meyler, L., *et al.*, Excerpta Medica Foundation, Amsterdam, pp. 229–36 (diuretics), 411–12 (corticosteroids), 428–9 (oral contraceptives).

REFERENCES

ABRAMSON, E. A., ARKY, R. A., and WOEBER, K. A. (1966) Effects of propranolol on the hormonal and metabolic responses to insulin-induced hypoglycaemia, *Lancet*, ii, 1386–8.

AURELL, M., CRAMER, K., and RYBO, G. (1966) Serum lipids and lipoproteins during long-term administration of an oral contraceptive, *Lancet*, i, 291–3.

BELTON, N. R., ETHERIDGE, J. E., JR., and MILLICHAP, J. G. (1965) Effects of convulsions and anticonvulsants on blood sugar in rabbits, *Epilepsia (Boston)*, 6, 243–9.

BLEREAU, R. P., and WEINGARTEN, C. M. (1964) Diabetic acidosis secondary to steroid therapy, *New Engl. J. Med.*, 271, 836.

BROWN, W. J., JR., and BROWN, F. K. (1967) Thiazide-induced alteration of carbohydrate tolerance in normal men, *Curr. ther. Res.*, 9, 200–7.

CLINCH, J., TURNBULL, A. C., and KHOSLA, T. (1969) Effect of oral contraceptives on glucose tolerance, *Lancet*, i, 857–8.

DICKSON, I. (1962) Glycosuria and diabetes mellitus following I.N.A.H. therapy, *Med. J. Aust.*, 49, 325–6.

DIGE-PETERSEN, H. (1966) Ethacrynic acid and carbohydrate metabolism, *Nord. Med.*, 75, 123–5.

DINON, L. R., KIM, Y. S., and VANDER VEER, J. B. (1958) Clinical experience with chlorothiazide (diuril) with particular emphasis on untoward responses. A report of 121 cases studied over a 15 month period, *Amer. J. med. Sci.*, 236, 533–45.

DIVITIISS, O. DE, GIORDANO, F., GALO, B., and JACONO, A. (1968) Tolbutamide and propranolol, *Lancet*, i, 749.

DOLLERY, C. T., PENTECOST, B. L., and SAMAAN, N. A. (1962) Drug-induced diabetes, *Lancet*, ii, 735–6.

DRASH, A., and WOLFF, F. (1964) Drug therapy in leucine-sensitive hypoglycemia, *Metabolism*, 13, 487–92.

ESBENSHADE, J. H., JR., and SMITH, R. J. (1965) Thiazides and pregnancy: A study of carbohydrate tolerance, *Amer. J. Obstet. Gynec.*, 92, 270–1.

FELDMAN, E., and DIAMOND, S. (1967) Ethacrynic acid. A non-diabetogenic diuretic, *Dis. Chest*, 51, 282–7.

FINNERTY, F. A. (1959) Discussions of special problems of therapy, in *Hypertension*, ed. Moyer, J. H., Philadelphia, p. 653.

GERSHBERG, H., JAVIER, Z., and HULSE, M. (1964) Glucose tolerance in women receiving an ovulatory suppressant‘ *Diabetes*, 13, 378–82.

GOLDNER, M. G., ZAROWITZ, H., and AKGUN, S. (1960) Hyperglycemia and glycosuria due to thiazide derivatives administered in diabetes mellitus, *New Engl. J. Med.*, 262, 403–5.

HAZZARD, W. R., SPIGER, M. J., BAGDADE, J. D., and BIERMAN, E. L. (1969) Studies on the mechanism of increased plasma triglyceride levels induced by oral contraceptives, *New Engl. J. Med.*, **280**, 471–4.

HOWELL, S. L., and TAYLOR, K. W. (1966) Effects of diazoxide on insulin secretion in vitro, *Lancet*, **i**, 128–9.

JONES, I. G., and PICKENS, P. T. (1967) Diabetes mellitus following oral diuretics, *Practitioner*, **199**, 209–10.

KERSHBAUM, A. (1963) Diabetogenic effect of fluorine-containing steroids, *Brit. med. J.*, **2**, 253.

KONIGSTEIN, R. P. (1965) Die Anwendung von Furosemid (Lasix) in der Geriatrie. Mit einem Beitrag zur sogenannten diabetogenen wirkung der Salidiuretika, *Wien. klin. Wschr.*, **77**, 93–7.

KOTLER, M. N., BERMAN, L., and RUBENSTEIN, A. H. (1966) Hypoglycaemia precipitated by propranolol, *Lancet*, **ii**, 1389–90.

KVAM, D. C., and STANTON, H. C. (1964) Studies on diazoxide hyperglycemia, *Diabetes*, **13**, 639–44.

LANCET (1969) Metabolic effects of oral contraceptives, leading article, *Lancet*, **ii**, 783–4.

LEBACQ, E., and MARCQ, M. (1967) A study of the mechanism of ethacrynic acid induced hyperglycemia, *Rev. franç. Étud. clin. biol.*, **12**, 160–2.

MADISON, J. F. (1964) Ketonuria after local steroids in necrobiosis lipoidica, *Arch. Derm.*, **90**, 477–8.

MATSUNAGA, F., KUBO, A., KATAKURA, G., et al. (1963) Steroid diabetes, diabetes mellitus appearing during treatment with pituitary-adrenal hormones, *J. Ther. (Tokyo)*, **45**, 1988–95.

MEADE, B. W., and ROSALKI, S. B. (1961) Neuropathy after thalidomide, *Brit. med. J.*, **2**, 1223.

MILLICHAP, J. G. (1965) Anticonvulsant drugs, in *Physiological Pharmacology*, Vol. 2, eds. Root, W. S., and Hofmann, F. S., New York, pp. 97–173.

MILLICHAP, J. G. (1969) Hyperglycemic effect of diphenylhydantoin, *New Engl. J. Med.*, **281**, 447.

OKUN, R., RUSSELL, R. P., and WILSON, W. R. (1963) Use of diazoxide with trichlormethiazide for hypertension, *Arch. intern. Med.*, **112**, 882–8.

PAROS, N. L. (1964) Side effect of oral contraceptives, *Brit. med. J.*, **1**, 630.

PENGELLY, C. R. (1965) Diabetes mellitus and cyclophosphamide, *Brit. med. J.*, **1**, 1312–13.

PETERS, B. H., and SAMAAN, N. A. (1969) Hyperglycemia with relative hypoinsulinemia in diphenylhydantoin toxicity, *New Engl. J. Med.*, **281**, 91–2.

PETERSON, W. F., STEEL, M. W., JR., and COYNE, R. V. (1966) Analysis of the effect of ovulatory suppressants on glucose tolerance, *Amer. J. Obstet. Gynec.*, **95**, 484–8.

REVENO, W. S., and ROSENBAUM, H. (1968) Propranolol and hypoglycaemia, *Lancet*, **i**, 920.

ROEDIGER, P. M., ALDEN, J., BEARDWOOD, D., and HUTCHISON, J. C. (1964) Benzothiadiazines and diabetes mellitus, II. Comparison of hyperglycemic effects of bendroflumethiazide and chlorothiazide in hypertensive patients with diabetes mellitus, *Curr. ther. Res.*, **6**, 670–6.

RUNYAN, J. W., JR. (1962) Influence of thiazide diuretics on carbohydrate metabolism in patients with mild diabetes, *New Engl. J. Med.*, **267**, 541–3.

SAMOLS, E., and MARKS, V. (1966) The treatment of hypoglycaemia with diazoxide, *Proc. roy. Soc. Med.*, **59**, 811–14.

SCHUBERT, G. E., and SCHULTE, H. D. (1963) Contribution to the clinical picture of steroid diabetes, *Dtsch. med. Wschr.*, **88**, 1175–88.

SELTZER, H. S., and ALLEN, E. W. (1965) Inhibition of insulin secretion in diazoxide diabetes, *Diabetes*, **14**, 439.

SHAPIRO, A. P., BENEDEK, T. G., and SMALL, J. L. (1961) Effects of thiazides on carbohydrate metabolism in patients with hypertension, *New Engl. J. Med.*, **265**, 1028–33.

SUGAR, S. N. J. (1961) Diabetic acidosis during chlorothiazide therapy, *J. Amer. med. Ass.*, **175**, 618–19.

SUSSMAN, K. E., STJERNHOLM, M. R., and VAUGHAN, G. D. (1967) Propranolol and hypoglycaemia, *Lancet*, **i**, 626.

SZABO, A. J., COLE, H. S., and GRIMALDI, R. D. (1970) Glucose tolerance in gestational diabetic women during and after treatment with a combination-type oral contraceptive, *New Engl. J. Med.*, **282**, 646–50.

TABACHNIK, I. I., GULBENKIAN, A., and SEIDMAN, F. (1964) The effect of a benzothiadiazine, diazoxide, on carbohydrate metabolism, *Diabetes*, **13**, 408–18.

TAYLOR, M. B., and KASS, M. B. (1968) Effect of oral contraceptives on glucose metabolism, *Amer. J. Obstet. Gynec.*, **102**, 1035–8.

TOIVONEN, S., and MUSTALA, O. (1966) Diabetogenic action of frusemide, *Brit. med. J.*, **1**, 920–1.

UNGER, R. H. (1966) Treatment of hypoglycemia associated with pancreatic and extrapancreatic tumours, *Mod. Treatm.*, **3**, 386–98.

VESSEY, M. P. (1970) Thrombosis and the Pill, *Prescribers' J.*, **10**, 1–7.

WAINE, H., FRIEDEN, E. H., CAPLAN, H. I., and COLE, T. (1963) Metabolic effects of Enovid in rheumatic patients, *Arthr. and Rheum.*, **6**, 796.

WALES, J. K., VIKTORA, J. F., and WOLFF, F. W. (1967) The effect of hydrochlorothiazide in normal subjects receiving high fat or high carbohydrate diets, *Amer. J. med. Sci.*, **254**, 499–505.

WILKINS, R. W. (1959) New drugs for the treatment of hypertension, *Ann. intern. Med.*, **50**, 1–10.

WOLFF, F. W., and PARMLEY, W. W. (1963) Aetiological factors in benzothiadiazine hyperglycaemia, *Lancet*, **ii**, 69.

WOLFF, F. W., PARMLEY, W. W., WHITE, K., and OKUN, R. (1963) Drug-induced diabetes. Diabetogenic activity of long-term administration of benzothiadiazines, *J. Amer. med. Ass.*, **185**, 568–74.

WOODBURY, D. M. (1952) Effects of chronic administration of anticonvulsant drugs alone and in combination with desoxycorticosterone on electroshock seizure threshold and tissue electrolytes, *J. Pharmacol. exp. Ther.*, **105**, 46–57.

WYNN, V., and DOAR, J. W. H. (1966) Some effects of oral contraceptives on carbohydrate metabolism, *Lancet*, **ii**, 715–19.

WYNN, V., and DOAR, J. W. H. (1969) Some effects of oral contraceptives on carbohydrate metabolism, *Lancet*, **ii**, 761–6.

WYNN, V., DOAR, J. W. H., and MILLS, G. L. (1966) Some effects of oral contraceptives on serum-lipid and lipoprotein levels, *Lancet*, **ii**, 720–3.

WYNN, V., DOAR, J. W. H., MILLS, G. L., and STOKES, T. (1969) Fasting serum triglyceride, cholesterol, and lipoprotein levels during oral contraceptive therapy, *Lancet*, **ii**, 756–60.

ZATUCHNI, J., and KORDASZ, F. (1961) The diabetogenic effect of thiazide diuretics, *Amer. J. Cardiol.*, **7**, 565–7.

12

DISTURBANCES OF WATER AND MINERAL BALANCE

DRUG-INDUCED SALT AND WATER RETENTION

Corticosteroids

Salt and water retention are so common in patients treated with corticosteroids as to be almost regarded as normal. The sodium and water retention caused by these steroids are causative factors in the weight gain, oedema and hypertension that frequently develop in treated patients. Cardiac failure has been reported and, as a sequel to this, hypervolaemia and concomitant hypertension.

In the past, corticosteroids were classified as either mineralocorticoids or glucocorticoids depending on the emphasis of their metabolic effects. Both properties were shared to a greater or lesser degree by all the older steroids although the sodium retaining properties of cortisone, deoxycorticosterone and aldosterone are far greater than those of, for example, prednisone and prednisolone and the newer steroid analogues, which have been specifically designed to avoid gross effects on salt and water metabolism (see D'Arcy, 1963).

Oral Contraceptives

Salt and water retention is a side-effect of combined oestrogen-progestogen oral contraceptive medication and leads to weight gain and oedema. This effect is almost certainly due to the oestrogen component since it has long been known that patients on oestrogen treatment frequently complain of fluid retention. The progestogen component probably plays little direct action in fluid retention since progestogens, in high dosage, are known to promote sodium excretion.

Worsening of existing hypertension has been associated with oral contraceptives, for example, Fuhr (1964) reported that *Anovlar* (norethisterone plus ethinyl-oestradiol) taken for 20 days in each cycle caused severe hypertensive encephalopathy in a woman already known to have hypertension and chronic pyelonephritis. However, recently hypertension has been reported as developing *de novo* during oral contraceptive medication in an increasing number of cases (Laragh *et al.*, 1967; Woods, 1967; Weinberger *et al.*, 1968; Harris, 1969; McEwan, 1969).

Walter and Lim (1969) studied cardiovascular dynamics in women receiving oral contraceptive therapy. They concluded that the blood-pressure pattern was determined by several factors involving a balance between increased cardiac output, the degree of

peripheral vasodilatation, increased fluid retention, and the interplay between the renal and adrenal hormonal system. Disruption of this balance could result in hypertension. Fluid retention is therefore certainly a factor of consequence in the development of a hypertensive state. Fortunately regular checks of blood pressure and patient's weight are now carried out at most family planning clinics in the management of oral oestrogen-progestogen contraception. These can do much to prevent the disruption of the balance that would otherwise lead to hypertension.

PHENYLBUTAZONE AND OXYPHEN-BUTAZONE (p-HYDROXYPHENYLBUTA-ZONE)

Weight gain and oedema due to sodium and fluid retention are common side-effects of phenylbutazone and its hydroxylated metabolite, oxyphenbutazone. Although there is considerable variation from patient to patient, oedema may occur in up to 10 per cent of patients; this usually occurs during the first days of treatment.

This fluid retention may precipitate cardiac failure and even fatal pulmonary oedema, especially in patients with cardiac disease. These cardiac complications are most likely to occur in the first 2 weeks of treatment (Shafar, 1965).

Mild to moderate hypertension can occur; Prescott (1968) has reviewed the literature and has cited cases of toxicity of both agents on the cardiovascular system.

CARBENOXOLONE SODIUM

Baron and Nabarro (1968) reported that administration of carbenoxolone sodium, 300 mg per day for 21 days, to four patients with peptic ulcer, resulted in weight gain due to sodium and chloride retention. Hypokalaemia without appreciable change in potassium balance was also observed.

Hypertension, oedema or potassium loss has been reported in up to 50 per cent of patients receiving 300 mg of carbenoxolone sodium daily (Doll *et al.*, 1965; Horwich and Galloway, 1965; Turpie and Thompson, 1965).

One case has been observed in which severe hypokalaemia, flaccid paralysis in all four limbs and myoglobinuria developed on the 38th day of therapy (Mohamed *et al.*, 1966). Another case in which sudden weakness in the lower limbs and back developed after

FIG. 12.1. *Structural relationship between some compounds causing salt and water retention*

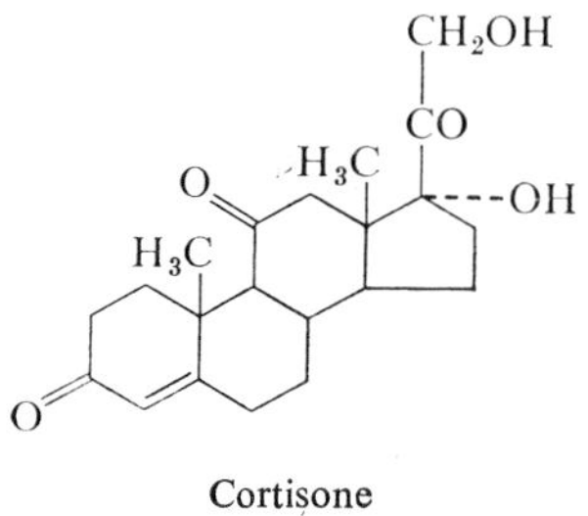

Cortisone

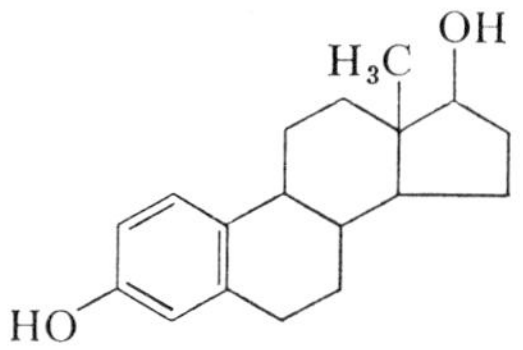

Oestradiol

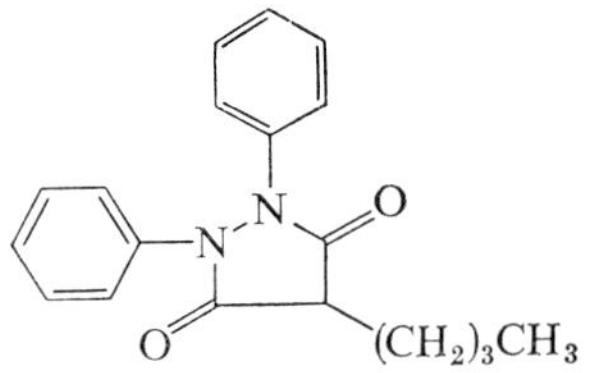

Phenylbutazone

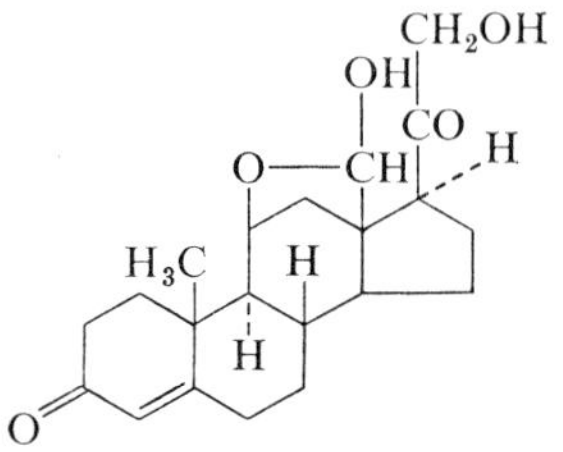

Aldosterone

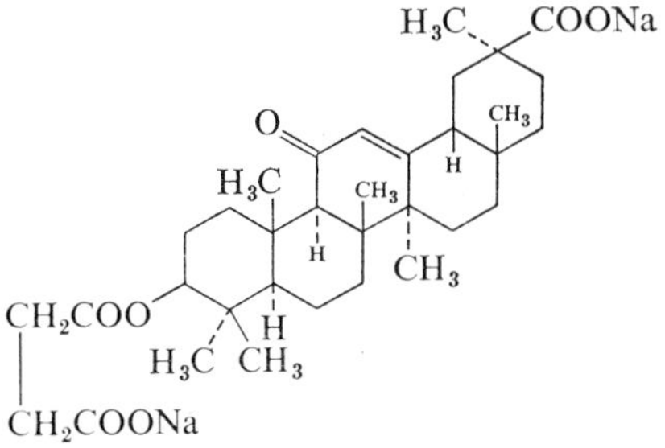

Carbenoxolone sodium
(disodium salt of glycyrrhetinic acid hydrogen succinate)

6 weeks' therapy of 200 mg/day of *Duogastrone* was also associated with marked hypokalaemia (Forshaw, 1969).

A formal metabolic study by Baron and associates (1969) of carbenoxolone sodium 300 mg/day was performed for 17 days on a woman with gastric ulcer who in a previous 21-day trial, on a 52-mEq sodium diet, showed weight gain, retention, and rise in plasma sodium and chloride concentrations, as well as hypokalaemia without change in potassium balance. In the second trial sodium intake was restricted to 26 mEq/day; while plasma electrolyte changes of lesser degree still occurred, there was no retention of water, sodium or chloride. Aldosterone secretion in the control period was 202 μg/24 hours, and fell to 74 μg/24 hours after carbenoxolone but plasma renin was unchanged.

These effects are thought to be due to an aldosterone-like action and certainly there is justification for this since carbenoxolone (glycyrrhetinic acid hydrogen succinate) has structural similarity to aldosterone. In the early days of their experimental study, the active isomers of glycyrrhetinic acid (a non-steroid triterpene) were all designated with a mineralocorticoid action, indeed control of Addison's disease with glycyrrhetinic acid was reported.

The present view, however, is that glycyrrhetinic acid and its derivatives powerfully inhibit the enzyme systems which inactivate intrinsic aldosterone and cortisol from the adrenal cortex, and that they exert their effect on water and electrolyte balance by this mechanism rather than by a direct mineralocorticoid action.

The results obtained by Baron and his associates (1969) in their second trial suggest that, with sodium deprivation, aldosterone secretion was suppressed by a mechanism which was not renin-mediated, possibly hypokalaemia.

A direct effect of carbenoxolone sodium on the adrenal cortex has been postulated by Mattingly and colleagues (1970) who investigated plasma 11-hydroxycorticoid levels after oral carbenoxolone sodium. They found increased levels in eight patients with duodenal ulcers and a similar rise was seen in one patient with sarcoidosis whose pituitary ACTH secretion had been acutely suppressed with dexamethasone. No such rise, however, was seen in three patients suffering from adrenal insufficiency. The authors concluded that carbenoxolone sodium acted directly on the adrenal cortex causing an increased production of corticosteroids.

FIGURE 12.1 illustrates the structural relationship between carbenoxolone, aldosterone, phenylbutazone and the oestrogen and corticosteroid nuclei, all of which produce mineralocorticoid effects.

DRUG-INDUCED DISORDERS OF CALCIUM METABOLISM

HEPARIN OSTEOPOROSIS

Six patients receiving heparin in daily doses of 150–300 mg for 6 months and longer, developed spontaneous fractures of vertebrae or ribs. Biopsy showed a soft bony matrix. In patients who received less than 100 mg heparin daily, no osteoporosis was found (Griffith *et al.*, 1965).

Jaffe and Willis (1965) reported a case of a 41-year-old man who received 200 mg heparin subcutaneously daily, over a period of 13 months, after which time it was observed that the patient had developed multiple fractures.

CORTICOSTEROID OSTEOPOROSIS

Administration of adrenal steroids leads to mobilization of calcium and phosphorus; osteoporosis is one of the common severe adverse effects of long-term treatment and occurs with all the adrenal steroids. An increased excretion of calcium has been demonstrated but the mechanism based on these changes is obscure.

Pathological fractures and vertebral collapse are most likely complications of steroid therapy where steroid-induced osteoporosis is superimposed on a senile osteoporosis.

Associated with the problem of osteoporosis is the occurrence of aseptic bone necrosis localized mainly to the femoral head. The presenting symptoms are always vague and involve pain in the hip, limitation of movement and slowly worsening symptoms. The following reports of cases illustrate the extent of this iatrogenic effect of corticosteroid therapy; other cases have been reviewed by De Lange and Doorenbos (1968).

Sutton *et al.* (1963) described eight male cases of aseptic bone necrosis of the femoral head; their ages ranged from 20–25 years. The range of dosage was 25–120 mg cortisone daily. The onset of pain and characteristic X-ray changes commenced from $1\frac{1}{2}$–29 months after starting therapy. Five of the eight had bilateral signs. One also had a destructive process of the humoral head.

Boksenbaum and Mendelson (1963) described the case of an 18-year-old woman who was treated for widespread pemphigus vulgaris before the birth of her first child. After a starting dose of 120 mg prednisolone daily, this was reduced to 75 mg. Thereafter, the patient was finally weaned off steroids and only took 15 mg intermittently for some days if new skin bullae appeared. After 2 years, typical bilateral aseptic necrosis of the femoral heads was diagnosed.

Velayos *et al.* (1964) reported nine patients who developed clinical and radiographic evidence of aseptic necrosis of the femoral head while on high dosage of corticoids. Two patients also had necrosis of the humoral head.

A 55-year-old woman who took 10–60 mg prednisolone daily for pemphigus, was reported by Epstein *et al.* (1965) to have developed bilateral necrosis of the head of the femur and the humerus.

Early recognition of symptoms of aseptic necrosis of the femoral and humoral heads may permit restoration with a regime of rest of the joint and cessation of steroid therapy. Unfortunately, this iatrogenic effect of corticoids is not restricted to systemic dosage since joint changes have been reported after intra-articular administration of corticosteroids (Le Ray Steinberg *et al.*, 1962); they include intra-articular fractures, secondary callus formation, cysts and active endochondrial ossification.

DIURETICS AND CALCIUM METABOLISM

In contrast to the increased excretion of calcium induced by heparin and corticosteroids, Lichtwitz and associates (1961) reported that the thiazide diuretic, hydroflumethiazide, reduced urinary calcium excretion. This was first noticed in a patient with Paget's disease who was given the drug in the hope that some relief of bone pain might follow changes in bone blood flow as a consequence of diuresis. The patient's symptoms were unaffected, but the urinary calcium loss per day fell to 50 per cent of the normal amount. It was subsequently shown by Lichtwitz *et al.* (1961) that such a fall in urinary calcium was due to increased tubular reabsorption of calcium and was a property of all thiazide diuretics. These findings have been confirmed and treatment with thiazide diuretics has been recommended for the control of idiopathic hypercalcinuria (Yendt *et al.*, 1966) and for immobilization osteoporosis (Rose, 1966).

However, in a recent publication, Parfitt (1969) has drawn attention to a hazard of using thiazide diuretics in treating osteoporosis or hypercalcinuria. Thiazides were given to a 21-year-old woman with idiopathic, juvenile osteoporosis treated with calciferol. Three to four days after commencing treatment, symptomatic hypercalcaemia developed (calcium level 12·6 mg/100 ml) and this was accompanied by a rise in blood urea. Restoration of previous calcium levels and disappearance of symptoms rapidly followed discontinuation of the drug.

Parfitt further examined ten other patients; pre-existing hypercalcaemia was exacerbated in two patients with primary hyperparathyroidism. In the other eight, the change in plasma calcium level did not correlate with the magnitude of the fall in output of urinary calcium, so that effects of thiazides, other than the hypocalcinuria, may have contributed to the hypercalcaemia. He concluded therefore that thiazide diuretics should be given with caution to actual or potential hypercalcaemic patients, and to those with diseases causing accelerated bone absorption in whom increased excretion of calcium by the kidney may be preventing or delaying the onset of hypercalcaemia.

Some experimental studies in animals and human volunteers have revealed further evidence of the nature and extent of the involvement of the thiazides in calcium metabolism. For example, Seitz and Jaworski (1964) reported a significant rise of 0·6 mg/100 ml in plasma calcium in seven normal subjects following thiazide therapy. This appeared to be a transient phenomenon and did not persist after the third day of therapy.

Kleeman *et al.* (1961) have suggested that thiazides potentiate the action of parathyroid hormone on both kidney and bone. In this context, it is of interest to note that hypoparathyroid patients are resistant to the hypocalcinuric action of thiazides (Parfitt, 1969).

Other studies of a related nature have shown that diuretics other than thiazides, e.g. frusemide, a monosulphamyl derivative, ethacrynic acid, a desulphamyl compound, and triamterene, an aminopteridine, do not provoke a fall in urinary calcium; indeed their effect is exactly the reverse and significant hypercalcinuria is produced by these diuretics. For example, Duarte (1967) showed that an increased clearance of ultrafilterable calcium occurred in dogs infused with frusemide, an effect directly opposite to that seen with thiazide diuretics. Hänze and Seyberth (1967) confirmed these findings of increased calcium clearance in their studies on normal volunteers given frusemide intravenously. They also observed similar effects with intravenous ethacrynic acid and oral triamterene.

Tambyah and Lim (1969) gave oral frusemide to 14 normal volunteers and found that significant hypercalcinuria occurred in all of them. This was not due to any change in glomerular filtration, but was due to a decreased tubular reabsorption of calcium.

The significance of hypercalcinuria caused by frusemide, ethacrynic acid, and triamterene, and the hypocalcinuria induced by thiazide diuretics in the pathogenesis of any clinical condition is uncertain. Nevertheless they could cause confusion in the diagnosis of parathyroid dysfunction and for this reason have been discussed in this context.

FIGURE 12.2 shows the structural differences in the formulae of hydrochlorothiazide, a parent member of the thiazide series, frusemide, ethacrynic acid, and triamterene.

FIG. 12.2. *Structural formulae of some diuretics with significant effects on calcium metabolism*

Ca_E = calcium excretion
Ca_R = calcium retention
Hydrochlorothiazide (Ca_R all thiazides)

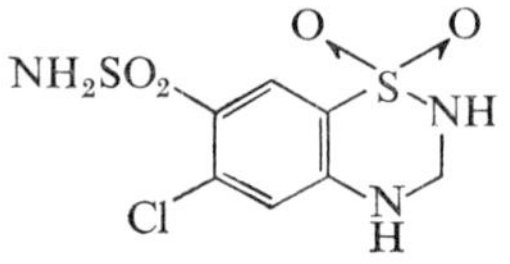

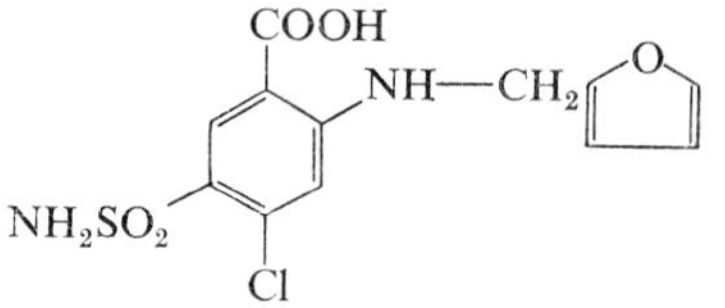

Frusemide (Ca_E)
(fursemide)

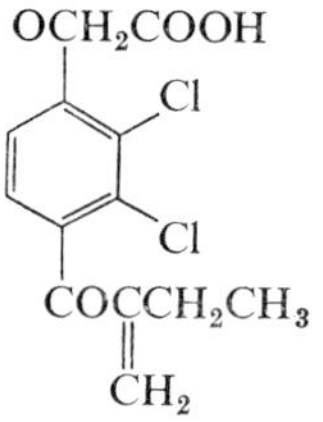

Ethacrynic acid (Ca_E)

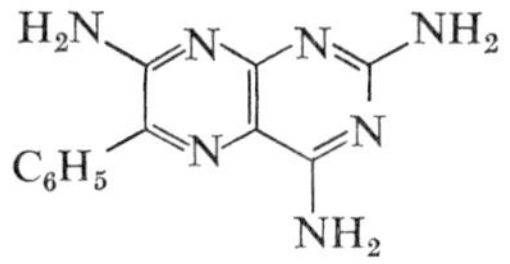

Triamterene (Ca_E)

RECOMMENDED FURTHER READING

BEYER, K. H., and BAER, J. E. (1961) Physiological basis for the action of newer diuretic agents, *Pharmacol. Rev.*, **13**, 517–62.

WILSON, G. M. (1963) Diuretics, *Brit. med. J.*, **1**, 285–92.

REFERENCES

BARON, J. H., and NABARRO, J. D. N. (1968) in *Symposium on Carbenoxolone Sodium*, eds. Robson, J. M., and Sullivan, F. M., London, p. 127.

BARON, J. H., NABARRO, J. D. N., SLATER, J. D. H., and TUFFLEY, R. (1969) Metabolic studies, aldosterone secretion rate, and plasma renin after carbenoxolone sodium, *Brit. med. J.*, **2**, 793–5.

BOKSENBAUM, M., and MENDELSON, C. G. (1963) Aseptic necrosis of the femoral head associated with steroid therapy, *J. Amer. med. Ass.*, **184**, 262–5.

D'ARCY, P. F. (1963) Steroid hormones and their synthetic analogues, *Medica Britannica*, **3**, 3–10, 35–42.

DE LANGE, W. E., and DOORENBOS, H. (1968) Hormones and synthetic substitutes, in *Side Effects of Drugs*, Vol. VI, eds. Meyler, L., and Herxheimer, A., Excerpta Medica Foundation, Amsterdam, pp. 383–421.

DOLL, R., HILL, I. D., and HUTTON, C. F. (1965) Treatment of gastric ulcer with carbenoxolone sodium plus oestrogens, *Gut*, **6**, 19–24.

DUARTE, C. G. (1967) Effects of furosemide and ethacrynic acid on the renal clearance of phosphate, ultrafiltrable calcium and magnesium, *Clin. Res.*, **15**, 357.

EPSTEIN, N. H., TUFFANELLI, D. L., and EPSTEIN, J. H. (1965) Avascular bone necrosis. A complication of long term corticosteroid therapy, *Arch. Derm.*, **92**, 178–80.

FORSHAW, J. (1969) Muscle paresis and hypokalaemia after treatment with Duogastrone, *Brit. med. J.*, **2**, 674.

FUHR, S. L. H. M. VAN DER (1964) Hypertensie-encefalopathie door Anovlar, *Ned. T. Geneesk*, **108**, 670.

GRIFFITH, G. C., NICHOLS, G., JR., ASHER, J. D., and FLANAGAN, B. (1965) Heparin osteoporosis, *J. Amer. med. Ass.*, **193**, 91–4.

HÄNZE, S., and SEYBERTH, H. (1967) Untersuchungen zur Wirkung der Diuretica Furosemid, Etacrynsaure und Triamteren auf der renale Magnesium und Calcium ausscheidung, *Klin. Wschr.*, **45**, 313–14.

HARRIS, P. W. R. (1969) Malignant hypertension associated with oral contraceptives, *Lancet*, **ii**, 466–7.

HORWICH, L., and GALLOWAY, R. (1965) Treatment of gastric ulceration with carbenoxolone sodium: Clinical and radiological evaluation, *Brit. med. J.*, **2**, 1274–7.

JAFFE, M. D., and WILLIS, P. W. (1965) Multiple fractures associated with long term heparin therapy, *J. Amer. med. Ass.*, **193**, 158–60.

KLEEMAN, C. R., BERNSTEIN, D., ROCKNEY, R., DOWLING, J. T., and MAXWELL, M. H. (1961) Studies on renal clearance of diffusable calcium and the role of the parathyroids in its regulation, *Yale J. Biol. Med.*, **34**, 1–30.

LARAGH, J. H., SEALEY, J. E., LEDINGHAM, J. G. G., and NEWTON, M. A. (1967) Oral contraceptives. Renin, aldosterone and high blood pressure, *J. Amer. med. Ass.*, **201**, 918–22.

LE RAY STEINBERG, C., DUTHIE, R. B., and PIVA, A. E. (1962) Charcot-like atrophy following intra-articular hydrocortisone, *Arthr. and Rheum.*, **5**, 659–60.

LICHTWITZ, A., PARLIER, R., HIOCO, D., PROUZET, CH., MIRAVET, L. F., and SÈZE, S. DE (1960) Hypocalcinuria caused by hydroflumethiazide, *Path. et Biol.*, **8**, 1873–7.

LICHTWITZ, A., PARLIER, R., SÈZE, S. DE, HIOCO, D., and MIRAVET, L. F. (1961) The hypocalcinuric effect of diuretic sulphonamides, *Sem. Hôp. Paris*, **37**, 2350–62.

MCEWAN, J. (1969) Oral contraceptives and hypertension, *Lancet*, **ii**, 594.

MATTINGLY, D., TYLER, C., and BILTON, E. (1970) Plasma 11-hydroxycorticoid levels after carbenoxolone sodium, *Brit. med. J.*, **3**, 498–500.

MOHAMED, S. D., CHAPMAN, R. S., and CROOKS, J. (1966) Hypokalaemia, flaccid quadruparesis and myoglobinuria with carbenoxolone, *Brit. med. J.*, **1**, 1581–2.

PARFITT, A. M. (1969) Chlorthiazide-induced hypercalcaemia in juvenile osteoporosis and hyperparathyroidism, *New Engl. J. Med.*, **281**, 55–9.

PRESCOTT, L. F. (1968) Antipyretic analgesic drugs, in *Side Effects of Drugs*, Vol. VI, eds. Meyler, L., and Herxheimer, A., Excerpta Medica Foundation, Amsterdam, pp. 101–39.

ROSE, G. A. (1966) Immobilisation osteoporosis: Study of extent, severity and treatment with bendrofluazide, *Brit. J. Surg.*, **53**, 769–74.

SEITZ, H., and JAWORSKI, Z. F. (1964) Effect of hydrochlorothiazide on serum and urinary calcium and urinary citrate, *Canad. med. Ass. J.*, **90**, 414–20.

SHAFAR, J. (1965) Phenylbutazone-induced pericarditis, *Brit. med. J.*, **2**, 795–7.

SUTTON, R. D., BENEDEK, T. G., and EDWARDS, G. A. (1963) Aseptic bone necrosis and corticosteroid therapy, *Arch. intern. Med.*, **112**, 594–602.

TAMBYAH, J. A., and LIM, M. K. L. (1969) Effect of frusemide on calcium excretion, *Brit. med. J.*, **1**, 751–2.

TURPIE, A. G. G., and THOMPSON, T. J. (1965) Carbenoxolone sodium in the treatment of gastric ulcer with special reference to side effects, *Gut*, **6**, 591–4.

VELAYOS, E., LEIDHOLT, J. D., and SMYTH, C. J. (1964) Steroid arthropathy, *Arthr. and Rheum.*, **7**, 758.

WALTER, W. A. W., and LIM, Y. L. (1969) Cardiovascular dynamics in women receiving oral contraceptive therapy, *Lancet*, **ii**, 879–81.

WEINBERGER, M. H., DOWDY, A. J., NOKES, G. W., and LUETSCHER, J. A. (1968) Reversible increases in plasma renin activity, aldosterone secretion and blood pressure in women taking oral contraceptive preparations, *Clin. Res.*, **16**, 150.

WOODS, J. W. (1967) Oral contraceptives and hypertension, *Lancet*, **ii**, 653–4.

YENDT, E. R., GAGNÉ, R. J., and COHANIM, M. (1966) The effects of thiazides in idiopathic hypercalciuria, *Amer. J. med. Sci.*, **251**, 449–60.

13

ENDOCRINE DYSFUNCTION

CORTICOSTEROID-INDUCED ADRENAL HYPOFUNCTION

Administration of corticosteroids for other than short periods of time results in suppression of adrenocortical activity and induces atrophy of the adrenal cortex. The patient is then at special risk and an adrenal insufficiency state can be caused by, for example, an omitted dose, a dose reduced below the physiological requirement or the exposure of the patient to a stressful episode when the cortex is unable to supply the endogenous cortisol required of it.

Surgical and anaesthetic trauma are perhaps the best examples of controlled stressful episodes, and historically the first report came in 1952 when a 34-year-old man who had been treated for 18 months with cortisone acetate for rheumatoid arthritis, had a cup arthroplasty on his hip. He developed irreversible shock and died (Fraser et al., 1952). Attention was drawn immediately to the fact that this man had died as a result of adrenocortical failure due to adrenal suppression by exogenous corticosteroids. Nevertheless, there were many subsequent reports in the early literature of severe shock developing not only in patients having corticosteroid therapy at the time of surgery, but also in those who had stopped treatment weeks or months before (Lewis et al., 1953; Salassa et al., 1953; Downs and Cooper, 1955; Harnagel and Kramer, 1955; Kittredge, 1955; Hayes, 1956; Hayes and Kushlan, 1956; Allanby, 1957; Plumer and Armstrong, 1957; Slaney and Brooke, 1957; Shneewind and Cole, 1959).

Prolonged administration of steroids reduces the weight of the adrenal glands and causes adrenal atrophy. The decrease in adrenal mass is accompanied by a loss of physiological sensitivity to pituitary corticotrophin (ACTH), which can be readily shown by a diminished output of adrenal steroids as compared with a normal gland after a standard dose of ACTH. This adrenal suppression is due to the administered steroids inhibiting the release of ACTH from the adenohypophysis, and is in keeping with the concept of a feedback homeostatic mechanism in which the circulating corticosteroid level regulates the rate of ACTH release from the pituitary (Sayers, 1950).

All corticosteroids cause pituitary inhibition of corticotrophin secretion; on a weight-for-weight basis some have a greater inhibitory action than others, but since the more potent ones are usually given in smaller dosage than the less potent parent steroids, cortisone and cortisol, the resultant degree of pituitary inhibition is about the same.

Adrenal weight reduction and histological changes are only a rough guide to the degree of suppression, which can be assessed more accurately by studying the response of the cortex to stimulation with a standard dose of corticotrophin and measuring the output of adrenocortical steroids. The degree of adrenocortical suppression may be more related to the duration of corticosteroid treatment than to the dosage. There are, however, wide individual variations in the response of patients' adrenals to corticosteroid dosage and this probably explains why some patients previously treated with steroids react badly to surgery or other stress while others do not.

In man there is little information on how long adrenal suppression persists after stopping treatment with corticosteroids, and such data as there are indicate a wide individual variation. Some patients may respond normally to corticotrophin within 4 days of stopping treatment, whereas Christy et al. (1956) found in a child of 11, who had had 75 mg of cortisone daily for a year, that 20 units of corticotrophin gel per day for 20 days failed to restore normal adrenal responsiveness.

Clinical experience also shows that there may be a very long delay before normal responsiveness returns. Patients who have stopped steroid treatment for as long as $4\frac{1}{2}$ to 24 months may develop irreversible shock after even minor surgical procedures, and this has led to the general adoption of special pre-operative preparation for any patient who has had steroid treatment.

Corticosteroids can cross the placental barrier and cause foetal adrenal failure. Bongiovanni and McPadden (1960), reviewed 260 pregnancies in which corticosteroids had been administered to the mothers. One case of adrenocortical failure was found; the mother had received 5,000 mg of cortisone during pregnancy. The baby was in a state of collapse for the first 72 hours after birth but eventually recovered.

A second case has been reported by Oppenheimer (1964); a male infant weighing 1·49 kg was born after 6 months' gestation. The mother suffered from Boeck's sarcoidosis and had been treated with high doses of prednisolone. The infant died shortly after birth. At autopsy, the adrenals were small, the outer zone showed necrosis, haemorrhage and cyst formation. In this infant the development and function of the adrenals had been arrested by the large doses of steroids given to the mother. After the child's birth, deprivation of the circulating maternal steroids precipitated adrenal insufficiency because of the hypoplastic cortex.

DRUG-INDUCED MYXOEDEMA

THALIDOMIDE

In 1959 Murdoch and Campbell studied the effects of thalidomide (2-phthalimidoglutarimide) on I^{131} uptake by the thyroid gland in nine euthyroid patients. The results from this investigation indicated that thalidomide had mild but definite antithyroid action. These workers did not advance any hypothesis to explain the mode of action of thalidomide's antithyroid activity but did issue a clear warning that it would be unjustified to use this drug as a long-term sedative or hypnotic.

Despite this relatively early work thalidomide was used in the very indications that these workers had warned against. Alexander (1961) described a case of myxoedema following long-term therapy with thalidomide, and Simpson (1962) described a further two cases of myxoedema induced by thalidomide; Lillicrap (1962) reported another case.

In the cases reported, the onset of the myxoedema occurred within 2 or 3 months of commencing therapy, and was described as of acute onset. Lillicrap's description is very detailed; 2 months after starting therapy the patient, a 49-year-old woman, complained of lethargy, intolerance of cold, rough dry skin and deepening of the voice. This patient was started on thyroid but continued to take thalidomide. One year later she stopped taking thyroid and her symptoms returned, and a month after stopping the thyroid the thalidomide was also stopped; it was then that her thyroid function began to improve and eventually returned to normal. This patient also developed the typical thalidomide-induced peripheral neuritis after 6 months on the drug; these symptoms did not disappear when thalidomide was stopped.

The thalidomide story is now very well known, but this aspect of thalidomide iatrogenesis is worthy of mention since if any series of cases were needed to illustrate lack of awareness of drug-induced disease, then certainly these present reports showed that the potential spectrum of thalidomide-induced disease was highlighted some 4 years before the appearance of the first reported clinical disaster.

SALICYLATES

Thyroid function may be depressed by salicylates; this has been demonstrated both in animal studies and in patients. Hetzel and associates (1963) showed that salicylates caused a fall in plasma-bound iodine while Myhill and Hales (1963) showed that there was a fall in plasma-bound iodine in six euthyroid and eight hyperthyroid subjects receiving 6·5 grams of calcium salicylate for four days.

The literature on this effect of salicylates has been reviewed by Prescott (1968). The general picture is that salicylates lower the plasma protein-bound iodine and they decrease the level of circulating pituitary thyroid stimulating hormone (TSH). This depression in TSH release corresponds with a rise in free circulating thyroxine which is caused by the salicylates displacing thyroxine from thyroid binding pre-albumin. The increased level of circulating free thyroxine is thought to act on the pituitary-thyroid feedback to reduce the output of TSH (Good et al., 1965; Marshal et al., 1965).

Of all the salicylates used in therapy, the dosage of para-aminosalicylic acid in tuberculosis is the greatest. It is therefore not surprising that Marchese et al. (1963) reported goitre with myxoedema as a rare complication of this therapy.

Generally, however, the effects of salicylates on thyroid function would seem to be of minor clinical importance although results of thyroid function tests may be influenced by concomitant salicylate ingestion.

PHENYLBUTAZONE

The administration of phenylbutazone may inhibit the uptake of iodine by the thyroid. The development of a non-toxic goitre in a man with psoriatic arthritis has been reported by Benedek (1962). The goitre was reversible and related to phenylbutazone therapy. It did not occur while he received either phenylbutazone or vitamin A separately, but occurred during each of two periods in which both drugs were administered. No effect on thyroid size and function was seen in two other men who received the same drugs in the same combination for a similar length of time. Therefore, it seemed likely that not only the combination of these drugs, each of which is known to cause hypothyroidism, but an idiosyncrasy was also involved in the above patient.

There have, however, been other cases in which phenylbutazone has been implicated in a thyroid-inhibiting action without involvement of vitamin A. These cases have been reviewed by Prescott (1968) and it would seem that the goitrogenic effects of phenylbutazone are more marked in patients with pre-existing thyroid enlargement.

Animal studies have confirmed the thyroid-inhibiting action of phenylbutazone and it is interesting to note that the lethal toxicity of phenylbutazone in these studies was reduced by about one-half by simultaneous administration of tri-iodothyronine (Eger and Fernholz, 1965); this may, however, have been due to increased metabolism of the phenylbutazone rather than to any reduction of toxicity due to thyroid inhibition.

IODIDE-CONTAINING THERAPEUTIC AGENTS

Administration of iodine salts may be associated on the one hand with the development of hyperthyroidism, and on the other with the appearance of myxoedema and the development of non-toxic goitre. The development of goitre is not uncommon (Begg and Hall, 1963; Frey, 1964; Helgason, 1964; Horden et al., 1964). Several cases of potassium iodide-induced goitres with or without hypothyroidism have been reported after prolonged ingestion of iodine-containing drugs. In particular the use of iodine-containing mixtures in chronic bronchitis and asthma has been incriminated. Frey

TABLE 13.1

IODINE-CONTAINING PREPARATIONS CURRENTLY AVAILABLE AS PRESCRIPTION OR
OVER-THE-COUNTER ITEMS IN THE UNITED KINGDOM
(Based on MIMS, Vol. 12, No: 6, 1970, and Extra Pharmacopoeia, 25th Edition, 1967)

PREPARATION	IODINE SOURCE	PRESCRIPTION OR OTHERWISE
Anaspasmne elixir	Potassium iodide 300 mg/5 ml	No prescription required
Brovonex elixir	Sodium iodide 333 mg/5 ml	No prescription required
Calcidrine syrup	Calcium iodide 200 mg/5 ml	Prescription required
Caphedrin Iodinata elixir	Iodine 10 mg/5 ml	Prescription required
Ephedrine compound elixir	Sodium iodide approx 53 mg/5 ml	No prescription required
Felsol powders	Iodine 12 mg/powder	No prescription required
Pefflan syrup	—	No prescription required
Trisan syrup	Potassium iodide 302.5 mg/5 ml	No prescription required
Potassium iodide and ammonia mixture B.P.C.	Potassium iodide 75 mg/5 ml	Prescription required
Stramonium and potassium iodide mixture B.P.C.	Potassium iodide 100 mg/5 ml	Prescription required

(1964) described five cases in adults where the dosage totalled 300 grams of potassium iodide per year for one patient and more than 500 grams per year for the other four. Discontinuation of iodide administration was followed by a return of thyroid condition to normal within 1 or 2 months, followed by a short period of slight thyroid hyperactivity. There was no relationship between the size of the thyroid gland and the severity of hypothyroidism.

In a survey of the incidence of non-toxic goitre it was found that in a group of 24 males with non-toxic goitre there were three drug-induced cases. All three patients had taken iodine-containing preparations for asthma over a period of years. One of the patients had, however, also taken the antithyroid drug, carbimazole (Horden *et al.*, 1964).

In one case the occurrence of a small thyroid adenoma was noted after continuous administration of iodide over a period of 3 years; the nodule disappeared completely following withdrawal of iodine (Siegal, 1964).

Twenty-three asthmatic patients who had taken powders containing iodopyrine with or without additional iodide in the form of mixtures or elixirs, were found by Begg and Hall (1963) to have goitre and hypothyroidism either alone or in combination. Iodine medication had continued regularly for 1 to 22 years and the thyroid disorder became evident after periods varying from 6 months to 20 years, most usually after 3 to 8 years of treatment. Several cases recovered when iodine medication was withdrawn and others improved with the aid of thyroid hormone.

Maternal ingestion of iodide has been implicated in the causation of congenital goitre since Parmelee and associates (1940) reported three cases of newborn infants with goitre. All three mothers had taken iodine-containing preparations throughout pregnancy; none of the mothers had goitre. Despite these reports congenital iodide goitres often with hypothyroidism are still occurring and iodide-containing preparations are still freely available to the general public in Great Britain.

Carswell *et al.* (1970) have reviewed the literature on iodide goitre in adults and children and have added eight cases of their own of congenital goitre and hypothyroidism due to maternal ingestion of iodide. These eight cases were seen in the Glasgow area in the past 14 years. There were four deaths, two of which were due to unrelated causes. Two of the survivors were mentally retarded, due presumably to foetal hypothyroidism. These authors strongly recommended that iodide-containing preparations should not be used during pregnancy and that they should cease to be available without prescription. TABLE 13.1 lists the iodide-containing preparations currently available as expectorants or cough suppressants or for use in hay fever.

Doctors should be aware of these risks and take the necessary steps to ensure that their asthmatic and bronchitic patients are warned of these dangers, and that their pregnant patients are especially questioned regarding such self-medication and advised accordingly.

OVARIAN CHANGES AFTER LONG-TERM ORAL CONTRACEPTION

Under the influence of oral contraceptives, the normal ovulatory cycle is changed to a non-ovulatory one. Vaginal bleeding following the discontinuation of oral contraceptive medication for several days between each cycle is, in fact, withdrawal bleeding and not a normal menstruation.

Plate (1968) reported on the histology of ovarian tissue from 11 women who had used ovulation inhibitors for contraception during 4–30 cycles; all the women were under 40 years of age and all had had regular menstruation before they started to use ovulation inhibitors. The specimens of ovarian tissue were obtained at operation in nine cases and post-mortem in two cases. The ovulation inhibitors used and the dosages per tablet were:

Lyndiol	5 mg lynoestrenol and 0·15 mg mes-tranol
Lyndiol 2·5	2·5 mg lynoestrenol and 0·075 mg mestranol
Gynovlar 21	3 mg norethisterone acetate and 0·05 mg ethinyloestradiol
Anovlar	4 mg norethisterone acetate and 0·05 mg ethinyloestradiol
Planovin	4 mg megestrol acetate and 0·05 mg ethinyloestradiol
Orthonovin	2 mg norethisterone and 0·1 mg mes-tranol

No corpora lutea were observed in any of the ovaries, but follicle growth or follicle maturation was present in nine women, hypothecosis in eight women, peri- or intra-follicular bleeding in four women and follicle cysts in 10 women.

The most conspicuous change was fibrosis which occurred in seven women and a thickened tunica albuginea in six women. As a result of this fibrosis, the follicles were sometimes imbedded completely in connective tissue. These changes were most marked in women who had been on oral contraceptive therapy for some considerable time.

Plate (1968) has also reviewed the literature on fibrotic changes associated with oral contraceptive medication. Ryan and colleagues (1964) found a 'focal cortical condensation of stroma in some degree' in about 50 per cent of 18 women investigated; O'Neil (1965) observed a 'definite Stein–Leventhal syndrome' in two women and Graudenz and Beirão de Almeida (1965) found moderate fibrosis, especially in the cortex, even after short-term use of ovulation inhibitors. In one of these patients the enlarged ovaries were reminiscent of the Stein–Leventhal syndrome. Other investigators found thickening of the tunica albuginea (Diddle *et al.*, 1966; Starup, 1967), while Van Roy (1966) described fibrotic granulations in the cortex. These changes were not, however, observed by all investigators, for example Linthorst (1966) did not find any thickening of the tunica albuginea in about 20 ovaries of patients who had been on ovulation inhibitors for a long time. In contrast others (Zussman *et al.*, 1967) found increased fibrosis in 10 patients who had been on oral contraceptives only for 1–3 cycles.

Plate (1968) questioned whether fibrosis occurred in the ovaries when ovulation was inhibited during pregnancy. He therefore examined the ovarian tissue of six women, five with full-term pregnancy and one who was seven months pregnant. There was slight fibrosis in four cases but there was no embedding of the follicles in fibrous tissue. No fibrosis was evident in the other two cases. None of the fibrosis seen in these cases was comparable with the degree of fibrosis seen after the use of oral contraceptives.

Plate (1968) also assumed that since, in the majority of women, regular menstruation returned after oral contraceptives were stopped, the fibrotic changes in the ovaries were reversible. To test this assumption he examined ovarian tissue from six patients who had ceased using oral contraceptives. The fibrosis of the stroma soon disappeared (within 2–5 cycles), and thickening of the tunica albuginea disappeared a little later. He found that the length of time for which oral contraceptives had been taken was of no great importance in this respect.

Having established these points, Plate (1968) then questioned whether fibrosis persists in cases in which amenorrhoea or anovulatory haemorrhage occurs after oral contraceptives have been stopped. Whitelaw *et al.* (1966) reported personal communications from a number of gynaecologists who observed amenorrhoea for up to 18 months after withdrawal of oral contraceptives. They observed that the relative frequency of anovulatory cycles and amenorrhoea after stopping oral contraceptive medication was much higher than had been suspected. The findings of other groups (referenced by Plate, 1968) were in general agreement. There was, however, little evidence in the literature to assist in determining what changes had taken place in the ovaries of women with such amenorrhoea or anovular bleeding. One such report by Lorrain (1966) cited a 22-year-old woman who was amenorrhoeic for 3 months after using *Enovid* for 3 months. Her ovaries were enlarged and contained follicle cysts with hyperthecosis, but no thickening of the tunica albuginea.

Plate (1968) summarized his study by concluding that, although in most cases the fibrotic ovarian changes induced by oral contraceptive medication were reversible, it would be unwise to assume that this was always the case. He therefore advocated that oral contraceptives should be withheld after a specific time (he suggested a year) and resumed only after a few ovulations had occurred. Shearman (1971) has described sixty-nine cases of secondary amenorrhoea of more than 12 months' duration were described after treatment with oral contraceptives. Two patients appeared to have undergone a premature menopause, and in the remainder the level of disturbance was hypothalamic. Galactorrhoea was the only other abnormal physical finding and was present in 11 women. Sixteen of 36 patients conceived after treatment with clomiphene citrate or human gonadotrophins, 19 improved spontaneously, and 25 continued to have amenorrhoea despite treatment.

VIRILIZING EFFECTS OF ANABOLIC STEROIDS

The various anabolic steroids have virilizing effects to a greater or lesser degree. These effects may disturb the menstrual pattern, may increase the libido in both sexes and cause failure of spermatogenesis. Boys may show precocious sexual development and in girls the clitoris may hypertrophy. Virilization of the voice is a troublesome early symptom reported after treatment with anabolic agents (De Lange and Doorenbos, 1968).

Fig. 13.1. *Structural relationship of some anabolic steroids*

PARENTS

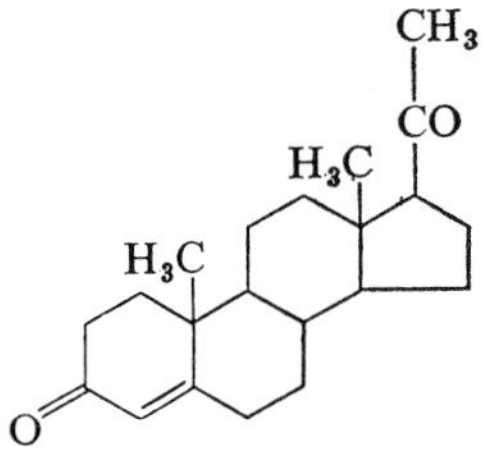

Progesterone

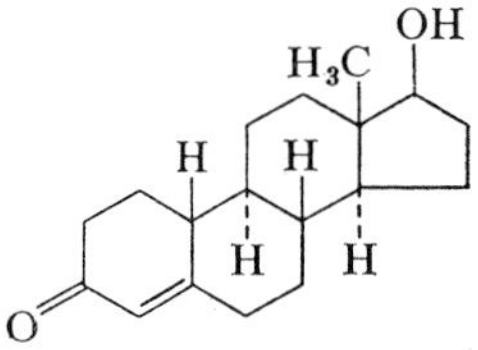

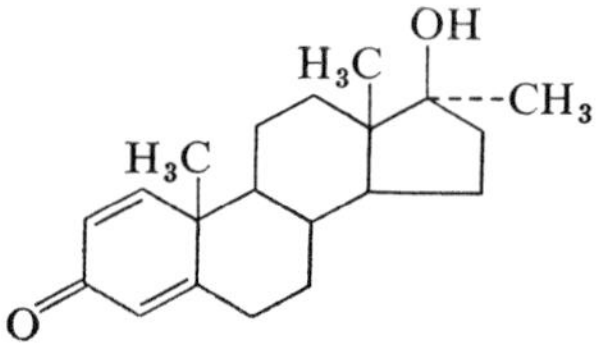

Methandienone (Methandrostenolone)
Anabolic +
Androgenic ±

Nandrolone
(19-Nortestosterone)

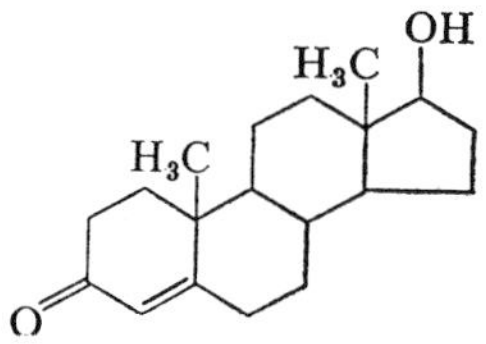

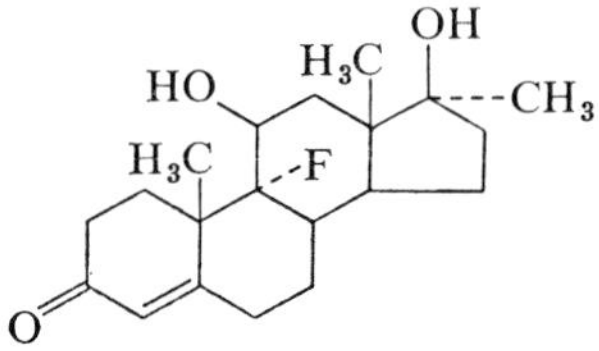

Fluoxymesterone
Anabolic +
Androgenic +

Testosterone

Stanolone
Anabolic +
Androgenic +

PROGENY

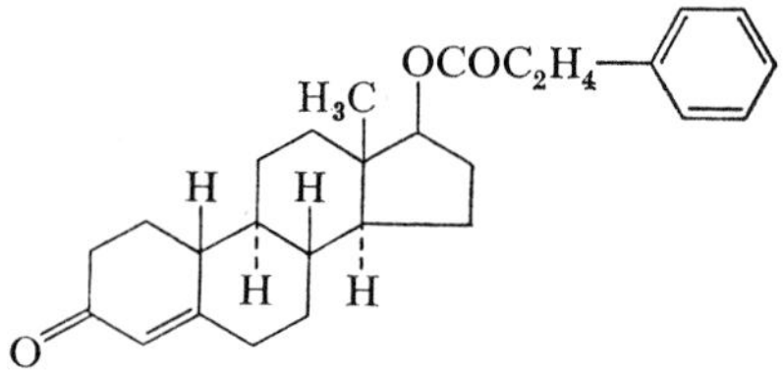

Nandrolone phenylpropionate
Nandrolone decanoate
Anabolic +
Androgenic ±

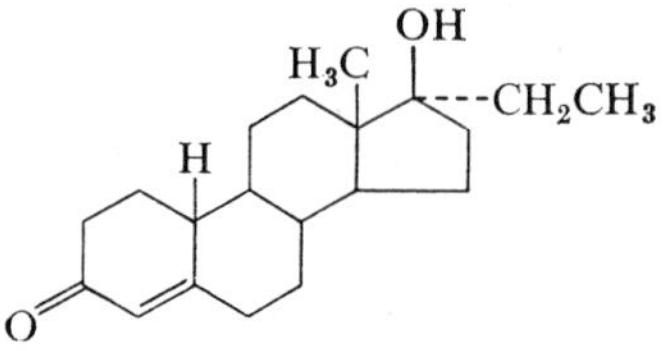

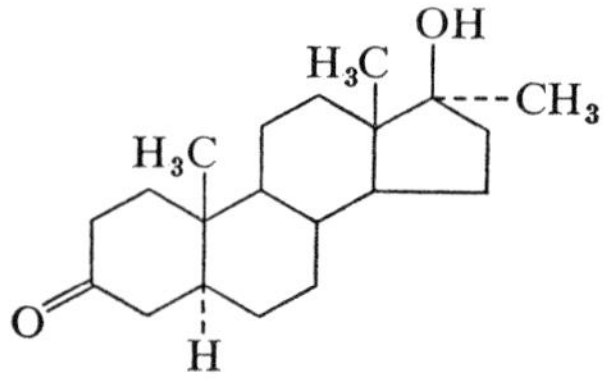

Mestanolone
Anabolic +
Androgenic ±

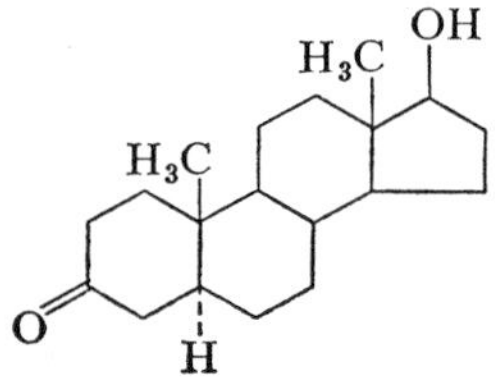

Norethandrolone
Anabolic +
Androgenic ±

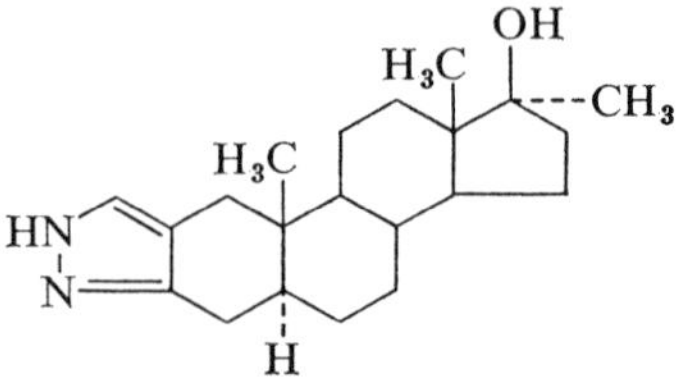

Stanozolol
(Androstanazole)
Anabolic +
Androgenic ±

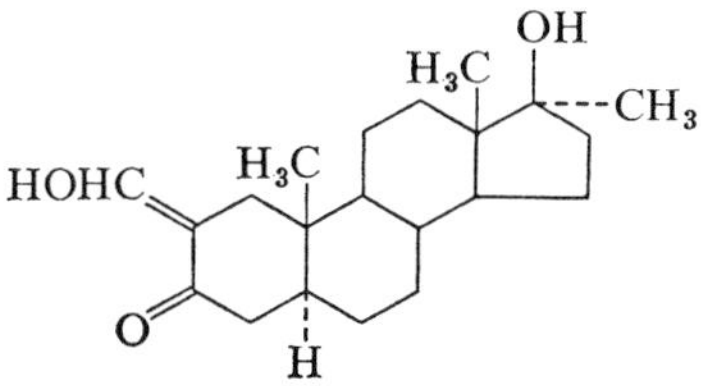

Oxymetholone
Anabolic +
Androgenic ±

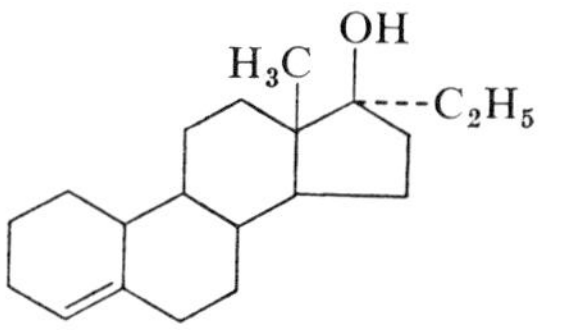

Ethyloestrenol (Ethylestrenol)
Anabolic +

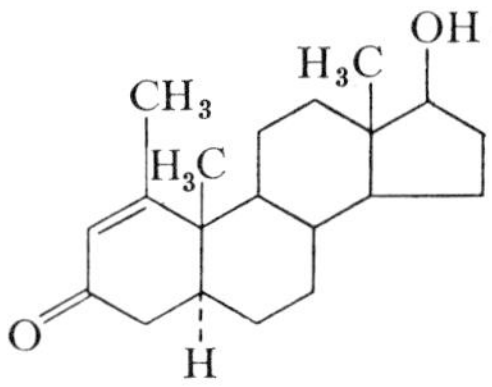

Methenolone
Methenolone 17-acetate
Methenolone 17-oenanthate
Anabolic +

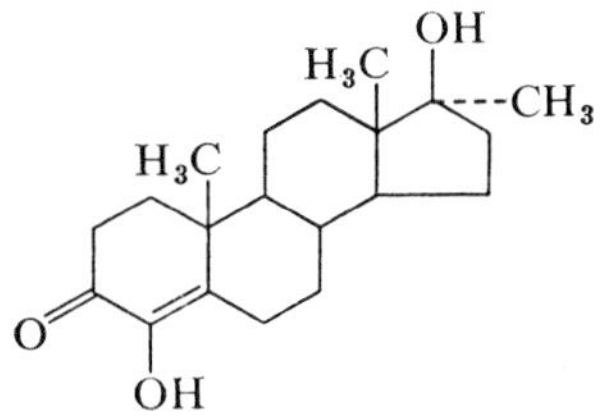

Oxymesterone (Oxymestrone)   Anabolic +

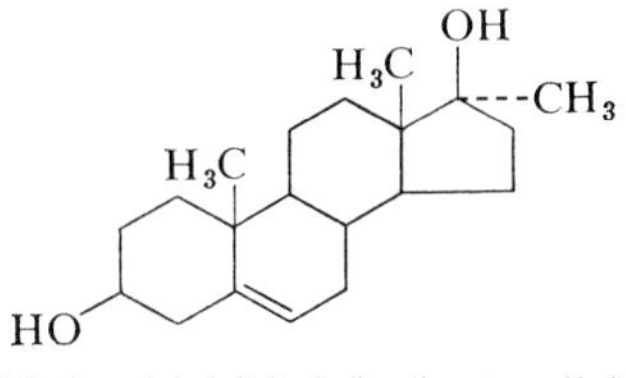

Methandriol (Methylandrostenediol)
Anabolic +
Androgenic ±

A special warning of these effects is especially pertinent since some anabolic agents in low dosage are included in some combination products whose proprietary names do not give any indication of the presence of such androgenic components.

The anabolic steroids have an interesting chemistry [FIG. 13.1] since structurally they resemble both androgen and progestogen and it is relevant in this context to review this in brief detail to illustrate where the virilizing action originates. This topic has been previously reviewed by D'Arcy (1963).

The anabolic effect of androgens was first demonstrated by Kochakian and Murlin (1935), who showed that extracts of male urine caused retention of nitrogen in dogs; later it was shown that testosterone had a similar effect in man (Kenyon et al., 1938). The use of testosterone and its esters as anabolic agents was, however, limited by androgenic effects and this has led to the development of compounds of high anabolic but low androgenic potency.

Most anabolic compounds are derivatives of 19-nortestosterone; some of these, although chemically related to the androgens, are pharmacologically purely progestogenic in their effects and, in many instances, have clinical application as oral progestogens as well as anabolic agents. This may be explained when it is recalled that ethisterone, an orally active substitute for progesterone, is chemically 17α-ethinyltestosterone.

Two such anabolic agents are nandrolone phenylpropionate and norethandrolone (17α-ethyl-19-nortestosterone); they have potent anabolic activity with little, if any, androgenic activity. Similarly methandrostenolone (1-dehydro-17α-methyltestosterone) is a potent anabolic agent without virilizing properties.

Other anabolic drugs are a halogenated testosterone compound, fluoxymesterone (9α-fluoro-11β-hydroxy-17α-methyltestosterone) and stanolone (androstane-17β-ol-3-one, androstanolone); with these, however, there is no dissociation of the primary and secondary effects since they both have potent anabolic and androgenic activities. The methyl derivative of stanolone, mestanolone (methylandrostanolone), however, appears to be more selectively anabolic (Harris, 1961).

Androstanazole, stanozolol (17β-hydroxy-17α-methylandrostano-(3,2-c)-pyrazole) is also a new anabolic agent, which in animal tests has shown potent anabolic but low androgenic activity (Clinton et al., 1959; Arnold et al., 1959); a further anabolic agent is oxymetholone (2-hydroxymethylene-17α-methyl-17-hydroxy-3-androstanone), which as shown by Myerson (1961) has potent anabolic activity in chronically ill malnourished patients, without any indication of androgenic activity or derangement of electrolyte balance.

More recent anabolic agents are, ethyloestrenol, methenolone, oxymesterone, and methylandrostenediol, which show a varied chemical structure although still confined to the basic 19-nortestosterone or progesterone moiety.

MAMMOTROPIC ACTION OF DRUGS

Drugs having a mammotropic action can be divided into two main types. Firstly, some drugs cause breast hypertrophy in men fairly commonly, notably digitalis, spironolactone, ethionamide, and griseofulvin.

This particular action of these drugs is rarely noticed or complained of in women patients, especially since none of these agents has ever been reported as inducing lactation. Drugs of this type are believed to exert their mammotropic action by mimicking oestrogen or progesterone at peripheral receptor sites.

The second group of drugs causes gynaecomastia in male patients and in women induces both mammary hypertrophy and galactorrhoea usually associated with amenorrhoea; this type of action is exhibited by reserpine, phenothiazine derivatives, methyldopa, chlordiazepoxide, imipramine, chlorprothixene, and thioridazine. A number of these compounds have an adrenolytic action and this group of drugs is thought to exert mammotropic action through the adrenergic mechanisms of the hypothalamo-pituitary link. Since surgical disruption of this link in pre-menopausal women has been shown to cause amenorrhoea and lactation (Ehni and Eckles, 1959), it is possible that these drugs produce a chronic pharmacological interruption of this link. Shearman (1971) has shown a similar effect with oral contraceptives.

GROUP 1

Digitalis

A relatively large number of cases of gynaecomastia have occurred in men on digitalis therapy, and in the majority of cases reported, therapy has been given in the form of digitalis leaf rather than digoxin or digitoxin (Conn, 1964). Cases of mammary adipose and glandular hypertrophy in women have only been reported on three occasions (Calov and Whyte, 1954; Bloch, 1961; and Capeller *et al.*, 1959). In these three instances, the patients were post-menopausal and were receiving digitalis leaf.

It is postulated that digitalis, or one of its metabolic products, has sufficient structural similarity to oestrogen [FIG. 13.2] for oestrogen-like effects to be produced under appropriate conditions. It is unlikely that this condition would be recognized in a plethora of endogenous oestrogen, hence it is only recognized when it occurs in men, or in women who are post-menopausal. It is not surprising therefore that only one case of mammotropic activity due to digitalis has been described in a pre-menopausal woman (Wolf, 1964).

Since oestrogen and digitalis are both metabolized and conjugated in the liver it has been suggested that a second condition necessary for the mammotrophic action of digitalis to become apparent is a disturbance of this hepatic metabolism, attributable to a concurrent circulatory disturbance of congestive heart failure. However, limited studies in men with digitalis-induced

FIG. 13.2. *Structural similarity between some mammotropic drugs and oestrogen or progesterone*

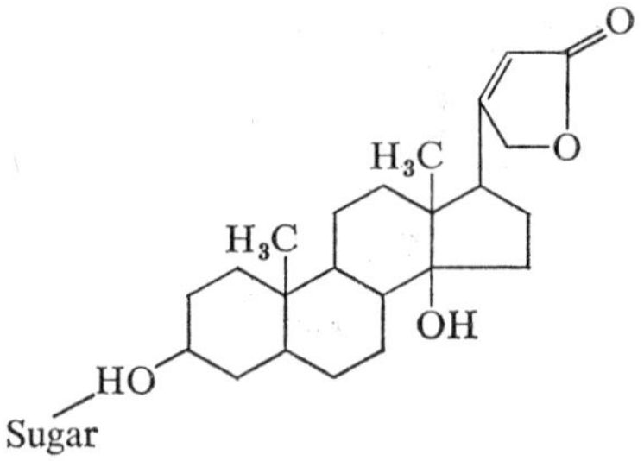

Basic structure of digitalis glycoside

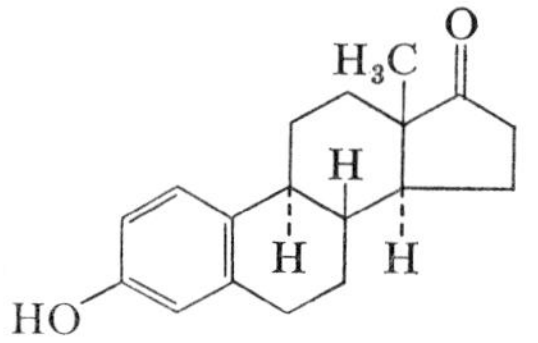

Oestrone

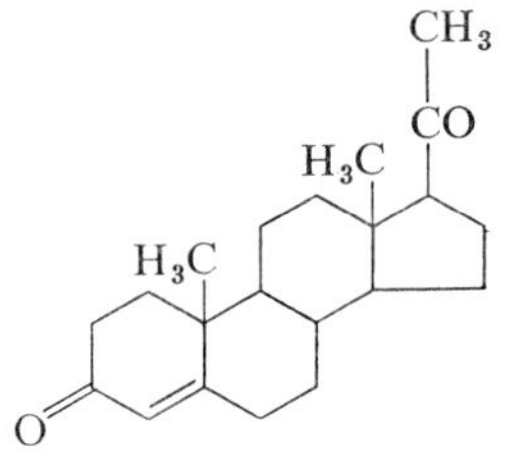

Progesterone

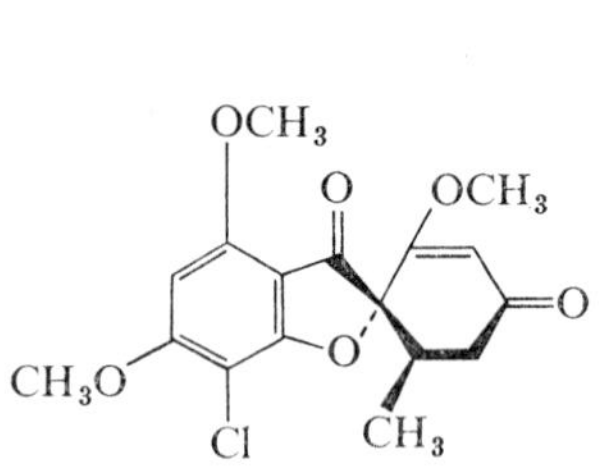

Griseofulvin

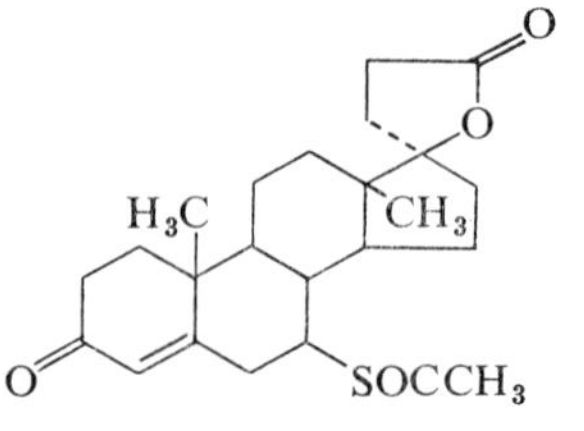

Spironolactone

gynaecomastia have failed to reveal any unusual or unexpected alteration of liver-function tests.

Spironolactone

Spironolactone was first incriminated as a cause of gynaecomastia by Smith (1962) and this was quickly followed by other reports of the same complication (Restifo and Farmer, 1962; Williams, 1962; Mann, 1963; Sussman, 1963).

Clark (1965) reported a series of 12 patients treated with spironolactone; four of the seven male patients and none of the five women complained of hypertrophy of the breast. The high incidence of gynaecomastia in this group of men indicates that it may be a common complication of spironolactone therapy. However, three of the four men with gynaecomastia had been treated with digitalis in addition to spironolactone, and digitalis may have potentiated a mammotropic action of spironolactone. Nevertheless, spironolactone has caused gynaecomastia without the synergistic action of digitalis.

The mammotropic action of spironolactone is thought to depend upon its structural similarity [FIG. 13.2] to progestational hormones (Sussman, 1963).

Ethionamide

Gynaecomastia was observed in 13 patients out of a total of 446 tuberculous patients tested with this drug (Gernez-Rieux et al., 1963).

Griseofulvin

Durand et al. (1964) described four patients in whom treatment with griseofulvin resulted in gynaecomastia, hyperpigmentation of the breast areolae, and of the external genitalia, hypertrophy of the clitoris and vaginal discharge. An oestrogenic activity of griseofulvin was postulated.

GROUP 2
Reserpine

Gynaecomastia was reported by Wilkins (1954) to have developed in male patients following administration of rauwolfia alkaloids and Khazan et al. (1962) described five cases of galactorrhoea in a series of 43 female patients treated with reserpine alone and 30 women treated with reserpine and chlorpromazine.

In animal studies Khazan et al. (1962) found that reserpine in adequate doses could induce lactation in adult female rats, and in these animals the morphological and histological changes in ovaries and uteri were similar to those encountered in normally lactating rats.

Phenothiazine Derivatives

Most of the phenothiazines used clinically have been reported as causing engorgement of the female breast with secretion of either milk or colostrum. The incidence of this mammotropic effect and secretion of colostrum occurs in some 10–15 per cent of patients receiving phenothiazine derivatives (Wright, 1955; Robinson, 1957). Robinson found that all the patients who lactated were below 43 years of age and were taking a dose of chlorpromazine in excess of 300–400 mg/day. Khazan et al. (1962) found that 33 women showed galactorrhoea in a series of 650 cases treated with chlorpromazine.

Khazan et al. (1962) studied the mammotropic action of phenothiazine derivatives on adult female rats 2–3 months old and weighing 120–150 grams. Each drug was injected subcutaneously into 10 female rats for 7 days. The relative effectiveness of the drugs was classified according to a mammotropic index ranging from 1 to 5. The most effective drugs in producing mammary hypertrophy (Grade 5) were trifluoperazine, prochlorperazine, perphenazine, and trifluupromazine.

Chlorpromazine and chlordiazepoxide were moderately effective (Grades 3 and 4).

Laevomepromazine, methopromazine, and iminopromazine showed less effect (Grades 1 and 2). This grading of mammotropic action in rats was borne out in Khazan's clinical experience.

Trifluoperazine was the most effective phenothiazine in producing mammary hypertrophy in the laboratory and this has also been borne out in clinical experience. Khazan et al. (1962) described the following case: 'A 20-year-old unmarried woman suffering from schizophrenia was given 20 mg/day Stelazine [trifluoperazine] for a period of 60 days. Prior to treatment she had regular menstrual cycles with no evidence of any endocrine disorders. It was noted that Stelazine caused enlargement of the breasts and very copious milk secretion, flowing almost freely from the breasts at the slightest pressure. The effect was much more intensive than that seen in all other cases treated with chlorpromazine or reserpine, and lactation ceased when the drug was withdrawn.'

Complications of the mammotropic actions of phenothiazines can occur. Whiffen (1963) described a case of a 26-year-old woman treated with chlorpromazine 300–400 mg daily for almost 5 years, who developed a non-tender mass in the left breast. On frozen section the lesion appeared to be a lipogranuloma, and on permanent section an increased number of ducts and acini were noted, some of which were slightly dilated and mildly inflamed. One segment of duct had lost its epithelial lining and there was a heavy infiltrate of lymphocytes, histiocytes and lipophagocytes. The appearance was of chronic mastitis with galactocoele formation. The excess mammary secretions had extravasated from the duct in this area and formed a lipogranuloma.

Methyldopa

Pettinger et al. (1963) described a series of 15 female patients who were treated for hypertension with α-methyldopa; five of these women commenced to lactate. These women were aged 33–47 years, four were premenopausal and one had undergone hysterectomy and oophorectomy. Relationship of the medication to lactation was verified when cessation of lactation occurred within 3 weeks in two subjects in whom the drug was discontinued; resumption of methyldopa therapy resulted in recurrence of lactation. Changing patients over to guanethidine (another sympatholytic drug) did not support a continuation of methyldopa-induced lactation.

Imipramine
Galactorrhoea, associated with swelling of the mammary glands, developed after a period of 6 months'

treatment with 75–100 mg imipramine daily in a 34-year-old woman. The lactation ceased on withdrawal of the drug, and recurred when therapy was recommenced (Khazan *et al.*, 1962).

Chlorprothixene and Thioridazine
These agents have also been reported as producing gynaecomastia in men, and lactation and amenorrhoea in women (Khazan *et al.*, 1962).

RECOMMENDED FURTHER READING

SANDLER, M., and BILLING, B., eds. (1970) The pill: Biochemical consequences, *J. clin. Path.*, **23**, Suppl., 1–82.

REFERENCES

ALEXANDER, I. R. W. (1961) Acute myxoedema, *Brit. med. J.*, **2**, 1434.

ALLANBY, K. D. (1957) Deaths associated with steroid hormone therapy, *Lancet*, **i**, 1104–10.

ARNOLD, A., BEYLER, A. L., and POTTS, G. O. (1959) Androstanazole, a new orally active anabolic steroid, *Proc. Soc. exp. Biol. (N.Y.)*, **102**, 184–7.

BEGG, T. B., and HALL, R. (1963) Iodide goitre and hypothyroidism, *Quart. J. Med.*, **32**, 351–62.

BENEDEK, T. G. (1962) Goitre formation as a result of phenylbutazone and vitamin A, *J. clin. Endocr.*, **22**, 959–62.

BLOCH, K. (1961) On pathogenesis of breast hypertrophy from digitalis therapy, *Z. Kreisl.-Forsch.*, **50**, 591–5.

BONGIOVANNI, A. M., and McPADDEN, A. J. (1960) Steroids during pregnancy and possible foetal consequences, *Fertil. and Steril.*, **11**, 181–6.

CALOV, W. L., and WHYTE, H. M. (1954) Oedema and mammary hypertrophy: Toxic effects of digitalis leaf, *Med. J. Aust.*, **1**, 556–7.

CAPELLER, D. VON, COPELAND, G. D., and STERN, T. N. (1959) Digitalis intoxication: A clinical report of 148 cases, *Ann. intern. Med.*, **50**, 869–78.

CARSWELL, F., KERR, M. M., and HUTCHISON, J. H. (1970) Congenital goitre and hypothyroidism produced by maternal ingestion of iodides, *Lancet*, **i**, 1241–3.

CHRISTY, N. P., WALLACE, E. Z., and JAILER, J. W. (1956) Comparative effects of prednisone and cortisone in suppressing the response of the adrenal cortex to ACTH, *J. clin. Endocr.*, **16**, 1059–74.

CLARK, E. (1965) Spironolactone therapy and gynecomastia, *J. Amer. med. Ass.*, **193**, 163–4.

CLINTON, R. O., MANSON, A. J., STONNER, F. W., BEYLER, A. L., POTTS, G. O., and ARNOLD, A. (1959) Steroidal [3, 2-c] pyrazoles, *J. Amer. chem. Soc.*, **81**, 1513–14.

CONN, H. L., JR., (1964) Digitalis therapy and gynecomastia, *J. Amer. med. Ass.*, **190**, 1018–19.

D'ARCY, P. F. (1963) Steroid hormones and their synthetic analogues, *Medica Britannica*, **3**, 3–10, 35–42.

DE LANGE, W. E., and DOORENBOS, H. (1968) Hormones and synthetic substitutes, in *Side Effects of Drugs*, Vol. VI, eds. Meyler, L., and Herxheimer, A., Excerpta Medica Foundation, Amsterdam, pp. 383–421.

DIDDLE, A. W., WATTS, G. E., GARDNER, W. H., and WILLIAMSON, P. J. (1966) Oral contraceptive medication. A prolonged experience, *Amer. J. Obstet. Gynec.*, **95**, 489–95.

DOWNS, J. W., and COOPER, W. G. (1955) Surgical complications resulting from ACTH and cortisone medication, *Amer. Surg.*, **21**, 141–6.

DURAND, P., BORRONE, C., SCARABICCHI, S., and RAZZI, A. (1964) Hyperpigmentation of breast areolae and external genitals with gynaecomastia following griseofulvin treatment, *Minerva med.*, **55**, 2422–5.

EGER, W., and FERNHOLZ, J. (1965) Über den thyreostatischen Effekt des Phenylbutazon und des Oxyphenbutazon unter dem Einfluss des Trijodthyronin, *Med. Pharmacol. exp. (Basel)*, **13**, 17–23.

EHNI, G., and ECKLES, N. E. (1959) Interruption of the pituitary stalk in the patient with mammary cancer, *J. Neurosurg.*, **16**, 628–52.

FRASER, C. G., PREUSS, F. S., and BIGFORD, W. D. (1952) Adrenal atrophy and irreversible shock associated with cortisone therapy, *J. Amer. med. Ass.*, **149**, 1542–3.

FREY, H. (1964) Hypofunction of the thyroid gland due to prolonged and excessive intake of potassium iodide, *Acta endocr. (Kbh.)*, **47**, 105–20.

GERNEZ-RIEUX, C., TACQUET, A., and MACQUET, V. (1963) Perfusions with ethionamide in the treatment of pulmonary tuberculosis, *G. ital. Chemioter.*, **10**, 87–98.

GOOD, B. F., HETZEL, B. S., and HOGG, B. M. (1965) Studies of the control of thyroid function in rats: Effects of salicylate and related drugs, *Endocrinology*, **77**, 674–82.

GRAUDENZ, M. G., and BEIRÃO DE ALMEIDA, A. (1965) Nor-esteróides anti-concepcionais. Estudo experimental baseado na histologia do útero, ovário e embrião, *Rev. Ginec. Obstet. (Rio de J.)*, **116**, 108–27.

HARNAGEL, E. E., and KRAMER, W. G. (1955) Severe adrenocortical insufficiency following joint manipulation, *J. Amer. med. Ass.*, **158**, 1518–19.

HARRIS, L. H. (1961) The protein anabolic action of mestanole, *J. clin. Endocr.*, **21**, 1099–1105.

HAYES, M. A. (1956) Surgical treatment as complicated by prior adrenocortical steroid therapy, *Surgery*, **40**, 945–50.

HAYES, M. A., and KUSHLAN, S. D. (1956) Influence of hormonal therapy for ulcerative colitis upon course of surgical treatment, *Gastroenterology*, **30**, 75–84.

HELGASON, T. (1964) Iodides, goitre and myxoedema in chronic respiratory disorders, *Brit. J. Dis. Chest*, **58**, 73–7.

HETZEL, B. S., GOOD, B. F., and WELLBY, M. L. (1963) Salicylate action and thyroidal autonomy in hyperthyroidism, *Lancet*, **ii**, 93–4.

HORDEN, R. M., ALEXANDER, W. D., and HARRISON, M. T. (1964) Non-toxic goitre in males, *Brit. med. J.*, **1**, 1419–21.

KENYON, A. T., SANDIFORD, I., BRYAN, A. H., KNOWLTON, K., and KOCH, F. C. (1938) Effect of testosterone propionate on nitrogen, electrolyte, water and energy metabolism in eunuchoidism, *Endocrinology*, **23**, 135–53.

KHAZAN, N., PRIMO, C., DANON, A., ASSAEL, M., SULMAN, F. G., and WINNIK, H. Z. (1962) The mammotropic effect of tranquillizing drugs, *Arch. int. Pharmacodyn.*, **141**, 291–305.

KITTREDGE, W. E. (1955) Potential hazards of cortisone in treatment of prostatic cancer: Report of a fatal case, *J. Urol.*, **73**, 585–90.

KOCHAKIAN, C. D., and MURLIN, J. R. (1935) Effect of male hormone on the protein and energy metabolism of castrate dogs, *J. Nutr.*, **10**, 437–59.

LEWIS, L., ROBINSON, R. F., YEE, J., HACKER, L. A., and EISEN, G. (1953) Fatal adrenal cortical insufficiency precipitated by surgery during prolonged continuous cortisone treatment, *Ann. intern. Med.*, **39**, 116–26.

LILLICRAP, D. A. (1962) Myxoedema after thalidomide ('Distaval'), *Brit. med. J.*, **1**, 477.

LINTHORST, G. (1966) The effects of oral contraceptives on the ovary, in *Social and Medical Aspects of Oral Contraception, Round-table Conference, Scheveningen, Netherlands,* ed. Dukes, M. N. G., Excerpta Medica Foundation, Amsterdam, pp. 95–7.

LORRAIN, J. (1966) Ovaries polykystiques à la suite d'un traitement au noréthynodrel, *Un. méd. Can.*, **95**, 1053.

MANN, V. M. (1963) Gynecomastia during therapy with spironolactone, *J. Amer. med. Ass.*, **184**, 778–80.

MARCHESE, M. J., BERTORELLO, M. C., and CARDOZO, E. (1963) Mixedema en el curso de tratamiento antituberculoso, *Rev. Asoc. méd. argent.*, **77**, 542–4.

MARSHALL, J. S., LEVY, R. P., and LEONARDS, J. R. (1965) The acute effect of salicylate administration on human thyroxine transport, *J. Lab. clin. Med.*, **66**, 1001.

MURDOCH, J. McC., and CAMPBELL, G. D. (1958) Antithyroid activity of N-phthalyl glutamic acid imide (K17), *Brit. med. J.*, **1**, 84–5.

MYERSON, R. M. (1961) Clinical and metabolic studies on a new anabolic steroid, oxymethalone, *Amer. J. med. Sci.*, **241**, 732–8.

MYHILL, J., and HALES, I. B. (1963) Salicylate action and thyroidal autonomy in hyperthyroidism, *Lancet*, **i**, 802–5.

O'NEIL, R. (1965) in *Recent Advances in Ovarian and Synthetic Steroids*, ed. Shearman, R. P., Sydney, p. 244.

OPPENHEIMER, E. H. (1964) Lesions in the adrenals of an infant following maternal corticosteroid therapy, *Bull. Johns Hopk. Hosp.*, **114**, 146–51.

PARMELEE, A. H., ALLEN, E., STEIN, I. F., and BUXBAUM, H. (1940) Three cases of congenital goitre, *Amer. J. Obstet. Gynec.*, **40**, 145–7.

PETTINGER, W. A., HORWITZ, D., and SJOERDSMA, A. (1963) Lactation due to methyldopa, *Brit. med. J.*, **1**, 1460.

PLATE, W. P. (1968) Ovarian changes after long-term oral contraception, in *Drug-Induced Diseases*, Vol. 3, eds.

Meyler, L., and Peck, H. M., Excerpta Medica Foundation, Amsterdam, pp. 235–8.

PLUMER, J. N., and ARMSTRONG, R. S. (1957) Adrenocortical failure following long term steroid therapy, *Ariz. Med.*, **14**, 202–5.

PRESCOTT, L. F. (1968) Antipyretic analgesic drugs, in *Side Effects of Drugs*, Vol. VI, eds. Meyler, L., and Herxheimer, A., Excerpta Medica Foundation, Amsterdam, pp. 101–39.

RESTIFO, R. A., and FARMER, T. A. (1962) Spironolactones and gynaecomastia, *Lancet*, **ii**, 1280.

ROBINSON, B. (1957) Breast changes in male and female with chlorpromazine and reserpine therapy, *Med. J. Aust.*, **2**, 239.

RYAN, G. M., CRAIG, J., and REID, D. E. (1964) Histology of the uterus and ovaries after long-term cyclic norethynodrel therapy, *Amer. J. Obstet. Gynec.*, **90**, 715–25.

SALASSA, R. M., BENNET, W. A., KEATING, F. R., and SPRAGUE, R. G. (1953) Post-operative adrenal cortical insufficiency, *J. Amer. med. Ass.*, **152**, 1509–15.

SAYERS, G. (1950) The adrenal cortex and homeostasis, *Physiol. Rev.*, **30**, 241–320.

SCHNEEWIND, J. H., and COLE, W. H. (1959) Steroid therapy in surgical patients, *J. Amer. med. Ass.*, **170**, 1411–21.

SHEARMAN, R. P. (1971) Prolonged secondary amenorrhœa after oral contraceptive therapy, *Lancet*, **ii**, 64–6.

SIEGAL, S. (1964) The asthma-suppressive action of potassium iodide, *J. Allergy*, **35**, 252–70.

SIMPSON, J. A. (1962) Myxoedema after thalidomide ('Distaval'), *Brit. med. J.*, **1**, 55.

SLANEY, G., and BROOKE, B. N. (1957) Postoperative collapse due to adrenal insufficiency following cortisone therapy, *Lancet*, **i**, 1167–70.

SMITH, W. G. (1962) Spironolactone and gynaecomastia, *Lancet*, **ii**, 886.

STARUP, J. (1967) The effects of gestagen and oestrogen treatment on the development of ovarian follicles: Laboratory observations, *Acta. obstet. gynec. scand.*, **46**, Suppl. 9, 15.

SUSSMAN, R. M. (1963) Spironolactone and gynaecomastia, *Lancet*, **i**, 58.

VAN ROY, M. (1966) cited by Plate, W. P. (1968).

WHIFFEN, J. D. (1963) Unusual surgical consideration of phenothiazine therapy, *Amer. J. Surg.*, **106**, 991–2.

WHITELAW, M. J., NOLA, V. F., and KALMAN, C. F. (1966) Irregular menses, amenorrhoea and infertility following synthetic progestational agents, *J. Amer. med. Ass.*, **195**, 780–2.

WILKINS, R. W. (1954) Clinical usage of Rauwolfia alkaloids, including reserpine (Serpasil), *Ann. N.Y. Acad. Sci.*, **59**, 36–44.

WILLIAMS, E. (1962) Spironolactone and gynaecomastia, *Lancet*, **ii**, 1113.

WOLF, H. L. (1964) Digitalis therapy and gynecomastia, *J. Amer. med. Ass.*, **190**, 1018.

WRIGHT, V. K. (1955) Complications of chlorpromazine treatment, *Dis. nerv. Syst.*, **16**, 114.

ZUSSMAN, W. V., FORBES, D. A., and CARPENTER, R. J., JR. (1967) Ovarian morphology following cyclic norethindrone mestranol therapy, *Amer. J. Obstet. Gynec.*, **99**, 99–105.

14

RENAL DISEASE

NATURE OF TOXIC EFFECTS ON THE KIDNEY

It is practically impossible to determine with any degree of accuracy the percentage of adverse reactions to drugs that involve the kidney. Zbinden (1963) thought about 2 per cent, and probably this is as good an estimate as any. What is certain, however, is that a large number of individual drugs has been implicated and that these drugs are representative of a whole range of therapeutic agents including analgesics, anti-inflammatory drugs, anticoagulants, antibiotics, antibacterials, anticonvulsants, hypoglycaemics, mercurial diuretics, uricosuric, and antimigraine agents. Perhaps the only property that these varied compounds have in common is that they pass through the kidneys.

Nephrotoxic reactions due to drugs can fall into one of three categories:

1. General hypersensitivity and idiosyncratic reactions with renal involvement.
2. Direct toxicity on the kidney.
3. Indirect toxicity on the kidney.

GENERAL HYPERSENSITIVITY AND IDIOSYNCRATIC REACTIONS

This type of reaction is neither dose nor dose-duration related; it occurs without warning, quite unpredictably after varying periods of exposure, and is most frequently generalized to include the skin, nervous system, liver and other body systems. Although renal involvement in hypersensitivity reactions is relatively uncommon, it is generally severe when it does occur.

Renal involvement in hypersensitivity reactions is most often manifest by glomerulopathy which causes nephrotic syndrome, or a syndrome which is difficult to differentiate clinically from post-streptococcal glomerulonephritis. Histologically diffuse or focal proliferative lesions of the glomeruli may be found, and basement-membrane thickening may occur or be the predominant lesion. Interstitial involvement is most striking at times and oedema and proliferation of lymphocytes, plasma cells and eosinophils typify this reaction. Acute tubular degeneration is an associated feature.

Fortunately in most instances the renal lesions of hypersensitivity reactions to drugs are not permanent and the syndrome is usually reversible after withdrawal of medication; corticosteroids or immunosuppressive therapy may be beneficial. In a relatively small number of cases, the renal lesion may, however, be progressive

or irreversible and fatal. In general, these changes due to hypersensitivity cannot be reproduced during the routine and exacting toxicological testing to which new drugs are now subjected during their development. As discussed in the Preface to this volume, hypersensitivity is an abnormal response on the part of the patient to an otherwise non-toxic drug. The potential hazard of such hypersensitivity reactions can therefore only be revealed by time and by clinical experience.

Fortunately both time and clinical experience have revealed that hypersensitivity reactions with renal involvement can be anticipated with a number of drugs including, for example, the following: NEPHROTIC SYNDROME: troxidone, paramethadione, penicillamine, bismuth and gold salts, mercurial diuretics, phenindione, and tolbutamide. NECROTIZING RENAL VASCULITIS: thiazide diuretics, sulphonamides, phenylbutazone, penicillin, tetracyclines, erythromycin, and quinine. ACUTE INTERSTITIAL NEPHRITIS: phenindione, and phenylbutazone. In addition a lupus-like syndrome has followed therapy with various agents including procainamide, phenytoin, and quinidine. Most patients with this 'acquired lupus' do not show evidence of severe renal involvement, and the syndrome is usually reversible on stopping the drug. However, some patients may exhibit arteriolar degenerative changes with fibrinoid necrosis similar to that of renal lesions seen in polyarteritis nodosa.

DIRECT TOXICITY

The following drugs are among those that have been incriminated as having direct toxic effects on the kidney. Antibiotics: penicillin, erythromycin, chloramphenicol, bacitracin, streptomycin, kanamycin, and neomycin; mercurial diuretics, bismuth salts, phenacetin, mannitol, and dextran.

Some drugs are toxic to the kidney at normal therapeutic dosage, others are only toxic when taken in excess or when the usual excretion pathway is blocked. With direct toxicity the extent of kidney damage resulting is usually dose related. The clinical syndromes of direct toxicity on the kidney include acute tubular necrosis, various degrees of tubular dysfunction including Fanconi syndrome, and progressive renal insufficiency. The histological picture is that of glomerulopathy, tubular degeneration or even papillary necrosis.

The direct toxic effects can be produced to a certain degree in experimental animals, and the majority of these effects will therefore have been revealed during the toxicological screening programme that precedes the introduction of the drug into the clinic; thus many of the toxic effects ought to be predictable to some degree in clinical practice. What are not so easy to predict, however, are those special circumstances which are capable of triggering off toxic sequelae at normal dosage.

INDIRECT TOXICITY

Drugs can have an indirect toxic effect on the kidney as a consequence of a primary extra-renal effect. For example, acute renal failure may result from primaquine-induced haemoglobinuria. In elderly men, antihistaminics, sedatives and ganglion-blocking hypotensives, may cause urinary retention with loss of renal function and attendant danger of pyelonephritis. Methysergide, taken for migraine, may induce hydronephrosis secondary to retroperitoneal fibrosis and ureteric obstruction.

In general these results are difficult to predict from animal studies although their pattern of development has been well established in the clinic. As might be expected there are no good correlations between dose administered and incidence and degree of the secondary toxic actions.

RENAL DAMAGE CAUSED BY ANALGESICS

PHENACETIN NEPHROPATHY

Phenacetin (acetophenetidin, para-acetophenetidin) was introduced into clinical medicine in 1887 and, in combination with aspirin, other analgesics, and caffeine has long been popular as an antipyretic and analgesic. Like most of the older drugs it has had peaks and troughs of popularity and mistrust. Undesirable effects on the blood have been well documented but since these side-effects are reversible, they gave little cause for undue concern. However, for almost the last 20 years there has been a steady stream of reports from many countries of a correlation of excessive consumption of phenacetin-containing analgesics with renal papillary necrosis and non-obstructive pyelonephritis, which may be fatal. The evidence, however, against phenacetin is largely circumstantial since the preparations concerned were analgesic mixtures and not a single substance. Since phenacetin was present in almost all the analgesic combinations implicated it has received most of the blame, although conclusive proof is far from certain (*Lancet*, leading article, 1968). Many of the clinical reports, although convincing, have been inadequately controlled and to confuse matters further experimental studies in animals given large doses of phenacetin have usually been negative or inconclusive (Shelley, 1967). Nor indeed has renal disease associated with the use of phenacetin alone been described in man.

What is absolutely clear, however, is that there is an undoubted association between papillary necrosis and heavy consumption of preparations containing not only phenacetin but also salicylates, phenazone (antipyrine), amidopyrine (aminopyrine, aminophenazone, dipyrine), caffeine, and codeine.

Renal papillary necrosis was hitherto a very rare condition seen almost exclusively in patients with diabetes mellitus or urinary tract obstruction (Mandel, 1952). The apparent incidence has, however, risen strikingly in recent years and papillary necrosis is now most often associated with analgesic abuse in the absence of other aetiological factors. In Australia abuse of analgesics is widespread and there renal papillary necrosis is said to be one of the commonest forms of renal disease (*Medical Journal of Australia*, Comments and Abstracts, 1968).

From an historical viewpoint it was from Europe that Spühler and Zollinger in 1953 first drew attention to the association between a high intake of analgesics and 'chronic interstitial nephritis', and although renal papillary necrosis was present in most of their cases they attached no particular significance to it. In the United States, Moolten and Smith in 1960 reported fatal nephritis in chronic phenacetin poisoning. Since then a vast international literature has accumulated from Scandinavia, Switzerland, Great Britain, Australia, Canada and the United States (for example: Schourup, 1957; Lindeneg et al., 1959; Reynolds and Edmondson, 1963; Sanerkin and Weaver, 1964; Dawborn et al., 1966; Koch et al., 1968). There have been several annotations and editorials (*British Medical Journal*, 1960; *Lancet*, 1963; *Journal of the American Medical Association*, 1963a, 1963b, 1964; *Canadian Medical Association Journal*, 1965; *Lancet*, 1968, 1969) and recent reviews (Haley, 1966; Prescott, 1966; Shelley, 1967; Gault et al., 1968) all associating renal disease with the intake of large quantities of analgesics. In their very comprehensive review on 'syndrome associated with the abuse of analgesics' Gault and his colleagues (1968) collected together reports of over 1,800 cases from more than 12 different countries; this gives an indication of the extent of the problem involved, a problem that is potentiated by the ready availability of many of these analgesic preparations without prescription.

Fortunately in some countries recognition of the possible role of phenacetin in the genesis of renal disease has resulted in legislation to control its sale. Phenacetin and its derivatives have been unobtainable, except on prescription, since 1961 in Sweden and Denmark and since 1963 in Switzerland.

Its sale in the United States has been prohibited since 1964 unless warning of possible kidney damage is given, although if a corollary may be made between this warning and that printed on cigarette packets it is doubtful whether this will achieve any real result. In 1965, legislation was enacted in Canada that requires a statement that injury may result from prolonged excessive intake and in Australia phenacetin can no longer be prescribed on the National Health Service (Gault et al., 1968).

Laudable and well-intentioned as such legislation surely is, it may have entirely missed the point of the whole exercise since with present knowledge it would seem unwise to ascribe renal damage due to analgesic abuse to a single agent since it would seem very probable that salicylates, other analgesics, caffeine or other ingredients of the multi-component analgesic-antipyretic preparation may contribute directly or indirectly to renal damage. Gault and colleagues (1968) have expressed a preference for the term 'analgesic nephropathy' rather than 'phenacetin nephritis', and with current knowledge this has our full support.

With regard to the precise mechanism by which 'analgesic abuse' damages the kidney, it must be admitted that, although a great deal has been written about chronic interstitial nephritis and papillary necrosis, their position with regard to analgesic nephropathy is confused. Kincaid-Smith (1967) has suggested that, in cases of analgesic abuse, the shrunken kidney of the so-called interstitial nephritis results from parenchymal atrophy which develops secondarily to cortical necrosis. She has described the pathological changes of analgesic nephropathy in detail and has commented that the macroscopic appearance of the kidney of analgesic abuse is quite different from that of chronic pyelonephritis.

When patients first show clinical evidence of renal disease, the kidneys are usually normal in size and renal body biopsy specimens are normal. Separation of papillae of the kidneys occurs over a period of weeks (Dawborn et al., 1966) and a specimen at this stage shows atrophy of cortical tubules with increased oedematous interstitial tissue. The small kidney found in the later stages usually shows a mixed picture with interstitial fibrosis, hyalinization of glomeruli, alternating hypertrophy and atrophy of tubules, and at times, superimposed pyelonephritis [see PLATE 4].

The rather complex microscopic picture produced by these changes has been discussed in full and interpreted by Kincaid-Smith (1967) in her paper. In summary of this interpretation, cortical changes were secondary to those in the medulla, the blockage of tubules in the necrotic papilla was followed by atrophy of related nephrons except when these were able to re-establish drainage to the newly formed calyceal cavity. Probably both acute and chronic papillary necrosis played a part in the pathogenesis of the renal lesion. Clinical episodes of sudden severe deterioration in function followed by the passage of papillae in the urine (Dawborn et al., 1966) represented clinical manifestations of acute necrosis.

Just how papillary necrosis occurs was obscure although the lesions in the medullary tubules which precede papillary necrosis in man, are very like those of the rabbit (Clausen, 1962, 1964) and similar to those of rats (Dawborn et al., 1964) on a high intake of phenacetin. The presence of prominent cast formation and tubular dilatation have suggested the possibility of precipitation of analgesic metabolites at a particular site in the loop of Henle due to high urinary concentration produced by the counter current mechanism. This combination of tubular lesions and reaction around interstitial casts was thought to be sufficient to impair blood supply via the vasa vasorum and cause papillary necrosis.

Since this view of the pathogenesis of chronic interstitial nephritis was first presented by Kincaid-Smith (1963), two other groups of workers (Burry et al., 1966; Sanerkin, 1966) have described similar pathological findings in association with a high intake of analgesics. Others have reported partial regeneration of the renal papillae if analgesic abuse is stopped early enough (Rapoport et al., 1962; Plass, 1964; Pearson, 1967).

The clinical picture of papillary necrosis due to analgesic abuse has been shown by Koch and associates (1968) to be different in many aspects from the papillary necrosis seen in patients without a history of analgesic abuse; indeed clinical and morphological findings seemed to distinguish two distinctly different syndromes.

With analgesic abuse, the papillary necrosis had a much better prognosis than that from other causes. With analgesic abuse there was a relatively higher incidence of peptic ulceration, but in both groups there was a preponderance of female patients.

The clinical course of the disease has been described by Koch et al. (1968). Firstly, there was sloughing of papillary tissue which could occur without any apparent symptoms (for example in 7 out of 15 in Koch's analgesic abuse group), although two cases found a 'big brown lump' in the urine. On other occasions (for example in 5 out of 15 of Koch's analgesic abuse group) papillary sloughing was dramatic and was accompanied by colic, oliguria, nausea and vomiting, followed some hours later by massive diuresis and haematuria.

In the second phase, symptoms were few or absent and renal function appeared normal with regard to creatinine clearance. The specific gravity was usually 1·010 at this stage, IVP showed calyceal clubbing and bacteriuria was common. With the analgesic abuse group there was also a strong association with anaemia and with acidosis.

The third stage was associated with renal insufficiency, rising blood urea, hypertension and death. Characteristically, progression into this third phase was longer in cases of analgesic nephropathy.

The implication of these findings in diagnosis means that a combination of peptic ulcer, psychoneurosis, anaemia, and headache or muscular pain in the middle-aged patient should certainly indicate prompt and careful examination of both the patient's drug habits and his urinary tract (Dawborn et al., 1966; Koch et al., 1968).

ANALGESIC ABUSE AND TUMOURS OF THE RENAL PELVIS

In the previous section, one aspect of analgesic abuse on renal function was emphasized. Unfortunately in recent months attention has been drawn to the possibility of another potentially lethal complication—namely, the development of transitional-cell tumours of the renal pelvis in patients with renal papillary necrosis (*Lancet*, leading article, 1969).

The first hint of such an association was raised by Hultengren and colleagues (1965) in Stockholm. They found four instances of renal pelvic carcinoma in 103 patients with renal papillary necrosis, and another two cases were found incidentally. Of this total of six cases, five were known to have taken phenacetin-containing analgesic preparations to excess.

In 1968, Bengtsson and associates from Göteborg reported a study of 242 patients with chronic non-obstructive pyelonephritis. Of these, 142 patients were classed as chronic abusers of drugs containing phenacetin. Seventy-nine per cent of all the patients were followed up for 1–11 years (mean 5·3 years). Out of the 142 analgesic abusers, 104 patients were followed up and, of these, eight developed transitional cell tumours of the renal pelvis. Bladder carcinoma was found in another two patients. Of the 100 control patients with non-obstructive pyelonephritis who had not taken analgesics, 88 were followed up; there were no tumours in this group. In the nearby department of surgery an additional 20 patients with renal pelvic carcinoma were seen over a period of eight years (1960–1967) and five of these patients had abused analgesics. Analgesic abusers developed tumours at a lower mean age than non-abusers, the lesions were less well differentiated, and the usual sex ratio was reversed with women predominating. Haematuria was the commonest presenting complaint.

Bengtsson *et al.* (1968) pointed out that in Sweden the average annual incidence of such tumours was 1 case per 183,000 inhabitants for the years 1960–1963, whereas in his series, eight cases were found in 104 patients with analgesic nephropathy followed up for an average of 5·3 years.

Angervall *et al.* (1969) reported 15 cases of renal pelvic carcinoma seen during 1960–1968 at the Jönkö-ping County Hospital, Sweden. Ten of these cases, possibly 12, admitted to having abused an analgesic preparation (Hjorton's powders) which contained phenacetin (500 mg), phenazone (500 mg) and caffeine (150 mg). Nine of these cases came from a small-arms factory at Huskvarna whose workers were notorious for heavy analgesic consumption. Two abusers had also developed a urinary bladder carcinoma.

The Huskvarna factory workers have been notorious for their heavy abuse of phenacetin-containing powders since the Spanish influenza pandemic in 1918 to 1919 until 1961, when these drugs were put on prescription. Grimlund (1963), medical officer at the factory, gave a comprehensive report on the findings among the 1,800 factory workers, mainly males, and the population in the town of Huskvarna (13,000). During a 10-year period, 1952 to 1961, there were 35 deaths from uraemia among the factory workers associated with analgesic abuse. The factory workers accounted for 80 per cent of the deaths from uraemia, although they accounted for only 14 per cent of the population. Patients dying

from obstructive uropathies, acute nephritis and diabetic nephropathy were excluded. The percentage of male deaths from uraemia was 78.

These results would suggest a causal link between analgesic abuse and renal pelvic tumours. In Sweden, analgesic abuse is obviously the commonest cause of renal pelvic tumours and this must be directly linked with world-wide analgesic abuse being the commonest cause of renal papillary necrosis. It has been suggested that chronic irritation at this site eventually leads to malignant change. The Swedish workers assume phenacetin to be the cause.

Although the evidence against analgesic abuse is very strong there may be other factors involved. All these cases have been reported in Sweden; possibly environmental factors play a role. The evidence against phenacetin is, however, circumstantial and in this respect one may question how these findings during the years 1960–1968 can be reconciled with the fact that since 1961 'over-the-counter' sales of products containing phenacetin and its derivatives have been banned in Sweden. Possibly, therefore, analgesics other than phenacetin are implicated. An alternative explanation, and one that has been put forward by Bengtsson and his colleagues, is that the apparent development of the tumour may take place long after the causative agent has been removed.

A further point of interest is that renal pelvic tumour is usually described as a predominantly male disease with a ratio of four men to one woman (Deming, 1963). However, in these Swedish studies the sex ratio has been reversed, but only in the analgesic-abuse groups, not in the non-analgesic abuse controls. For example: the six patients with tumours in the series of Hultengren *et al.* were all women; in the Bengtsson *et al.* studies, six of the eight patients with tumours were women; all had a history of analgesic abuse. Since women are more prone to take analgesic drugs, especially for menstrual pain, this would tend to strengthen a causal relationship between analgesic abuse and tumour growth and if it is true that tumour development may take place long after the causative agent has been removed then surely women who take excessive amounts of analgesics at monthly intervals from puberty to menopause are at special hazard; a special hazard that embraces renal papillary necrosis, non-obstructive pyelonephritis, blood dyscrasias, gastroduodenal ulceration and haemorrhage, and renal pelvic tumour.

RENAL FAILURE DUE TO AMIDOPYRINE (AMINOPYRINE)

Aminopyrine, a very near chemical relative of phenazone, is an analgesic and antipyretic although it is no longer used extensively, mainly because of its toxic effects on the bone-marrow which produce leucopenia, neutropenia and agranulocytosis, and sometimes result in death.

A single case of renal failure caused by aminopyrine has been described by Eknoyan and Matson (1964). A

37-year-old woman with Hodgkin's disease, after being given various other drugs, was given aminopyrine, 600 mg thrice daily, for fever. Her fever abated but her urine output dropped and urine analysis showed hyaline and granular casts. Mannitol and stoppage of aminopyrine re-established urine output at about 500 ml every eight hours. Because of persistent fever she was given aminopyrine in a dose of 300 mg four times daily, but again developed anuria. Despite withdrawal of the aminopyrine and treatment for acute renal failure, her condition worsened and she died 11 days later. The patient had previously shown renal damage during a brief course of amphotericin B.

This case was the first reported of acute renal failure caused by aminopyrine and at the time drew attention to the need for greater discrimination in the use of the drug, especially in patients whose renal function had been damaged previously.

SALICYLATE NEPHROTOXICITY?

Salicylates cause renal irritation, and cells, casts and albumin appear in the urine. The effect is proportional to the dose, and the presence of casts in the urine can lead to the erroneous diagnosis of renal disease. If the patient continues to take salicylates the renal effect passes off in about a week. There is no evidence that permanent renal damage occurs.

It must not be forgotten, however, that aspirin and phenacetin are a popular combination in many analgesics. Although phenacetin has been incriminated as the toxic offender in this partnership, salicylates can certainly not be excluded from possibly a supportive role, especially in instances of frank analgesic abuse.

Prescott (1968) has reviewed salicylate toxicity, and has commented that impaired renal function, oliguria and anuria with renal tubular necrosis may occur with overdosage of salicylates, and degenerative tubular lesions are often present in fatal cases of poisoning. Albuminuria, haematuria, increased cells and casts in the urine and impaired renal function are often known to follow large doses of salicylates which are still within the accepted therapeutic range.

Renal papillary necrosis and chronic interstitial nephritis have been described in patients taking salicylates alone or salicylates in combination with caffeine. Although these numbers are very small in comparison with the reports of nephrotoxicity resulting from mixed analgesic preparations containing phenacetin, they are indicative of potential salicylate nephrotoxicity (Harvald, 1963; Olafsson et al., 1966; Lawson and Maclean, 1966).

One should be careful not to 'miss the wood for the trees' even if the trees are willows; it is quite reasonable to assume that one drug can influence the nephrotoxic potential of another, and this may be done in a variety of ways; even simply by altering the direction or rate of metabolism. With a nephrotoxic combination of phenacetin and salicylates, it seems a little naive to assume that phenacetin is solely responsible. A very recent paper by Nanra and Kincaid-Smith (1970) reporting the results of experimental studies in rats adds new evidence to this argument. Nearly half the rats gavage-fed with aspirin and aspirin-containing mixtures developed papillary necrosis in 20 weeks. This incidence was similar to that found in rats on A.P.C. mixtures with high and low concentrations of p-chloracetanilide, an impurity of phenacetin. Aspirin alone produced necrosis in 7 out of 19 rats (36·8 per cent) whereas phenacetin in the same dose had failed to cause any renal damage over 6 to 9 months of dosage. The authors have suggested that, if these experimental results can be related to man, they suggest that aspirin and not phenacetin may be the major factor in analgesic nephropathy in patients taking A.P.C. mixtures.

NEPHROPATHY DUE TO PHENINDIONE SENSITIVITY

Experimental studies in animals have shown that the anticoagulant phenindione, a member of the indanediones, may affect the kidney. Soulier and Gueguen (1947) produced glomerular damage, and Jaques et al. (1950) produced tubular necrosis.

In clinical practice an increasing number of sensitivity reactions to phenindione have been reported since its introduction in 1947. Transient albuminuria is often noted during the first few days of therapy (Coon et al., 1953) although Goodman and Gilman (1955) were of the opinion that this was of no consequence and could be disregarded. However, renal sensitivity reactions, although rare, are usually severe and most often fatal.

Kirkeby (1954) reported the first fatal case with renal involvement; he thought the underlying pathology was a lower-nephron nephrosis which appeared after 5 weeks of therapy. Burns and Desmond (1958) reported a case of severe sensitivity in a man who died of myocardial infarction after 4 weeks of therapy. The kidneys showed round-cell infiltration of the interstitial tissues.

Brooks and Calleja (1960) reported one case of albuminuria and 'toxic nephritis' which developed about 5 weeks after phenindione treatment had started and disappeared within 2 weeks of cessation of therapy. Tait (1960) noted the development of a nephrotic syndrome 7 weeks after treatment was begun. Observation of this patient for 10 months led him to believe that the renal damage caused by phenindione was permanent.

Barritt and Jordan (1960) reported a fatal case of anuria which came on some weeks after a second course of phenindione; the lesion was considered to be an extensive renal tubular necrosis. The Postgraduate Medical School of London (1960) reported a well-documented case of renal hypersensitivity to phenindione in a patient with pulmonary hypertension, who died despite dialysis. Acute renal failure developed after 2 months' treatment. Ante-mortem renal biopsy and necropsy sections of the kidney showed interstitial oedema, plasma-cell infiltration, and damage to the proximal tubular epithelium. The presence of mitotic figures in these cells was thought to indicate that the renal lesion was reversible. The glomeruli were normal.

Perkins (1962) from Manchester reported three further cases of phenindione sensitivity bringing the total reported in the literature at that time up to 138 cases. In an extensive analysis of reports he identified cases from 1947 to 1962. Common manifestations of all these cases were rash, pyrexia, diarrhoea, granulocytopenia, and stomatitis, in decreasing order of frequency. Hepatic and renal damage occurred, renal involvement having the worst prognosis. Many of the reported reactions were severe, and six deaths were attributed to drug reaction. He suggested that some toxic effects of phenindione might be due to inhibition of oxidative phosphorylation.

Galea *et al.* (1963) described a case, in Australia, of a 47-year-old man who suffered from angina and was given phenindione prophylactically. On the 25th day of treatment pruritis developed and phenindione was discontinued after 31 days due to the development of a skin rash. Six weeks after commencing treatment the patient was oliguric and had a blood urea of 468 mg/100 ml. Despite dialysis the patient died 16 days after the onset of anuria.

At autopsy the kidneys were greatly enlarged, the combined weight was 680 grams (normal 320 grams). The glomeruli showed thickening of the basement membrane and polymorphs, plasma cells and eosinophils were found in the glomerular tufts. The tubules, both proximal and distal, showed cloudy swelling, granular degeneration and frank necrosis. Early regeneration was indicated by the presence of mitotic figures. Casts blocked many of the tubes. There was gross oedema of the interstitial tissue with cellular infiltration by plasma cells and eosinophils.

Since the latter publication, other investigators have reported acute oliguria or anuria associated with phenindione treatment (for example: Baker and Williams, 1963; Pearce, 1963; Smith, 1965; Menon and Burrell, 1966; Guedon *et al.*, 1966). Smith (1965) has also reported nephrotic azotaemia.

In some of the cases described in this section, earlier signs of sensitivity to phenindione, especially skin eruptions, have preceded the onset of renal reactions. Galea and colleagues (1963) were of the opinion that when phenindione is used, it should be stopped immediately on the appearance of a rash or persistent albuminuria, especially when accompanied by an unexplained fever. They also emphasized a further practical point in that severe renal reactions occurred after the 4th week of therapy; they recommended therefore that these reactions be looked for especially in patients who had been treated for periods longer than that. They also emphasized that reactions could develop up to 25 days after phenindione treatment had been stopped.

Perkins (1962) has suggested that when a phenindione sensitivity reaction develops, or is suspected, and further anticoagulant therapy is desirable, warfarin sodium or nicoumalone (acenocoumarol) may be used, although he warned that there could be cross-sensitization between these two 4-hydroxycoumarin derivatives and phenindione.

NEPHROTOXICITY OF ANTIBIOTICS

In a comprehensive review, Kunin (1967) has listed those antibiotics in current clinical use which are potentially nephrotoxic. They are: neomycin, kanamycin, paromomycin, bacitracin, the polymyxins (polymyxin B, and colistin), the tetracyclines, and amphotericin B. In the early days of streptomycin, this antibiotic was also regarded as nephrotoxic although the drug now commercially available does not appear to have this property.

In general terms, patients with underlying renal disease appear to be particularly sensitive to most of these antibiotics, probably because ordinary therapeutic doses rapidly accumulate in the blood of uraemic patients and rise to toxic levels. Fortunately with each of these antibiotics, the nephrotoxicity appears to be reversible providing medication is stopped early enough.

It is convenient in discussing these antibiotics to classify them into groups depending on their molecular structures. This has the added advantage of revealing 'structure-toxicity' relationships and also predicting where 'cross-sensitivity-toxicity' relations might be expected to occur. Toxic side-effects of therapy other than nephrotoxic are included in these descriptions since the former may well precede the latter and give timely warning of a greater danger to follow unless treatment is stopped.

AMPHOTERICIN B

Amphotericin B is a heptaene member of the large family of polyene antifungal antibiotics. It has high activity against a wide range of yeast-like fungi, but apart from its tetraene relative, nystatin, it is the only polyene antibiotic to have achieved general clinical use in the treatment of systemic fungal disease.

Amphotericin B is insoluble and is poorly absorbed after oral administration. It does, however, form salts of sufficient solubility in water to provide solutions for therapeutic use. When given by injection side-effects are common and frequent; indeed the *British Medical Journal* in To-Day's Drugs (1964) characterized it with 'no other antibiotic so regularly causes severe side-effects'. Fever and nausea are liable to follow each injection and necessitate control with sedatives and antihistaminics; there has been a number of reports of nephrotoxicity (Rhoades *et al.*, 1961; Bell *et al.*, 1962; Takacs *et al.*, 1963; Butler *et al.*, 1964a).

Doses of this drug necessary to treat systemic fungal infections decrease the clearance of inulin, the mean clearance of para-aminohippuric acid (PAH) and the maximum concentrating ability of the kidney. These functions generally return towards normal after dosage is stopped, but progressive and fatal renal disease can occur. In studies on the dog, Butler *et al.* (1964*b*) have shown that injection of amphotericin B causes marked renal vasoconstriction which in turn causes depression of glomerular filtration, and tubular transport of PAH.

Nystatin (fungicidin) has not been reported to have nephrotoxicity; indeed clinically the toxic spectrum of this antibiotic has been nothing more than trivial side-effect. This is, of course, due to its low solubility and poor absorption from the intestine.

KANAMYCIN, NEOMYCIN, AND PAROMOMYCIN

These three antibiotics are chemically related members of the aminoglycoside family which includes streptomycin. They are produced by species of *Streptomyces* and all have a similar broad spectrum of antibacterial activity with particular effect against *Mycobacteria*. Paromomycin is also active against *Entamoeba histolytica*.

The three antibiotics are all bases and are used therapeutically as the sulphates, which are freely soluble. They have almost identical pharmacological behaviour, and even their toxic effects are similar, but the wide variations in the ease with which these are produced are mainly responsible for differences in their mode of use.

All three cause pain and irritation at the site of injection and are apt to cause damage to the eighth cranial nerve and the kidneys. Neomycin and paromomycin are so toxic in both these respects that their systemic use is rarely justified. Neomycin has a remarkably wide range of local uses, whilst paromomycin is now only used orally for temporary or long-term suppression of bowel flora, for the treatment of various forms of acute enteritis and of intestinal amoebiasis.

The renal lesion produced by these antibiotics primarily involves the proximal convoluted tubules. Clinical manifestation includes decreases in glomerular filtration rate (fall in inulin or creatinine clearance), the clearance of PAH and the maximal tubular concentration; less often, proteinuria and microscopic haematuria occur. Kanamycin sulphate is ordinarily given in doses of 0·5 gram, intramuscularly, twice daily. Larger doses may be used in severe infections, but the dose should be reduced to 1 gram/day as the patient improves.

BACITRACIN AND POLYMYXINS

These are polypeptide antibiotics, closely related and all derived from bacterial, as opposed to fungal, sources. They are products of organisms of the genus *Bacillus*.

Bacitracin has its main action against Gram-positive cocci and although a successful antibiotic in this respect its main toxic effect is on the kidney. Parenteral treatment always causes albuminuria with casts, and if treatment is continued it may then lead to oliguria and a rise in blood urea. The lesion responsible is degeneration of the epithelium of the proximal and distal convoluted tubules. Abnormalities in function and urinary sediment have been noted in patients receiving doses of 400 to 4,000 units/day. Results of almost all renal function tests are abnormal, including decreases in clearance in inulin and PAH, maximum tubular reabsorption rate for glucose and maximum tubular excretory capacity for PAH. Proteinuria and urinary casts are found but haematuria is rare. If treatment is stopped early enough the lesion can resolve completely. Pre-existing renal disease enhances the danger of nephrotoxicity.

Two polymyxins are available in the clinic, polymyxin B sulphate which is actually a mixture of polymyxins B_1 and B_2, and colistin sulphate or sulphomethate which is identical with polymyxin E. There is also a sulphomethyl derivative of polymyxin B for injection use. The polymyxins have activity against Gram-negative organisms.

The sulphates of polymyxins produce intense pain when injected intramuscularly. They also tend to cause dizziness and disturbances of sensation, numbness and paraesthesiae, mainly affecting the face. These defects have been largely overcome by the use of the sulphomethyl (methane sulphonate) derivatives.

The only serious toxic effect of the polymyxins is on the renal tubules. Polymyxin B is rather more toxic than polymyxin E and the sulphates are more toxic than their sulphomethyl derivatives. This gradation of toxicity interestingly enough matches the gradation in antibacterial activity.

Nephrotoxicity with the polymyxins is much less than that with bacitracin. Normal dosage in a patient with normal kidneys presents no hazard and does not cause albuminuria. However, greater caution is required in the presence of the damaged kidney, but, even so, renal function has repeatedly been seen actually to improve during treatment for pyelonephritis with polymyxin (*British Medical Journal*, Today's Drugs, 1968). When renal function is grossly impaired the dose interval may have to be widened.

TETRACYCLINES

A variety of cases of nephrotoxicity due to tetracyclines has been described; these may be classified into three groups. Firstly, those who show transient uraemia following tetracycline treatment; secondly, those who develop extreme toxicity, even death, in which hepatic dysfunction is most prominent, but who also demonstrate functional and histological abnormalities of the kidney and other organs (pancreas, brain); and finally, those cases with nephropathy due to degradation products of tetracycline, in which there is a severe derangement of tubular, and to a lesser extent, glomerular function, such changes being reversible.

It is not intended in this particular discussion to differentiate between individual tetracyclines; as a family they differ only in minutiae of molecular structure and they all have much the same spectra of activity and toxicity.

Transient Uraemia

Transient uraemia is particularly common when tetra-cyclines are given to patients who have had pre-existing renal impairment.

In a retrospective study Solomon *et al.* (1965) reported 22 patients who were azotaemic, did not have oliguria and received tetracycline treatment for 30 or more days. Twenty patients had increased blood urea nitrogen (BUN) levels rising steadily from 5 days after the onset of tetracycline therapy until it was stopped. Thereafter BUN levels remained at the same level for approximately 5 days, and then declined in all cases. The inorganic phosphorus also increased. The rising BUN was associated with symptoms of uraemic syndrome, vomiting, twitching and lethargy.

Shils (1963) examined the metabolic effects of tetracycline in patients with, and without, renal disease. The tetracycline, in doses of 0·4 to 2 grams caused a significant increase in BUN in eight patients with obvious renal disease and azotaemia prior to the treatment, with return to pre-treatment levels several days after the treatment stopped. Five of the patients had an accompanying rise of the inorganic phosphorus but no significant changes of the serum creatinine and serum uric acid were noted. Serum tetracycline concentrations were high (12–31 μg/ml) at the end of the antibiotic administration in patients with renal disease receiving more than 0·5–1 gram per day. Eight patients without renal disease treated similarly, demonstrated no change of the blood urea nitrogen. All patients who developed azotaemia complained of nausea, vomiting, weakness and malaise. Urinary nitrogen excretion paralleled the rising blood urea.

Extreme Toxicity with Hepatic and Renal Involvement

Kunelis *et al.* (1965) reported on 16 patients who developed fatty liver of pregnancy. Twelve of these were given tetracycline intravenously for the treatment of pyelonephritis just before the development of this syndrome. Eight patients died in coma or shock after a clinical course characterized by jaundice, rises in the BUN, low serum bicarbonate levels and occasional elevations of serum lactate and serum amylase levels. In all these patients there was extensive and fine vacuolization of the hepatic cells. Renal tissue was examined in five of these patients and areas of circumscribed cortical necrosis were evident, often surrounded by lymphocytes and histiocytes. These lesions were considered to be toxic in origin rather than due to pyelonephritis.

Dowling and Lepper (1964) reported on three non-pregnant patients who received intravenous tetracycline for infections and also developed the fatty liver syndrome. Two of these patients had serum tetracycline levels above 80 μg/ml during therapy. Winterling and Goldman (1965) described the case of a 66-year-old castrated man who had received stilboestrol for the treatment of prostatic carcinoma. Eight days after

starting treatment with parenteral tetracycline (2 to 3 grams daily) for cholangitis, the patient developed severe acidosis, azotaemia, and died. The liver showed extensive and fine vacuolization, and in the kidneys there was extensive fine vacuolization of the tubular epithelium, focal hyaline droplet degeneration, as well as necrosis of tubular epithelial cells.

It appears that fatal complications are more likely to occur in those patients who have received large amounts of tetracycline intravenously. Most of the reported patients were pregnant women who were treated for acute pyelonephritis (Schultz *et al.*, 1963; Dowling and Lepper, 1964; Gough and Searcy, 1964; Kunelis *et al.*, 1965; Lew and French, 1966); however, fatal complications also occurred in non-pregnant patients (Bateman *et al.*, 1952; Lepper *et al.*, 1953; Faloon *et al.*, 1957; Kunin *et al.*, 1959). The symptoms were nausea, vomiting, jaundice, azotaemia, acidosis, abdominal pain, intestinal haemorrhage, hypotension and finally death in shock or coma. In most of the reported cases hepatic abnormalities were emphasized; however, in a large number of the patients renal abnormalities were found (Schultz *et al.*, 1963; Kunelis *et al.*, 1965; Winterling and Goldman, 1965).

Nephropathy due to Degradation Products of Tetracycline

Degraded products of tetracycline cause a fairly characteristic syndrome; this was first reported by Ehrlich and Stein (1963) and Gross (1963). Abnormalities similar to those seen in the Fanconi syndrome were recognized by Gross (1963) and Frimpter *et al.* (1963). Fourteen cases have been described in the literature and they all have characteristic clinical histories.

Twelve of the fourteen cases were female; the ages ranged in both sexes from 6½ to 54 years. Symptoms occurred 1 to 7 days after ingestion of tetracycline. Nausea and vomiting occurred firstly in all but two (Fulop and Drapin, 1965) followed by lethargy in nine; dehydration and weakness were common. Two had Kussmaul's respiration (Wegienka and Weller, 1964; Mavrommatis, 1965). Aminoaciduria, albuminuria and glycosuria were invariably present. One patient lost 7 grams of protein in the urine during the seventh day of his illness (Mavrommatis, 1965). Urinary proteins had the electrophoretic composition seen predominantly in glomerular diseases (Butler and Flynn, 1958; Butler *et al.*, 1962; Rice *et al.*, 1964). The urinary sediments revealed moderate numbers of white blood cells, occasional red blood cells and casts. In two cases the urine was positive for Bence-Jones protein (Frimpter *et al.*, 1963; Mavrommatis, 1965). No case was fatal and all recovered normal renal function within one month.

Renal biopsies were taken on two of the cases. Two weeks after the initial symptoms one case had both tubular and glomerular damage. The tubular cells displayed desquamation, cast formation and obstruction of the tubular lumina, as well as marked hyaline and granular changes and irregular cytoplasmic vacuolization. Occasional foci of haemosiderinophages were seen. Apical portions of the epithelial cells were frequently shredded, while the nuclei stained poorly. Occasional mitotic figures in the tubules suggested regeneration. The glomerular tufts were swollen and their basement membranes were thickened. In the other case striking vacuolization of the distal tubular epithelium was found on biopsy approximately 2 weeks after onset. One week later a repeat biopsy showed hyper-cellularity of the glomerular tufts, with prominent capillary loops and basement-membrane thickening. Fine hyaline droplets were present in the cells of the proximal convoluted tubules and there were signs of epithelial regeneration in the distal tubules.

Frimpter *et al.* (1963) and Gross (1963) have commented that in their cases the tetracycline capsules were mostly outdated. In two cases, the patients had used capsules that had been carried on extensive trips abroad. Frimpter *et al.* (1963) were able to obtain some of the unused capsules and saw that they contained a hard black plug. Analysis by the manufacturer showed that approximately 23·7 per cent of the original 250 mg of tetracycline hydrochloride in each capsule had degraded to anhydrotetracycline and that 61·6 per cent was present as epianhydrotetracycline. These two degradation products are likely to form under adverse storage conditions especially in the presence of moisture and acid. Manufacturers no longer include citric acid in the formulation for this reason. Frimpter *et al.* (1963) stressed that these degradation products of tetracycline were responsible for the Fanconi syndrome, and that there was no evidence that fresh or pure tetracycline hydrochloride caused such toxicity.

Lindquist and Fellers recreated this syndrome in rats by injecting them intraperitoneally with old tetracycline (Fellers and Lindquist, 1964; Lindquist and Fellers, 1966). They observed glycosuria, aminoaciduria and hypophosphataemia. Morphological changes of the tubules were first noted at 3 days with progressive loss of stainable mitochondria and brush borders. At 7 days there were marked alterations of proximal convoluted tubules. Yet function and morphology returned to normal in 14 days in spite of continued administration of degraded tetracycline.

Deteriorated tetracycline was shown to contain anhydrotetracycline and epianhydrotetracycline in various proportions. It was the latter compound that appeared to be the most toxic.

Similar experimental studies in rats and dogs by Benitz and Diermeier (1964) also showed that tetracycline was degradated by heat, moisture and low pH and that of these degradation products, the epianhydrotetracycline (anhydro-4-epi-tetracycline) produced abnormal urinary findings similar to the Fanconi-type syndrome seen in man.

The conclusions to be drawn from these latter studies are obvious and certainly tetracyclines are nephrotoxic when taken in outdated and degraded form. However,

the range of nephrotoxicity discussed in the other two sections (transient uraemia—extreme toxicity with hepatic and renal involvement) cannot be explained by this occurrence. Tetracyclines are intrinsically nephrotoxic and they are retained in the presence of uraemia. If they are required to treat patients with concomitant renal failure, they can be used with caution if given in reduced doses.

CEPHALORIDINE AND CEPHALOTHIN

Cephaloridine and cephalothin are semi-synthetic derivatives of cephalosporin C, one of three antibiotics extracted from a *Cephalosporium* fungus isolated from a sewer outfall off the coast of Sardinia. Although structurally related to the penicillins, these derivatives have a different chemical nucleus, namely 7-cephalosporanic acid instead of 6-aminopenicillanic acid.

Cephaloridine and cephalothin are not destroyed by penicillinase, they have a wide spectrum of bactericidal activity and have to be given by injection as they are poorly absorbed orally.

As a group the cephalosporins (cephalosporin P, cephalosporin N (adicillin), cephalosporin C and its two derivatives cephaloridine and cephalothin) share the low toxicity of the penicillins. Initially it was thought that the cephalosporins did not show cross-hypersensitivity with the penicillins; however, Manten (1968) has reviewed the recent literature which generally suggests now that anaphylactic reactions to the initial injection of cephalosporin C derivatives (cephaloridine and cephalothin) may sometimes occur in patients known to be penicillin-hypersensitive. Allergic reactions have been reported in persons not sensitive to penicillin.

Reports of renal dysfunction have been associated with cephaloridine and cephalothin. Steinbrunn and Haemmerli (1966) reported that one out of nine patients developed proteinuria whilst receiving 12–24 grams of cephalothin daily by intravenous infusion. Another patient given enormous doses (24 grams daily) became anuric.

Ballingall and Turpie (1967) also described a case of proteinuria following treatment with cephaloridine. The patient was left with a continuous proteinuria after the first course of therapy. A second course of treatment was followed by a rapid deterioration of renal function culminating in anuria.

High doses of cephaloridine (up to 6 grams daily) given to patients with poor renal function may raise the blood urea; hyaline and granular casts may also be formed (Foord and Snell, 1966).

Cephalexin is a new cephalosporin antibiotic which is well absorbed when given orally; absorption has been claimed to approach 100 per cent and it was thought that this antibiotic would have little or no effect on the intestinal bacterial flora. However, Gaya and associates (1970) gave oral cephalexin to 18 patients with urinary tract infections. Absorption was variable and between 29 and 89 per cent of the total daily dose (0·5–1 gram four times a day) was excreted in the urine in 24 hours.

A significant number of patients became faecal carriers of *Pseudomonas aeruginosa*, compared with a control group who received no antibiotic. Four of the cephalexin-treated patients acquired a strain of *Ps. aeruginosa* known to be present in food from the hospital diet kitchen and one patient developed a urinary tract infection with this strain.

SULPHONAMIDES AND THE KIDNEY

Sulphonamides may be generally classified into two groups; those that are well absorbed and those that are poorly absorbed. It is with the former group that crystalluria may occur during sulphamide therapy.

The well-absorbed sulphonamides are rapidly and completely absorbed from the small intestine; elimination is almost entirely via the kidneys. Most sulphonamides are acetylated and usually the acetyl derivative is less soluble than the parent molecule, especially at low pH. The ratio of free to acetylated compound varies with the sulphonamide. If a large amount of insoluble acetylated sulphonamide is excreted in a small volume of acid urine there is a real risk of crystalluria.

A few sulphonamides are excreted as the glucuronide, which is very soluble, thus there is no danger of crystalluria with these. In recent years, a number of long-acting (slowly-excreted) sulphonamides have been introduced; again with these there is no danger of crystalluria because of their slow rate of excretion. The second group mentioned earlier, the poorly absorbed sulphonamides present no problem since they are not sufficiently well absorbed to cause kidney damage. FIGURE 14.1

FIG. 14.1. *Classification and structural formulae of some of the sulphonamides in common use*

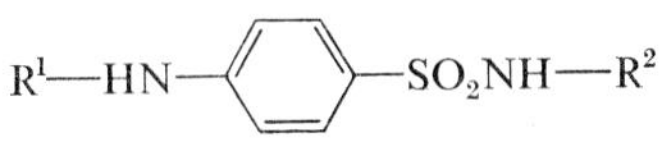

R¹—HN—⟨benzene ring⟩—SO₂NH—R²

Basic structure of sulphonamide

GROUP 1. SHORT-ACTING (readily and rapidly absorbed)

R¹   R²

H

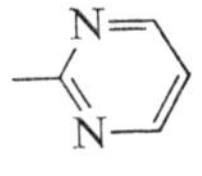

Sulphadiazine
(Sulphapyrimidine)

H

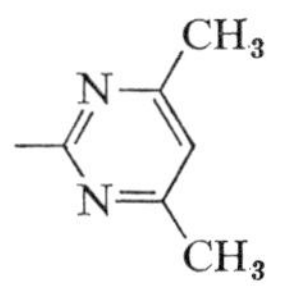

Sulphadimidine
(Sulphamethazine

R¹   R²

H

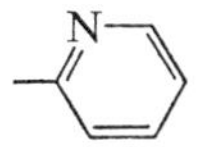

Sulphapyridine

H

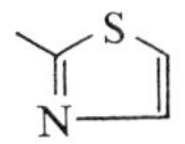

Sulphathiazole

H

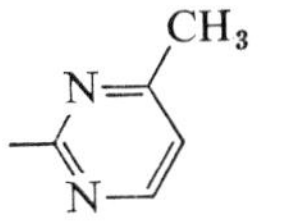

Sulphamerazine
(Sulfamethyldiazine)

GROUP 2. LONG-ACTING (well absorbed, slowly excreted, extensively bound to plasma protein)

R¹   R²

H   CO—⟨benzene ring⟩—OCH(CH₃)₂

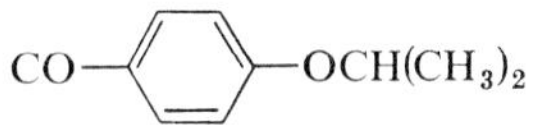

Sulphaproxyline

H

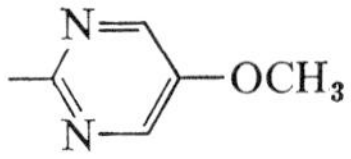

Sulphamethoxydiazine
(Sulfametin)
(Methoxypyrimal)
(Sulfamonomethoxine)

H

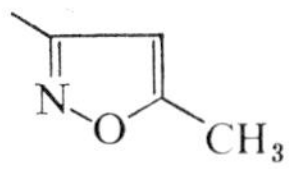

Sulphamethoxazole
(Sulfamethoxizole)
(Sulfisomezole)

H

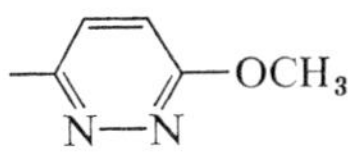

Sulphamethoxypyridazine
(Sulfamethoxypyrazine)

H

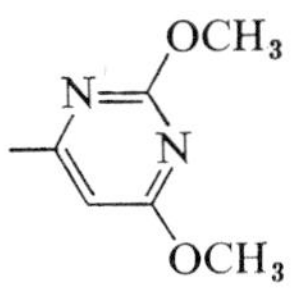

Sulphadimethoxine

R^1	R^2

H C_6H_5

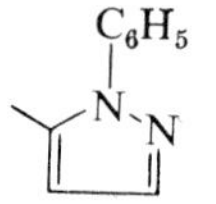

Sulphaphenazole

GROUP 3. INTESTINAL (poorly absorbed)

R^1	R^2

$HOOCCH_2CH_2CO$

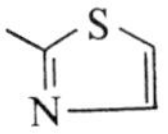

Succinylsulphathiazole

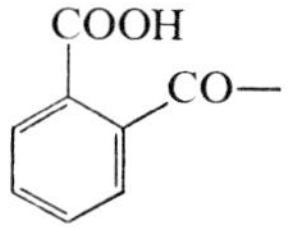

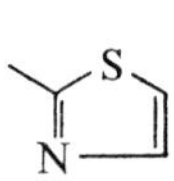

Phthalylsulphathiazole
(Phthalylsulfonazole)

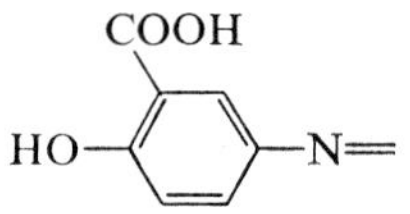

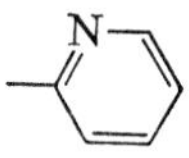

Sulphasalazine
(Salicylazosulfapyridine)

H $-\overset{NH}{\overset{\|}{C}}NH_2$

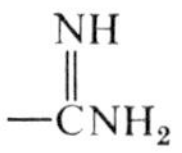

Sulphaguanidine
(Sulfanilylguanidine)

GROUP 4. URINARY

R^1	R^2

H

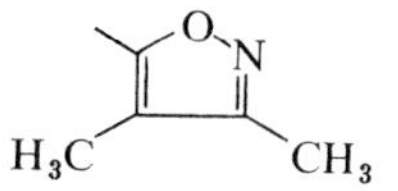

Sulphafurazole
(Sulfisoxazole)
(Sulfafurazole)

H

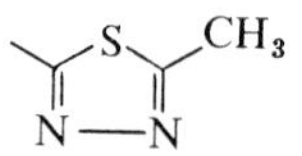

Sulphamethizole
(Sulfamethylthiadiazole)

shows the division of the available sulphonamides into the categories that have been mentioned.

Crystalluria may be symptomless if very mild, but may cause renal pain, haematuria, oliguria and eventually anuria. If detected before anuria develops, copious fluid should be given and the urine rendered alkaline with potassium or sodium bicarbonate.

Anuria due to crystals must be distinguished from that due to renal tubular necrosis which can also occur. The renal tubular necrosis, which is a hypersensitivity phenomenon, is likely to recur on any subsequent occasion that the patient is exposed to sulphonamides.

The treatment of sulphonamide anuria therefore depends on whether it is due to tubular necrosis or crystalluria. In the case of anuria due to crystalluria, ureteric catheterization or nephrostomy should be performed; in the case of renal tubular necrosis the anuria is treated in the usual way.

NEPHROTIC SYNDROME CAUSED BY URICOSURIC AGENTS

Prolonged administration of a uricosuric agent together with abundant intake of fluids and alkalization of the urine is useful in the prevention and treatment of uratic renal lesions in the patient suffering from gout. Vigorous uricosuria from over-zealous dosage together with inadequate fluid may produce a momentary 'flash colic', a true renal colic with urate crystalluria and haematuria. Apart from these logically predictable renal complications of gout and its therapy, which are largely related to urate deposition, renal tubular toxicity has been described in connexion with probenecid and phenylbutazone.

PHENYLBUTAZONE

Oliguria and anuria are rare complications of phenylbutazone therapy. The first cases were reported by Kling (1952) and Feldman (1952).

Meiers and Wetzels (1964) reviewed the effects of phenylbutazone on renal function. Water retention and weight gain were universal, and seemed to reach a maximum between 3 to 7 days of therapy. Phenylbutazone also caused sodium and chloride retention but did not alter potassium excretion. Glomerular filtration was unaffected. Tubular reabsorption of uric acid was inhibited as was the tubular secretion of para-aminohippuric acid, para-aminosalicylic acid and phenol red. These facts suggested a tubular locus for the action of phenylbutazone, although all tubular transfer mechanisms could not be affected since glucose absorption continued to be normal.

Bloch et al. (1966) reviewed the literature and found 50 cases of renal complications of phenylbutazone therapy. They also reported a personal case of phenylbutazone-induced nephropathy in which acute toxic renal tubular failure was produced on the third day of therapy with a treatment of 600 mg intramuscularly per day. They emphasized the rarity of this complication and also felt that this effect was unrelated to dosage.

Thiele et al. (1967) reviewed the changes produced by a total of 18 drugs on the renal tubules and commented that phenylbutazone produced glomerular and distal convoluted tubular damage, but spared the proximal tubules. Baumgartner et al. (1967) described a single case of renal necrosis which was attributed to phenylbutazone. This woman aged 61 years was treated for ileo-sacral pain with a drug combination of aminophenazone and phenylbutazone. She reacted by developing oliguria, uraemia, nausea and haemorrhagic vesicles on the lips. The patient died 6 weeks later because of irreversible renal failure. Autopsy showed bilateral renal cortical necrosis of the Shwartzmann-Sanorelli type.

Lesions produced by phenylbutazone would, therefore, appear to be of two basic types. The first, and more common, a distal tubular lesion sometimes associated with glomerular damage; the second, acute cortical necrosis.

PROBENECID

Ferris and co-workers (1961) reported the first case of probenecid-induced nephropathy. Six years later Sokol et al. (1967) reported a further case. Their patient was a 34-year-old man suffering from gout. He was started on probenecid 0·5 gram twice daily. Eight weeks later he complained of marked facial oedema, headaches and dizziness. He denied taking any medicaments other than probenecid.

Laboratory investigations showed abundant albumin in the urine; blood urea was normal as also his anti-streptolysin titre. He was admitted to hospital and treated with diuretics and prednisone, and within 14 days the nephrotic syndrome had cleared and no protein appeared in the urine.

Kidney biopsy taken during the active phase of the nephrotic syndrome showed normal glomerular and tubular structure, but precipitated protein was revealed in Bowman's spaces and in the convoluted tubules.

Four weeks after discharge from hospital the patient resumed probenecid therapy 0·5 gram twice daily. After a further 5 weeks of treatment, oedema of the hands and face developed and there was profound albuminuria. Probenecid was immediately discontinued and the oedema and proteinuria subsided over a period of 2 weeks.

Scott and associates (1966) also reported a case but this was different from the previous two described in that the nephrotic syndrome occurred about 1 year after treatment with probenecid had started. The patient had severe oedema and proteinuria. All signs and symptoms remitted after the drug was stopped. Meyler (1968) records that this complication had been reported earlier in three cases prior to 1963.

MISCELLANEOUS DRUGS CAUSING IATROGENIC NEPHROPATHY

TROXIDONE (TRIMETHADIONE)

In 1948 Barnett and co-workers recorded that some patients with petit mal developed a nephrotic syndrome that seemed to be due to the administration of the anti-convulsant, trimethadione. Heymann (1967) stated that he knew of 37 cases that confirmed Barnett's observations; four of these cases were fatal.

In four patients in the literature (Barnett et al., 1948; Haugen, 1957; Lubowitz, 1966) readministration of the drug was followed by recurrence of nephrotic syndrome that had previously subsided when trimethadione therapy had been discontinued.

Heymann (1967) advises that every patient receiving oxazolidinedione derivatives (i.e. trimethadione, paramethadione and aloxidone) should have regular urine checks every 2 to 3 weeks, and, because the renal lesion may become manifest even as long as $5\frac{1}{2}$ years after commencing treatment, these regular examinations should not be discontinued. Steroids have a place in the treatment of trimethadione-induced nephrotic syndrome and Heymann suggested that they be commenced if the nephrotic syndrome had not resolved within 2 weeks of stopping trimethadione dosage.

The American Medical Association Registry on Adverse Reactions records that 26 of the total of 37 cases of trimethadione-associated nephrotic syndrome occurred after 1960.

D-PENICILLAMINE

Jaffe et al. (1968) described two patients, given the chelating agent d-penicillamine for rheumatoid arthritis and scleroderma who developed renal damage. In one patient a renal biopsy had been obtained before treatment was begun and this permitted comparison with subsequent biopsies taken after the toxicity appeared. The changes found by electron microscopy in both patients were those of membranous transformation-electron-dense deposits on the epithelial surface of the basement membrane and fusion of epithelial foot processes. Immunofluorescent staining was positive with antisera to IgG and complement. Both patients improved after the drug was discontinued, and the intensity of immunofluorescent staining diminished. The nephropathy was thought to be due to an immunological mechanism.

Earlier, Sternlieb (1966) had described eight incidences of nephrotic syndrome in patients receiving the racemate (dl-penicillamine) for hepatolenticular degeneration; it was suggested then that this might be due to the presence of the l-isomer. However, Rosenberg and Hayslett (1967) later described nephrotic syndrome in three of 18 cystinuric patients treated with the d-isomer of the drug.

TOLBUTAMIDE

The nephrotic syndrome has been described as a rare complication of the sulphonylurea hypoglycaemics (*British Medical Journal*, 1963; Arnold and Lauener, 1964).

Moore (1962) described the case of a 62-year-old man with diabetes of 10 years duration who was changed from insulin therapy to tolbutamide. On the 19th day of tolbutamide therapy he showed a weight gain of 10 lb and complained of nausea, orthopnoea, and oedema. A diagnosis of heart failure or diabetic nephropathy was made. Tolbutamide was continued combined with digitalis and diuretics but with no response. Four days after admission to hospital the tolbutamide was suspected and promptly discontinued and steroid therapy instituted. The patient recovered rapidly.

MERCURIAL DIURETICS (MERSALYL, MERCURAMIDE WITH THEOPHYLLINE, CHLORMERODRIN, MERCAPTOMERIN)

The first case of nephrotic syndrome due to mercurials was reported by Sprunt (1930), and this was followed by other reports (Tarr and Jacobson, 1932; Rosenthal, 1933; Waife and Pratt, 1946; Bruno, 1948; Preedy and Russell, 1953).

However, considering the use of both injected and oral mercurial diuretics before the advent of the oral thiazide diuretics, the incidence of nephrotic syndrome compared with total usage was very slight. Indeed there may have been a tendency to overlook the risk.

The possible risk was, however, raised again by Burston and co-workers (1958) who described a single case of the nephrotic syndrome following the administration of mersalyl. This case was fatal. Riddle and her associates (1958) reported the nephrotic syndrome complicating congestive heart failure in five patients who received mercurial diuretics by injection (mersalyl, mercuramide with theophylline, mercaptomerin) or orally (chlormerodrin) for long periods.

Three cases were fatal and pathological findings suggested that the renal lesions were due to mercury. These workers commented that the most useful evidence of tubular damage was persistence of albuminuria despite a satisfactory diuresis in response to mercurial therapy, and emphasized that early recognition of the condition was of the utmost importance if fatal outcome was to be avoided.

RETROPERITONEAL FIBROSIS DUE TO METHYSERGIDE

In 1959, Sicuteri reported on the effectiveness of methysergide in the prevention of migraine, but in 1964, Graham, reporting on his experience in treating 500 patients with methysergide, commented that two patients developed retroperitoneal fibrosis. Utz *et al.* (1965) reported three cases of patients on methysergide who subsequently developed retroperitoneal fibrosis, and Weiss and Hinman (1966) reported a further case.

Graham (1968) collected information on a series of 55 cases of retroperitoneal fibrosis which had either been reported directly to him or had been reported in the literature up until 1 October, 1967. The ages of these patients ranged from 26–75 years with an average age of 49 years. The sex distribution was in favour of females 3:2, a reversal of the ratio in 'idiopathic' retroperitoneal fibrosis which is quoted as 3:1 or 2:1 in favour of men. This probably reflects the fact that migraine, and hence the use of methysergide, is more prevalent in women.

The smallest dosage of methysergide used by any patient who developed retroperitoneal fibrosis was 2 mg daily taken over 21 months. The shortest duration of treatment before the diagnosis of retroperitoneal fibrosis was made over 7 months.

The signs and symptoms of drug-induced retroperitoneal fibrosis and the laboratory findings were the same as in the 'idiopathic' form. Although this disorder caused malaise, backache, fatigue, weight loss and low grade fever for months as initial symptoms, the presenting symptoms were those resulting from fibrotic obstruction in the retroperitoneal space of the ureters, great vessels, lymphatics or bowel. Thus, constipation, dysuria, hydrocele and thrombophlebitis or intermittent claudication provided the first indication of the already established fibrotic process. An intravenous pyelogram was found to be the best diagnostic aid, and this usually showed medial deviation of the ureters at the level of the 4th or 5th lumbar vertebrae in the early cases, and, in more advanced cases, hydro-ureter and hydronephrosis were revealed.

With two exceptions, cessation of methysergide therapy was associated with partial or complete regression of the signs, symptoms and X-ray evidence of the disease process in 28 patients treated conservatively. Those who were treated by omission of methysergide therapy fared as well as 25 patients in whom surgical measures were employed. Patients taking methysergide or ergotamine for their migraine after surgical treatment, had traumatic post-operative courses at times requiring repeat operations.

Clinical and pathological evidence suggested that steroids might alleviate the condition by reducing the inflammatory process, although they were not effective if methysergide therapy continued.

The pathological process in methysergide-induced retroperitoneal fibrosis consisted of an inflammatory non-specific response. Several phases of this response were observed in different areas of the same surgical biopsy specimen. There was a suggestion that the early lesion might consist of infiltration of fat by lymphocytes followed by plasma cells and eosinophils of the walls of small arteries and veins with intimal proliferation and subsequent obliteration of their lumen.

RECOMMENDED FURTHER READING

GAULT, M. H., RUDWAL, T. C., ENGLES, W. D., and DOSSETOR, J. B. (1968) Syndrome associated with the abuse of analgesics, *Ann. intern. Med.*, **68**, 906–25.

HALEY, T. J. (1966) Is phenacetin the cause of 'analgesic nephrotoxicity'?, *J. New Drugs*, **6**, 193–202.

KINCAID-SMITH, P. (1967) Pathogenesis of the renal lesion associated with the abuse of analgesics, *Lancet*, **1**, 859–62.

KUNIN, C. M. (1967) Nephrotoxicity of antibiotics, *J. Amer. med. Ass.*, **202**, 204–8.

OKUN, D. E. (1968) Drug induced renal disease, *Practitioner*, **201**, 461–6.

PRESCOTT, L. F. (1966) The nephrotoxicity of analgesics, *J. Pharm. Pharmacol.*, **18**, 331–53.

SHELLEY, J. H. (1967) Phenacetin through the looking glass, *Clin. Pharmacol. Ther.*, **8**, 428–71.

WEIR, R. J., TREE, M., and FRASER, R. (1970) Effect of oral contraceptives on blood pressure and on plasma renin, renin substrate, and corticosteroids, *J. clin. Path.*, **23**, Suppl. (Ass. Clin. Path.), **3**, 49–54.

REFERENCES

ANGERVALL, L., BENGTSSON, U., ZETTERLUND, C. G., and ZSIGMOND, M. (1969) Renal pelvic carcinoma in a Swedish district with abuse of a phenacetin-containing drug, *Brit. J. Urol.*, **41**, 401–5.

ARNOLD, C. R., and LAUENER, R. W. (1964) Oral hypoglycaemic drugs, *Canad. med. Ass. J.*, **91**, 395–6.

BAKER, S. B. DE C., and WILLIAMS, R. T. (1963) Acute interstitial nephritis due to drug sensitivity, *Brit. med. J.*, **1**, 1655–8.

BALLINGALL, D. L., and TURPIE, A. G. C. (1967) Cephaloridine toxicity, *Lancet*, **ii**, 835–6.

BARNETT, H. L., SIMONS, D. J., and WELLS, R. E. (1948) Nephrotic syndrome occurring after tridione therapy, *Amer. J. Med.*, **4**, 760–4.

BARRITT, D. W., and JORDAN, S. C. (1960) Anticoagulant drugs in the treatment of pulmonary embolism. A controlled trial, *Lancet*, **i**, 1309–12.

BATEMAN, J. C., BARBERIO, J. R., GRICE, P., KLOPP, C. T., and PIERPONT, H. (1952) Fatal complications of intensive antibiotic therapy in patients with neoplastic disease, *Arch. intern. Med.*, **90**, 763–73.

BAUMGARTNER, H., SCHEITLIN, W., and RECHENBERG, H. K. VON (1967) Beidseitige Nierenrindennekrose nach pyrazolan behandlung, *Dtsch. med. Wschr.*, **92**, 1075–7.

BELL, N. H., ANDRIOLE, V. T., SABESIN, S. M., and UTZ, J. P. (1962) On the nephrotoxicity of amphotericin B in man, *Amer. J. Med.*, **33**, 64–9.

BENGTSSON, U., ANGERVALL, L., EKMAN, H., and LEHMANN, L. (1968) Transitional cell tumours of the renal pelvis in analgesic abusers, *Scand. J. Urol. Nephrol.*, **2**, 145–50.

BENITZ, K. F., and DIERMEIER, H. F. (1964) Renal toxicity of tetracycline degradation products, *Proc. Soc. exp. Biol. (N.Y.)*, **115**, 930–5.

BLOCH, M. H., GORINS, A., and MEYEROVITCH, A. (1966) Les accidents renaux de la Phenylbutazone, *Presse méd.*, **74**, 2671–4.

BRITISH MEDICAL JOURNAL (1960) Renal risks of phenacetin, editorial, *Brit. med. J.*, **1**, 714–15.

BRITISH MEDICAL JOURNAL (1963) Oral hypoglycaemic agents, in *Today's Drugs*, *Brit. med. J.*, **1**, 521–2.

BRITISH MEDICAL JOURNAL (1964) Anti-fungal antibiotics, in *Today's Drugs*, British Medical Association, London, pp. 47–51.

BRITISH MEDICAL JOURNAL (1968) Bacitracin and polymyxins, in *Today's Drugs*, *Brit. med. J.*, **3**, 106–7.

BROOKS, R. H., and CALLEJA, H. B. (1960) Dermatitis, hepatitis and nephritis due to pheninidione (phenylindanedione), *Ann. intern. Med.*, **52**, 706–10.

BRUNO, M. S. (1948) Fatal toxic nephrosis following administration of mercurial diuretics, *New Engl. J. Med.*, **239**, 769–73.

BURNS, C., and DESMOND, F. B. (1958) Sensitivity to Dindevan (phenylindanedione): Report of a case with review of literature, *N.Z. med. J.*, **57**, 283–91.

BURRY, A. F., DEJERSEY, P., and WEEDEN, D. (1966) Phenacetin and renal papillary necrosis: Results of a prospective autopsy investigation, *Med. J. Aust.*, **1**, 873–9.

BURSTON, J., DARMADY, E. M., and STRANACK, F. (1958) Nephrosis due to mercurial diuretics, *Brit. med. J.*, **1**, 1277–9.

BUTLER, E. A., and FLYNN, F. V. (1958) The proteinuria of renal tubular disorders, *Lancet*, **ii**, 978–80.

BUTLER, E. A., FLYNN, F. V., HARRIS, H., and ROBSON, E. B. (1962) A study of urine proteins by two-dimensional electrophoresis with special reference to proteinuria of renal tubular disorders, *Clin. chim. Acta.*, **7**, 34–41.

BUTLER, W. T., BENNETT, J. E., ALLING, D. W., WESTLAKE, P. T., UTZ, J. P., and HILL, G. J. (1964a) Nephrotoxicity of amphotericin B: Early and late effects in 81 patients, *Ann. intern. Med.*, **61**, 175–87.

BUTLER, W. T., HILL, G. J., SZWED, C. F., and KNIGHT, V. (1964b) Amphotericin B renal toxicity in the dog, *J. Pharmacol. exp. Ther.*, **146**, 47–56.

CANADIAN MEDICAL ASSOCIATION JOURNAL (1965) Analgesic abuse and kidney damage, editorial, *Canad. med. Ass. J.*, **92**, 84–5.

CLAUSEN, E. (1962) Nephrotoxic effect of phenacetin and acetylsalicylic acid in animal experiments, *Acta med. scand.*, **172**, 419–26.

CLAUSEN, E. (1964) Histological changes in rabbit kidneys induced by phenacetin and acetylsalicylic acid, *Lancet*, **ii**, 123–4.

COON, W. W., DUFF, I. F., HODGSON, P. E., and DENNIS, E W. (1953) Therapeutic evaluation of new anticoagulant phenylindanedione, *Ann. Surg.*, **138**, 467–75.

DAWBORN, J. K., FAIRLEY, K. E., KINCAID-SMITH, P., and KING, W. E. (1966) The association of peptic ulceration, chronic renal disease and analgesic abuse, *Quart. J. Med.*, **35**, 69–83.

DAWBORN, J. K., KINCAID-SMITH, P., and McLAREN, J. (1964) The effect of aspirin and phenacetin on ascending infection in the rat kidney, *Aust. Ann. Med.*, **13**, 217–21.

DEMING, C. L. (1963) Tumours of the kidney, in *Urology*, Vol. II, ed. Campbell, M. F., Philadelphia, p. 895.

DOWLING, H. F., and LEPPER, M. H. (1964) Hepatic reactions to tetracycline, *J. Amer. med. Ass.*, **188**, 307–9.

EHRLICH, L. I., and STEIN, H. S. (1963) Abnormal urinary

finding following administration of Achromycin V, *Paediatrics*, **31**, 339.

EKNOYAN, G., and MATSON, J. L. (1964) Acute renal failure caused by aminopyrine, *J. Amer. med. Ass.*, **190**, 934–5.

FALOON, W. W., DOWNS, J. J., DUGGAN, K., and PRIOR, J. R. (1957) Nitrogen and electrolyte metabolism and hepatic function and histology in patients receiving tetracycline, *Amer. J. med. Sci.*, **233**, 563–72.

FELDMAN, H. A. (1952) Proceedings of annual meeting, discussion, *Ann. rheum. Dis.*, **11**, 299.

FELLERS, F. X., and LINDQUIST, R. L. (1964) Mechanism of induced nephropathy by old tetracycline, *Fed. Proc.*, **23**, 573.

FERRIS, T. F., MORGAN, W. S., and LEVITIN, H. (1961) Nephrotic syndrome caused by probenecid, *New Engl. J. Med.*, **265**, 381–3.

FOORD, R. D., and SNELL, E. S. (1966) Clinical experiences with Cephaloridin, *Praxis*, **55**, 978–85.

FRIMPTER, G. W., TIMPANELLI, A. E., EISENMENGER, W. J., STEIN, H. S., and EHRLICH, L. J. (1963) Reversible 'Fanconi syndrome' caused by degraded tetracycline, *J. Amer. med. Ass.*, **184**, 111–13.

FULOP, M., and DRAPIN, A. (1965) Potassium depletion secondary to nephropathy apparently caused by 'outdated tetracycline', *New Engl. J. Med.*, **27**, 986–9.

GALEA, E. G., YOUNG, L. N., and BELL, J. R. (1963) Fatal nephropathy due to phenindione sensitivity, *Lancet*, **i**, 920–2.

GAYA, H., ADNITT, P. I., and TURNER, P. (1970) Changes in gut flora after cephalexin treatment, *Brit. med. J.*, **3**, 624–5.

GAULT, M. H., RUDWAL, T. C., ENGLES, W. D., and DOSSETOR, J. B. (1968) Syndrome associated with the abuse of analgesics, *Ann. intern. Med.*, **68**, 906–25.

GOODMAN, L. S., and GILMAN, A. (1955) *Pharmacological Basis of Therapeutics*, 2nd ed., New York, p. 1518.

GOUGH, G. S., and SEARCY, R. L. (1964) Additional case of fatty liver disease with tetracycline therapy, *New Engl. J. Med.*, **270**, 157–8.

GRAHAM, J. R. (1964) Methysergide for prevention of headache: Experience in five hundred patients over three years, *New Engl. J. Med.*, **270**, 67–72.

GRAHAM, J. R. (1968) Fibrosis associated with methysergide therapy, in *Drug-Induced Diseases*, Vol. 3, eds. Meyler, L., and Peck, H. M., Excerpta Medica Foundation, Amsterdam, pp. 249–69.

GRIMLUND, K. (1963) Phenacetin and renal damage at a Swedish factory, *Acta med. scand.*, **174**, Suppl. 405, 1–26.

GROSS, J. M. (1963) Fanconi syndrome (adult type) developing secondary to ingestion of outdated tetracycline, *Ann. intern. Med.*, **58**, 523–8.

GUEDON, J., CORBIN, J. L., VUAGNAT, P., and CHAPMAN, A. (1966) Néphropathie interstitielle aiguë avec anurie transitoire secondaire à une intolérance a la phénindione, *J. Urol. Néphrol.*, **72**, 901–8.

HALEY, T. J. (1966) Is phenacetin the cause of 'analgesic nephrotoxicity'?, *J. New Drugs*, **6**, 193–202.

HARVALD, B. (1963) Renal papillary necrosis. A clinical survey of sixty-six cases, *Amer. J. Med.*, **35**, 481–6.

HAUGEN, N. N. (1957) Tridione nephropathy, *Acta med. scand.*, **159**, 375–80.

HEYMANN, W. (1967) Nephrotic syndrome after use of trimethadione and paramethadione in petit mal, *J. Amer. med. Ass.*, **202**, 893–4.

HULTENGREN, N., LAGERGREN, C., and LJUNGQVIST, A. (1965) Carcinoma of the renal pelvis in renal papillary necrosis, *Acta chir. scand.*, **130**, 314–20.

JAQUES, L. B., GORDON, E., and LEPP, E. (1950) New prothrombopenic drug, phenylindanedione, *Canad. med. Ass. J.*, **62**, 465–70.

JAFFE, I. A., TRESER, G., SUZUKI, Y., and EHRENREICH, T. (1968) Nephropathy induced by D-penicillamine, *Ann. intern. Med.*, **69**, 549–56.

JOURNAL OF THE AMERICAN MEDICAL ASSOCIATION (1963a) Kidney disease and abuse of analgesics, editorial, *J. Amer. med. Ass.*, **184**, 494.

JOURNAL OF THE AMERICAN MEDICAL ASSOCIATION (1963b) Analgesic abuse and renal toxicity, editorial, *J. Amer. med. Ass.*, **184**, 495–6.

JOURNAL OF THE AMERICAN MEDICAL ASSOCIATION (1964) Analgesic abuse and the kidney—a commentary, editorial, *J. Amer. med. Ass.*, **190**, 238–9.

KINCAID-SMITH, P. (1963) The association between chronic renal disease, peptic ulceration and analgesic abuse. A clinico-pathological study, *Excerpta med. (Amst.)*, **67**, 91–2.

KINCAID-SMITH, P. (1967) Pathogenesis of the renal lesion associated with the abuse of analgesics, *Lancet*, **i**, 859–62.

KIRKEBY, K. (1954) Agranulocytosis following treatment with phenylindanedione, *Lancet*, **ii**, 580–1.

KLING, D. H. (1952) Proceedings of annual meeting, discussion, *Ann. rheum. Dis.*, **11**, 299.

KOCH, B., IRVINE, A. H., MCIVER, J. R., and LIEPA, E. (1968) Renal papillary necrosis and abuse of analgesics, *Canad. med. Ass. J.*, **98**, 8–15.

KUNELIS, C. T., PETERS, J. L., and EDMONDSON, H. A. (1965) Fatty liver of pregnancy and its relationship to tetracycline therapy, *Amer. J. Med.*, **38**, 359–77.

KUNIN, C. M. (1967) Nephrotoxicity of antibiotics, *J. Amer. med. Ass.*, **202**, 204–8.

KUNIN, C. M., SEARLE, B. R., MERRILL, J. P., and FINLAND, M. (1959) Persistence of antibiotics in blood of patients with acute renal failure, I. Tetracycline and chlortetracycline, *J. clin. Invest.*, **38**, 1487–97.

LANCET (1963) Renal papillary necrosis and phenacetin, annotation, *Lancet*, **i**, 1106.

LANCET (1968) Phenacetin, leading article, *Lancet*, **ii**, 717–18.

LANCET (1969) Analgesic abuse and tumours of the renal pelvis, leading article, *Lancet*, **ii**, 1233–4.

LAWSON, A. A. H., and MACLEAN, N. (1966) Renal disease and drug therapy in rheumatoid arthritis, *Ann. rheum. Dis.*, **25**, 441–9.

LEPPER, M. H., WOLFE, C. K., ZIMMERMAN, H. J., CALDWELL, E. R., JR., SPIES, H. W., and DOWLING, H. F. (1953) Effects of large doses of aureomycin on human liver, *Arch. intern. Med.*, **88**, 271.

LEW, H. T., and FRENCH, S. W. (1966) Tetracycline nephrotoxicity and nonoliguric acute renal failure, *Arch. intern. Med.*, **118**, 123–8.

LINDENEG, O., FISCHER, S., PEDERSEN, J., and NISSEN, N. I. (1959) Necrosis of the renal papillae and prolonged abuse of phenacetin, *Acta med. scand.*, **165**, 321–8.

LINDQUIST, R. L., and FELLERS, F. X. (1966) Degraded tetracycline nephropathy. Functional, morphologic, and histochemical observations, *Lab. Invest.*, **15**, 864–76.

LUBOWITZ, H. (1966) Trimethadione nephrosis, *J. Amer. med. Ass.*, **195**, 151.

MANDEL, E. E. (1952) Renal medullary necrosis, *Amer. J. Med.*, **13**, 322–7.

MANTEN, A. (1968) Antibiotic drugs, in *Side Effects of Drugs*, Vol. VI, eds. Meyler, L., and Herxheimer, A., Excerpta Medica Foundation, Amsterdam, pp. 263–314.

MAVROMMATIS, F. (1965) Tetracycline nephrotoxicity: Case report with renal biopsy, *J. Amer. med. Ass.*, **193**, 191–4.

MEDICAL JOURNAL OF AUSTRALIA (1968) Renal papillary

necrosis and analgesic abuse, comments and abstracts, *Med. J. Aust.*, **1**, 227–8.

MEIERS, H. G., and WETZELS, E. (1964) Phenylbutazone and renal function, *Arzneimittel-Forsch.*, **14**, 252–8.

MENON, I. S., and BURRELL, N. S. (1966) Phenindione sensitivity complicating anticoagulant therapy, *J. Indian med. Ass.*, **47**, 552–4.

MEYLER, L. (1968) Drugs used in the treatment of gout, in *Side Effects of Drugs*, Vol. VI, eds. Meyler, L., and Herxheimer, A., Excerpta Medica Foundation, Amsterdam, pp. 507–8.

MOOLTEN, S. E., and SMITH, I. B. (1960) Fatal nephritis in chronic phenacetin poisoning, *Amer. J. Med.*, **28**, 127–34.

MOORE, M. J. (1962) Renal toxicity with nephrotic-like edema resulting from tolbutamide, *Amer. Practit.*, **13**, 350–4.

NANRA, R. S., and KINCAID-SMITH, P. (1970) Papillary necrosis in rats caused by aspirin and aspirin-containing mixtures, *Brit. med. J.*, **3**, 559–61.

OLAFSSON, Ó., GUDMUNDSSON, K. R., and BREKKAN, Á. (1966) Migraine, gastritis and renal papillary necrosis. A syndrome in chronic non-obstructive pyelonephritis, *Acta med. scand.*, **179**, 121–8.

PEARCE, J. M. S. (1963) Nephropathy and phenindione sensitivity, *Lancet*, **i**, 1158–9.

PEARSON, H. H. (1967) Residual renal defects in non-fatal phenacetin nephritis, *Med. J. Aust.*, **2**, 308–13.

PERKINS, J. (1962) Phenindione sensitivity, *Lancet*, **i**, 127–30.

PLASS, H. F. R. (1964) Renal papillary necrosis associated with analgesic abuse, *Ann. intern. Med.*, **60**, 111–14.

POSTGRADUATE MEDICAL SCHOOL OF LONDON, (1960) A case of pulmonary hypertension, *Brit. med. J.*, **2**, 1219–24.

PREEDY, J. R. K., and RUSSELL, D. S. (1953) Acute salt depletion associated with the nephrotic syndrome developing during treatment with a mercurial diuretic, *Lancet*, **ii**, 1181–4.

PRESCOTT, L. F. (1966) The nephrotoxicity of analgesics, *J. Pharm. Pharmacol.*, **18**, 331–53.

PRESCOTT, L. F. (1968) Antipyretic analgesic drugs, in *Side Effects of Drugs*, Vol. VI, eds. Meyler, L., and Herxheimer, A., Excerpta Medica Foundation, Amsterdam, pp. 101–39.

RAPOPORT, A., WHITE, L. W., and RANKING, G. N. (1962) Renal damage associated with chronic phenacetin overdosage, *Ann. intern. Med.*, **75**, 970–80.

REYNOLDS, T. B., and EDMONDSON, H. A. (1963) Chronic renal disease and heavy use of analgesics, *J. Amer. med. Ass.*, **184**, 435–44.

RHOADES, E., MUCHMORE, H. G., and HAMMERSTEN, J. F. (1961) Pulmonary cryptococcosis. Report of a case treated with Amphotericin B, *Dis. Chest*, **39**, 535–8.

RICE, E. C., ANDERSON, W. S., and CLARK, G. R. (1964). Reversible Fanconi syndrome associated with degradation products of tetracycline (case report), *Clin. Proc. Child. Hosp. (Wash.)*, **20**, 223–8.

RIDDLE, M., GARDNER, F., BESWICK, I., and FILSHIE, I. (1958) The nephrotic syndrome complicating mercurial diuretic therapy, *Brit. med. J.*, **1**, 1274–7.

ROSENBERG, L. E., and HAYSLETT, J. P. (1967) Nephrotoxic effects of penicillamine in cystinuria, *J. Amer. med. Ass.*, **201**, 698–9.

ROSENTHAL, M. (1933) Anatomic lesions of fatal mercurial ntoxication from salyrgan, *Arch. Path.*, **15**, 352–66.

SANERKIN, N. G. (1966) Chronic phenacetin nephropathy (with particular reference to the relationship between renal papillary necrosis and 'chronic interstitial nephritis'), *Brit. J. Urol.*, **38**, 361–70.

SANERKIN, N. G., and WEAVER, C. M. (1964) Chronic phenacetin nephropathy ('chronic interstitial nephritis') with papillary necrosis, *Brit. med. J.*, **1**, 288.

SCHOURUP, K. (1957) Necrosis of the renal papillae; postmortem series, *Acta path. microbiol. scand.*, **41**, 462–78.

SCHULTZ, J. C., ADAMSON, J. S., JR., WORKMAN, W. W., and NORMAN, T. D. (1963) Fatty liver disease after intravenous administration of tetracycline in high dosage, *New Engl. J. Med.*, **269**, 999–1004.

SCOTT, J. T., HALL, A. P., and GRAHAME, R. (1966) Allopurinol in treatment of gout, *Brit. med. J.*, **2**, 321–7.

SHELLEY, J. H. (1967) Phenacetin through the looking glass, *Clin. Pharmacol. Ther.*, **8**, 427–71.

SHILS, M. E. (1963) Renal disease and the metabolic effects of tetracycline, *Ann. intern. Med.*, **58**, 389–408.

SICUTERI, F. (1959) Prophylactic and therapeutic properties of 1-methyl-lysergic acid butanolamide in migraine, *Int. Arch. Allergy*, **15**, 300–7.

SMITH, K. (1965) Acute renal failure in phenindione sensitivity, *Brit. med. J.*, **2**, 24–6.

SOKOL, A., BASHNER, M. H., and OKUN, R. (1967) Nephrotic syndrome caused by probenecid, *J. Amer. med. Ass.*, **199**, 43–4.

SOLOMON, M., GALLOWAY, N. C., and PATTERSON, R. (1965) The kidney and tetracycline toxicity, *Missouri. Med.*, **62**, 283–6.

SOULIER, J. P., and GEUGUEN, J. (1947) Hypothrombinemia (anti-K) effect of phenylindanedione. Experimental study in rabbit; application to human therapy, *C.R. Soc. Biol. (Paris)*, **141**, 1007–11.

SPRUNT, D. H. (1930) Renal damage following administration of Merbaphen (novasurol). Report of nine cases, *Arch. intern. Med.*, **46**, 494–501.

SPÜHLER, O., and ZOLLINGER, H. N. (1953) Chronic interstitial nephritis, *Z. klin. Med.*, **151**, 1–50.

STEINBRUNN, W., and HAEMMERLI, U. P. (1966) Clinical investigation of a new antibiotic Cefalothin, *Dtsch. med. Wschr.*, **91**, 2003–7.

STERNLIEB, I. (1966) Penicillamine and the nephrotic syndrome. Results in patients with hepatolenticular degeneration, *J. Amer. med. Ass.*, **198**, 1311–12.

TAIT, G. B. (1960) Neuropathy during phenindione therapy, *Lancet*, **ii**, 1198–9.

TAKACS, F. J., TOMKIEWICZ, Z. M., and MERRILL, J. P. (1963) Amphotericin B nephrotoxicity with irreversible renal failure, *Ann. intern. Med.*, **59**, 716–24.

TARR, L., and JACOBSON, S. (1932) Toxicity of Mersalyl (salyrgan). A clinical and anatomic study, *Arch. intern. Med.*, **50**, 158–66.

THIELE, K. G., MUEHRIKE, R. C., and BERNING, H. (1967) Nierenerkrank ungen durch Medikamente, *Dtsch. med. Wschr.*, **92**, 1632–5.

UTZ, D. C., ROOKE, E. D., SPITTELL, J. A., and BARTHOLOMEW, L. G. (1965) Retroperitoneal fibrosis in patients taking methysergide, *J. Amer. med. Ass.*, **191**, 111–14.

WAIFE, S. O., and PRATT, P. T. (1946) Fatal mercurial poisoning following prolonged administration of mercurophylline, *Arch. intern Med.*, **78**, 42–8.

WEGIENKA, L. C., and WELLER, J. M. (1964) Renal tubular acidosis caused by degraded tetracycline, *Arch. intern. Med.*, **115**, 232–5.

WEISS, J. M., and HINMAN, F. (1966) Reversible retroperitoneal fibrosis with ureteric obstruction associated with the ingestion of Sansert, *J. Urol. (Baltimore)*, **95**, 771–5.

WINTERLING, A. N., and GOLDMAN, R. L. (1965) Hepatic and renal lesions in a case of tetracycline toxicity during long-term estrogen therapy after orchidectomy, *Calif. Med.*, **102**, 314–16.

ZBINDEN, G. (1963) Experimental and clinical aspects of drug toxicity, *Advanc. Pharmacol.*, **2**, 1–112.

15

DISEASE OF THE NERVOUS SYSTEM

Drug-induced disorders of the nervous system are not common, although a large number of drugs are capable of producing these effects. For convenience in this discussion, these complications of therapy have been classified as either peripheral or central nervous disorders.

PERIPHERAL NERVOUS DYSFUNCTION

DRUG-INDUCED NEUROPATHY

Thalidomide

Despite the fact that this drug has been withdrawn from the market for reasons only too well known, its mention in this present context is fully justified since, apart from its teratogenic effects, it serves as a very good example of a drug which induces peripheral neuropathy.

Early in 1960 isolated reports were received by Burley, of Distillers Company (Biochemicals) Limited, from various parts of Great Britain describing symptoms and signs suggestive of peripheral neuritis occurring in patients receiving thalidomide regularly for periods of six months or more (Burley, 1961). Florence, however, gave the first report in the literature in December 1960; four patients had developed polyneuritis while on thalidomide presumably as a toxic effect of the drug. Kuenssberg and colleagues reported five similar cases in January 1961. However, it was not until the more detailed report of Fullerton and Kremer appeared in September 1961 that the association of thalidomide and resulting neuropathy became fully realized in Great Britain. The *British Medical Journal* soon carried an Editorial and a number of case reports, including personal experience, rapidly followed (Brown, 1961; Cahill, 1961; Heathfield, 1961; Pirrie, 1961; Powell-Tuck, 1961; Yorke *et al.*, 1962).

Articles on thalidomide first appeared in West German literature in May 1961 (Scheid *et al.*, 1961; Broser, 1962) and several authors mentioned the predominance of women in their series (Scheid *et al.*, 1961; Simpson, 1961; Voss, 1961). It is not known whether this predominance of reports in women reflected increased susceptibility or merely increased ingestion of thalidomide. The majority of these women patients were in the age group 35–75 years, although the total range was from 22 to 80 years. The dosage of thalidomide varied from 25 mg to 400 mg a night, but in most cases the dosage was not excessive. Symptoms were noted after 2 to 20 months of medication; there did not appear to be any firm relationship between onset of symptoms, dosage and duration of treatment. For example, symptoms of peripheral neuritis developed in one patient who took 50 mg per night for 3 months, whereas another patient on 200–300 mg a night went for 18 months before symptoms appeared (Scheid *et al.*, 1961).

One physician (Brown, 1961) took 25 mg a night for 12 months and developed numbness and some loss of tactile sensibility in the fingers of both hands, and to a lesser extent in both feet. Many people, of course, took the drug for a long time without signs of neuropathy. The nature of the neuropathy appeared to be sensory changes, which appeared first in the feet and later in the hands. The distribution was generally a stocking-glove pattern. The paraesthesia had various descriptions; hyperaesthesia was less common than hypoaesthesia. Other descriptions used were hyperalgia, hypoalgia, muscle pain and tenderness, numbness, 'pins and needles', burning, tightness, thickness, and sand in the skin. Coldness, pallor and intolerance to cold were noted, as well as red palms. Leg cramps were a common experience, and muscular fasciculation was less common. An associated finding of brittle fingernails was also recorded. Other sensory changes—such as disturbances of vibration, position and temperature—were rarely noted. Motor manifestations appeared much later than sensory changes. These were usually recognized as weakness, although early recognition of palsy of the dorsiflexors and plantarflexors of the feet had been noted. Ataxia and cerebellar symptoms were mentioned. Deep tendon reflexes were recorded as increased, normal, decreased or absent. The plantar response was generally normal. Nerve-conduction tests revealed some abnormalities in motor-nerve velocity and sensory-nerve potential (Fullerton and Kremer, 1961; Simpson, 1961). Muscle biopsies in two patients showed changes characteristic of denervation (Fullerton and Kremer, 1961).

The nature of thalidomide neuropathy was suspected to be something other than just peripheral neuritis, possibly involvement of the posterior columns (Broser, 1961). Three investigators examined cerebrospinal fluid; two of these considered their findings to be normal (Scheid *et al.*, 1961) but the third reported protein to be in the range of 25–100 mg per 100 ml (Fullerton and Kremer, 1961).

There were no reports on progression of neuropathy after thalidomide was withdrawn and most investigators noted improvement of the condition when the drug was stopped; several cases of exacerbation of the neuropathy after reinstitution of thalidomide are recorded (Broser, 1962).

The cause of thalidomide-induced peripheral neuropathy has never been clearly elucidated; a number of suggestions have been made and some of these have been supported by laboratory findings. For example, Ford-Robertson (1962) observed that about 25 per cent of patients on thalidomide developed a glossitis; within a few days from the start of dosage there was rapid denudation of the mucous membranes, and in some cases this extended to the fauces and buccal areas. The development of mouth lesions was controlled by oral dosage of vitamin B complex. It has been suggested that in some way thalidomide interferes with the action of certain of the B vitamins, and that as a result of this antagonism foetal damage can occur, and that in the adult there may be a link between this effect and the polyneuritis seen during treatment (Evered and Randall, 1963). Other drugs have been implicated in vitamin B complex deficiency, notably the tetracyclines and with these antibiotics, teratogenic disturbances have also been reported. Congenital cataracts were described in the infants of eight mothers who had received drugs during pregnancy; tetracycline had been taken by three of these eight mothers (Harley *et al.*, 1964). Although this report is inclusive, tetracyclines have been associated, in both animal studies and clinical reports, with teratogenic changes associated with osteogenesis and odontogenesis (Manten, 1968). Obviously the implication of the B vitamin deficiencies in drug-induced polyneuritis and possibly teratogenicity is worthy of further thought and study.

Nitrofurantoin

Nitrofurantoin is a member of a group of chemically related furan derivatives [FIG. 15.1] synthesized in the mid-1940s which have an unfortunately collective history of toxic side-effects. Nitrofurazone, an early member of this series, is used topically as an anti-infective agent; hypersensitivity reactions are fairly common (Laurence, 1963). Furazolidone has a broad antimicrobial spectrum which includes shigellae and salmonellae; it is used in bowel infections. Toxic effects include vomiting, headache and rashes, and the drug may induce susceptibility to hypertensive attacks from exogenous amines, such as tyramine in cheese and wine, changes that are characteristic of those observed following administration of MAO inhibitors. There is also one report of deafness with tinnitus associated with the use of furazolidone (Van Der Grient, 1968). Furaltadone (furmethonol), a systemic antimicrobial, was withdrawn from the market in the early 1960s in view of its neurotoxic and other adverse effects.

Nitrofurantoin was introduced into the clinic in 1953 and since then has been widely used in the treatment of urinary-tract infections, particularly those resistant to other agents. It is a synthetic antimicrobial agent with an antibacterial spectrum similar to that of chloramphenicol; it owes its use also to the fact that when taken by mouth it is rapidly absorbed and excreted into the urine and since some 40 per cent of

FIG. 15.1. *Structural formulae of furan derivatives in current or previous clinical use*

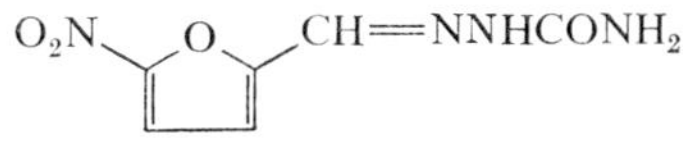

Nitrofurazone

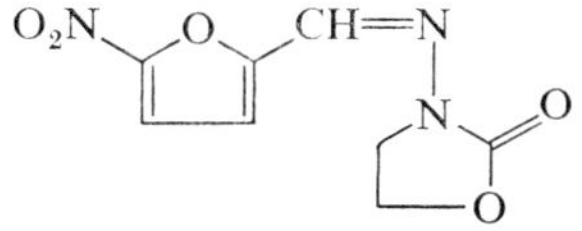

Furazolidone

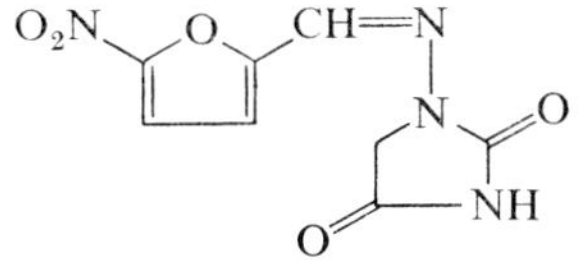

Nitrofurantoin

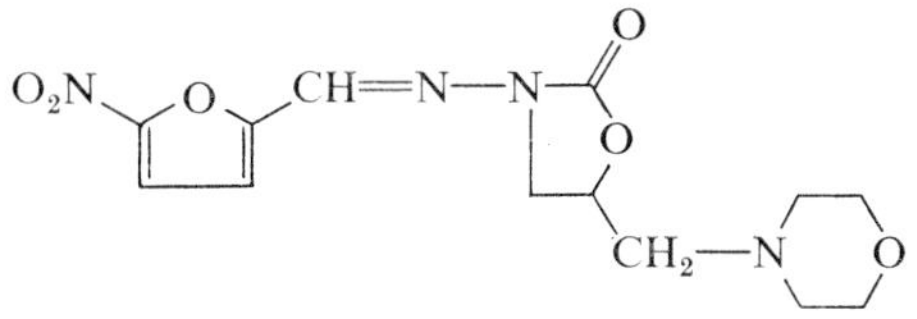

Furaltadone
(furmethonol)
(nitrofurmethone)
Withdrawn from clinical use

the amount taken finds its way into the urine it can be used as a urinary tract antiseptic.

The most frequently occurring side-effects have been easily reversible anorexia, nausea, vomiting and diarrhoea due to the gastric irritant action of the drug. Less commonly there have been reports implicating nitrofurantoin as the cause of skin rashes, eosinophilia, leucopenia, haemolytic anaemia, megaloblastic anaemia due to folic acid deficiency, and pulmonary infiltration.

In addition to these complications of medication, numerous cases of peripheral neuropathy attributable to nitrofurantoin have been reported from all parts of the world (Larsen and Bertelsen, 1956; Olivarius, 1956; Palmlov and Tunevall, 1956; Falk *et al.*, 1957; Briand and Tygstrup, 1959; Hafstrom, 1959; Collings, 1960; Ellis, 1962; Loughbridge, 1962; Martin *et al.*, 1962; Uesu, 1962; Willett, 1963; Heffelfinger *et al.*, 1964; Roelsen, 1964; Rubinstein, 1964; Beverungen *et al.*, 1965; Vickers, 1965; Herndon and Fox, 1966; Morris, 1966).

The symptoms of the neuropathy usually began with distal paraesthesias and dysaesthesias, more often in the lower extremities than in the upper limb, and progressed, over a matter of days, to produce a weakness and sensory loss. All the symptoms and neurological findings began distally and spread centripetally. Sensations of pain, light touch and vibration were impaired in a 'glove and stocking' distribution; joint position-sense usually remained unimpaired. Weakness and muscle wasting ascended the limbs in a like manner, leaving a flaccid paresis and diminished deep tendon reflexes. The plantar reflexes consistently remained normal.

Autopsy or nerve-muscle biopsies showed that the neuropathological lesions involved Wallerian degeneration of the peripheral nerves with interstitial oedema but no inflammatory cells (Collings, 1960; Herndon and Fox, 1966; Loughbridge, 1962; Morris, 1966). Herndon and Fox (1966) observed swelling of the anterior horn cells of the spinal cord with eccentrically placed nuclei, and marked chromatolysis.

Most of the reported cases occurred in patients with impaired renal function which would cause increased blood levels of nitrofurantoin (Loughbridge, 1962) but in at least two cases, renal function was normal. The symptoms began after taking doses of nitrofurantoin in doses of 200–500 mg/day for periods of time ranging from 1 day to 4 years in patients aged from 9–83 years.

The prognosis of the neuropathy was generally one of improvement when the drug was discontinued, sensory function recovering more rapidly than motor function. However, once muscle wasting occurred following neuropathy, recovery of motor function was generally incomplete.

In animal studies, Behar and colleagues (1965) have produced experimental neuropathy with very high doses of nitrofurantoin given over a period of 2–6 days. When compared with control animals, the treated groups exhibited a progressively increased chronaxie, decreased conduction velocity and axonal dystrophy.

The mechanism of nitrofurantoin neuropathy is uncertain although Loughbridge (1962) showed that the compound caused a reversible inhibition of the conversion of pyruvate and coenzyme A to acetyl CoA, a metabolic block which could be relevant to the picture of clinical toxicity.

Although the mechanism of toxicity is uncertain, it is well established that polyneuritis is directly related to the blood levels of nitrofurantoin obtained, and in patients with impaired renal function this blood level will rise to potentially toxic levels. Behar *et al.* (1965) showed that normal patients on a dosage level of 300 mg nitrofurantoin orally per day had blood levels of 1·8–2·2 μg/ml; however, in patients with a blood urea above 45 mg/100 ml, this blood level of drug rose to 5·1–6·5 μg/ml. Nitrofurantoin should therefore not be prescribed for patients with impaired renal function; not only is the patient exposed to toxicity hazards but the drug is also ineffective, since, in most cases, an insufficient amount of the drug is excreted and concentrations in the urine are too low to exert bacteriostatic activity (Hubmann and Bremer, 1965).

Since the incidence of neuropathy induced by nitrofurantoin appears to be directly related to blood levels of the drug, it is important in this context to draw attention to potential dangers of the drug in the foetal circulation. Nitrofurantoin crosses the placental barrier and enters the foetal circulation in experimental animals; foetal degradation of the drug is less than or equal to that of the maternal tissues and foetal kidneys do not excrete nitrofurantoin (Buzard and Conklin, 1964).

Imipramine

Imipramine is an iminodibenzyl derivative chemically related to the phenothiazine series [FIG. 15.2] with

FIG. 15.2. *Structural similarity between imipramine, amitriptyline and the phenothiazines*

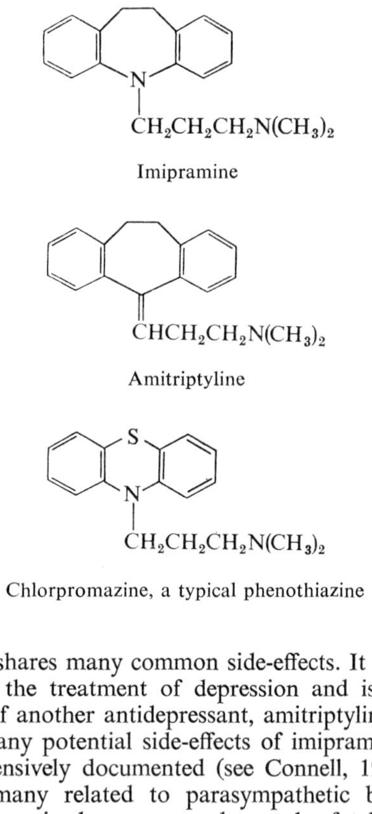

Imipramine

Amitriptyline

Chlorpromazine, a typical phenothiazine

which it shares many common side-effects. It is widely used for the treatment of depression and is a close relative of another antidepressant, amitriptyline.

The many potential side-effects of imipramine have been extensively documented (see Connell, 1968) and include many related to parasympathetic blockade. Over-dosage is dangerous and may be fatal; this is especially so with young children even with relatively small doses of the drug (Giles, 1963).

Sensory paraesthesias have been reported in 5 per cent of cases treated with imipramine (Freyhan, 1959). Tremors of diverse types, but especially of the tongue and hands, were seen in 30 per cent of patients (Sharp, 1960) while muscular twitching and myoclonic episodes were observed in 14 per cent. Grand mal seizures have also been reported in patients receiving over 300 mg imipramine per day.

Six cases of motor neuropathy have been reported in the literature. Collier and Martin (1960) described three

TABLE 15.1
ANTIBIOTICS IMPLICATED IN PRODUCING NEUROMUSCULAR BLOCKADE IN MAN

Antibiotic	Source	Chemistry	Neuromuscular Block
Neomycin sulphate	Streptomyces fradiae	Aminoglycoside	Curare-like
Streptomycin sulphate	Streptomyces griseus	Aminoglycoside	Curare-like
Dihydrostreptomycin sulphate	Streptomyces griseus	Aminoglycoside	Curare-like
Kanamycin sulphate	Streptomyces kanamycetius	Aminoglycoside	Depolarizing
Viomycin sulphate	Streptomyces floridae, S. punaceus, S. vinaceus	Aminoglycoside	Curare-like
Polymyxin B sulphate	Bacillus polymyxa	Polypeptide	Depolarizing
Colistin sulphate	Bacillus species	Polypeptide	Depolarizing
Colistin methanesulphonate			

cases in elderly women on daily doses of imipramine of 75 mg, 200 mg and 300 mg. Onset of symptoms ranged from the 10th to the 48th day of treatment; neurological findings were confined to flaccidity of the lower limbs, absent knee and ankle jerks. After imipramine treatment was stopped the neurological symptoms disappeared. Saavedra et al. (1960) described two cases of unilateral, peroneal nerve palsy; one was a man aged 57 years and the other a woman aged 59 years, both of whom were taking 300 mg of imipramine per day. Neither patient showed any improvement in the neuropathy on follow-up after cessation of imipramine therapy. Miller (1963) reported a single case of a 66-year-old woman who developed bilateral peroneal nerve palsy 41 days after commencing treatment with imipramine, 150 mg/day, and 22 days after its discontinuation. Follow-up after 5 and 8 weeks showed some recovery but the patient continued to require a walking brace.

It would seem from these reports that elderly patients are more prone to peripheral neuropathy following imipramine treatment, and that the neuropathy is a localized lesion affecting the lower limb, particularly the peroneal nerve. Polyneuritis has also been reported after the use of amitriptyline (Isaacs and Carlish, 1963).

DRUG-INDUCED NEUROMUSCULAR BLOCK

Antibiotics

The neuromuscular blocking action of neomycin sulphate was first reported by Pridgen in 1956, who noted respiratory depression following the instillation of this antibiotic into the peritoneal cavity. Engel and Denson (1957) reported respiratory depression in four infants who had received 1 gram of neomycin intraperitoneally. Other reports soon followed (e.g. Pittinger and Long,

1958; Pittinger et al., 1958), and the treatment of this condition with cholinesterase inhibitors and/or calcium was advocated. This complication has also been seen with oral and intrapleural administration of neomycin. It is more apt to occur when the antibiotic is used in excessive amounts or when it is used in conjunction with ether anaesthesia or with d-tubocurarine.

Other antibiotics have also been implicated in neuromuscular blocking activity [TABLE 15.1]; Timmerman and associates (1959) screened a number of antibiotics on the sciatic nerve-gastrocnemius muscle preparation of the anaesthetized rabbit and showed that streptomycin sulphate, dihydrostreptomycin sulphate, polymyxin B sulphate, kanamycin sulphate and neomycin sulphate produced neuromuscular blockade in the rabbit at various dosage levels. The blocking action of these five antibiotics, with the exception of polymyxin B sulphate, was enhanced by the simultaneous administration of d-tubocurarine chloride. Neostigmine methylsulphate antagonized the neuromuscular blockade, produced by neomycin, streptomycin and dihydrostreptomycin but tended to enhance the neuromuscular blocking action of polymyxin and kanamycin. Other antibiotics tested, tetracycline hydrochloride, ristocetin, oleandomycin, erythromycin, bacitracin and penicillin G, showed no neuromuscular blocking activity.

Other investigators have shown that viomycin and colistin have weak neuromuscular blocking properties; that due to viomycin can be reversed by anticholinesterase whereas that produced by colistin, at least under clinical conditions, is not antagonized by neostigmine (Barlow and Groesbeek, 1966; Pohlmann, 1966), nor counteracted by the cholinesterase inhibitor edrophonium.

These results would suggest that neomycin, viomycin, streptomycin and dihydrostreptomycin have a curare-like neuromuscular blocking action, whereas polymyxin

B, colistin and kanamycin have a depolarizing neuro-muscular blocking action. Neomycin, viomycin, streptomycin and dihydrostreptomycin, have a common aminoglycoside structure and are all derived from species of actinomyces [TABLE 15.1]; it is not surprising therefore that they all share neuromuscular blocking activity of the same type. Kanamycin, however, would seem to be the odd one out since it is also an aminoglycoside but has a depolarizing, not a curare-like. action.

Polymyxin B is one of a family of polypeptide antibiotics, the polymyxins, derived from bacterial species [TABLE 15.1]; they form a separate group of antibiotics with characteristic microbiological, pharmacological and toxicological features. Polymyxin E is identical with colistin; it is therefore not surprising that colistin and polymyxin B have neuromuscular blocking properties of the same type.

Streptomycin and dihydrostreptomycin have produced neuromuscular blockade when used intraperitoneally, and patients on prolonged intramuscular therapy of 1 gram of streptomycin per day have developed muscular weakness, fatigability and blurred vision, though secondary to this effect. Continued therapy has been made possible by the concomitant administration of oral neostigmine. Hokkanen (1964) reported that patients with myasthenia gravis were unusually sensitive to the blocking effect of streptomycin. Kanamycin also has produced respiratory depression when given intravenously or intraperitoneally. This effect responded favourably to neostigmine in one instance and calcium gluconate in another.

The polypeptide antibiotics, polymyxin A, polymyxin B, and colistin seem to have an unusually high potential for producing neurological side-effects, and many reports of the neurotoxicity of parenteral colistin or polymyxin B have been published (see Manten, 1968). The symptoms of intoxication vary from minor neurological dysfunctions, such as circumoral tingling, numbness and tingling in the limbs, to severe episodes such as convulsions, apnoea and ultimately death. These polypeptides are all nephrotoxic and initially circumoral numbness, ataxia, and bizarre behaviour was noted to occur in patients with impaired renal function where significant accumulation of the drug was thought to occur. Some patients have progressed to generalized muscular weakness and apnoea. However, occasionally marked neuromuscular blockade occurs even with normal 'therapeutic' blood levels of colistin methanesulphonate resulting from doses of the order of 75 mg twice daily or every 12 hours (Gold and Richardson, 1965, 1966). In these patients there was normal renal function and no obvious predisposing factor; premonitory signs were minimal or absent. The block was only partially reversed by edrophonium (10 mg i.v.); limb weakness improved but not that of facial muscles. After colistin was withdrawn, the myasthenia disappeared.

It has been suggested that the nephrotoxic and neurotoxic actions of colistin are due to drug-induced potassium-losing nephropathy and hypokalaemia. However, in a study of drug-induced decrease of plasma potassium and sodium in relation to coexistent nervous disturbance in three patients, the disturbances did not resemble those observed in either azotaemic or hypokalaemic patients. A direct action of colistin on the nervous system has therefore been suggested (Baron *et al.*, 1967).

Some investigators have reported a slight neuromuscular blocking effect for tetracycline and chloramphenicol. However, most studies have been negative in this regard, and for the present at least, tetracycline and chloramphenicol may be considered free of this hazard.

The key to the successful treatment of antibiotic-induced neuromuscular blockade, especially of respiratory muscles, is early recognition of the occurrence. Once it is established that a patient is developing neuromuscular blockade, immediate supportive therapy should be commenced. Since the greatest danger is respiratory depression, anoxia, and cardiac arrest, the patient's respiratory function must be closely monitored, and he should be intubated and ventilated at the first signs of distress. If adequate ventilation has been assured, or if muscular weakness is only minimal, the physician may attempt to hasten recovery by the following methods. Calcium gluconate, 10 to 200 mg, should be given by slow intravenous infusion to minimize its cardiac effect. If improvement does not occur edrophonium, 10 mg, can be given intravenously over one minute carefully observing the patient for signs of improvement over the next 10 minutes. If a favourable effect is noted, neostigmine, 1–2 mg, intramuscularly every 4 hours should be given as the action of edrophonium is fleeting. Atropine 0·4 to 0·6 mg, may be given with the neostigmine if one wishes to minimize the muscarinic effects of salivation, increased bronchial secretions, and gastrointestinal cramps of the latter medication (personal communication, Creese, 1969).

Suxamethonium

Suxamethonium (succinylcholine, diacetylcholine) was introduced in 1949 by Bovet and his colleagues. It is a potent neuromuscular blocking agent of the depolarizing type with very brief duration. This is because suxamethonium is rapidly hydrolyzed and inactivated by pseudocholinesterase present in the serum. It is used when only a brief period of muscle relaxation is needed or it may be given by intravenous drip to produce prolonged neuromuscular blockade.

Suxamethonium is a very useful muscle relaxant although there have been reports since its early use of prolonged apnoea and muscular pain and stiffness in some cases.

Bourne *et al.* (1952) and Evans *et al.* (1952, 1953) drew attention to the prolonged apnoea in man after suxamethonium in the presence of low plasma serum-pseudocholinesterase. Lehmann and Ryan (1956) observed a familial incidence of low pseudocholinesterase in the absence of overt disease and Lehmann and Simmons (1958) described suxamethonium apnoea in two brothers who had low plasma-pseudocholinesterase levels and both had, one of them repeatedly, a prolonged muscular paralysis following the injection of suxamethonium. Kaufman *et al.* (1960) recorded the first observation of suxamethonium apnoea in an infant; the family was studied in detail and there was a deficiency of pseudocholinesterase in one paternal and in one maternal grandparent. The parents had normal values for pseudocholinesterase although these were in the lower end of the normal range. Parbrook and Pierce (1960) compared the incidence of muscular pain and stiffness after the use of suxamethonium and suxethonium for dental in-patient anaesthesia and found no significant difference in the incidence or character of the post-operative pain or stiffness. Telfer *et al.* (1964) described the case histories of seven patients who possessed an atypical form of pseudocholinesterase; six of these patients presented as prolonged response to suxamethonium. The familial incidence of the occurrence of an atypical cholinesterase was demonstrated in each of these cases.

This prolonged peripheral neuromuscular block commonly presenting as prolonged apnoea has been attributed over the years to one or more of the following mechanisms:

Succinylmonocholine and Choline Block. Suxamethonium (succinylcholine chloride or bromide) is normally rapidly hydrolyzed by pseudocholinesterase to succinylmonocholine and choline. The succinylmonocholine in turn is hydrolyzed to succinic acid and choline [Fig. 15.3]. Succinylmonocholine and choline each have a weak depolarizing action; however, effective concentrations of these two metabolites are unlikely to accumulate unless massive doses of suxamethonium have been given, for example 1·5–2 grams (Wylie and Churchill-Davidson, 1960).

Dual Block. After an intravenous injection of suxamethonium, certain subjects develop a non-depolarizing block at the motor end-plate following the original depolarizing block. This is usually seen after multiple doses of suxamethonium, although occasionally, it may appear even after a single injection. Patients with myasthenia gravis are particularly prone to develop this type of response (Churchill-Davidson, 1955). This type of block is temporarily improved by edrophonium and is reversed by neostigmine.

Deficiency of Pseudocholinesterase. Plasma pseudocholinesterase is responsible for the rapid destruction of suxamethonium, therefore any reduction in pseudocholinesterase activity or plasma level of the enzyme will prolong the duration of the neuromuscular blockade. Production of pseudocholinesterase is depressed in certain pathological conditions including liver disease, severe malnutrition and hyperproteinaemia other than that due to renal disease. The action of the enzyme is inhibited by organophosphorous compounds such as

FIG. 15.3. *Metabolic fate of succinylcholine (suxamethonium)*

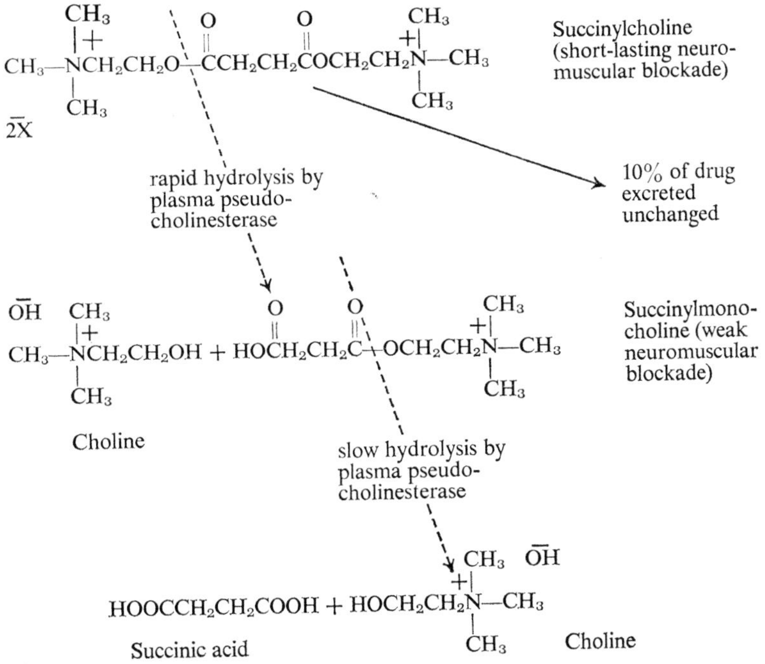

are used in nerve gases and insecticides. A commoner cause of a transient inactivation of pseudocholinesterase is the excessive administration by the anaesthetist or surgeon of drugs with anticholinesterase activity such as cocaine, procaine, and lignocaine. Some ganglionic blocking agents, trimetaphan camsylate and phenactropinium chloride (phenacylhomatropinium chloride), are also powerful cholinesterase inhibitors (Lehmann and Simmons, 1958).

There may also be a genetically determined deficiency of the enzyme (Allot and Thompson, 1956; Lehmann and Ryan, 1956; Kalow and Staron, 1957; Lehmann and Simmons, 1958). Complete absence of pseudo-cholinesterase has been reported (Hart and Mitchell, 1962).

Presence of an Atypical Form of Pseudocholinesterase. Some people who are abnormally sensitive to suxamethonium have been shown to have an atypical form of pseudocholinesterase in their serum (Kalow, 1956, 1959). This atypical enzyme hydrolyzes suxamethonium at a much slower rate than does the normal or usual type of serum-cholinesterase, and consequently the apnoea which the drug induces is excessively prolonged. The genetics of the condition have been reviewed by Lehmann and Liddell (1962).

Patients with an atypical form of pseudocholinesterase do not present any other recognizable abnormality, and they usually present as cases of prolonged apnoea following a single injection of suxamethonium. A technique has, however, been developed to detect the presence of this atypical enzyme (Kalow and Genest, 1957; Kalow and Staron, 1957) by determining what is known as the 'dibucaine number'. This is the percentage inhibition of enzyme activity produced by the inhibitor dibucaine under certain standardized conditions. In the test, the activity of the enzyme (usual pseudocholinesterase, or atypical pseudocholinesterase) in the presence and in the absence of dibucaine (10^{-5} M) is measured by following the rate of hydrolysis of the substrate benzoylcholine (5×10^{-5} M) spectrophotometrically at 240 mμ. The reaction is carried out at pH 7·4 in phosphate buffer.

With this technique most people show a dibucaine number of about 80 (normal homozygotes), those with atypical pseudocholinesterase may be classified as dibucaine number 40–75 (heterozygotes) or dibucaine number 30 or below (abnormal homozygotes). The intermediate group (heterozygotes) have a mean dibucaine number of about 62 and are believed to synthesize both the 'usual' and 'atypical' forms of the enzyme. They do not generally show an abnormal response to suxamethonium.

Evidence, either experimental or clinical, has been presented for each, or for combinations of, these four theories. Current opinion is that prolonged apnoea after suxamethonium is due to quantitatively or qualitatively deficient pseudocholinesterase (Lealock *et al.*, 1966; Mone and Mathie, 1967). Qualitative defects of

pseudocholinesterase activity are due to genetic abnormalities. Four allelic genes seem to control the inheritance of pseudocholinesterase: one normal, two atypical, and one silent allelic gene. They form pseudocholinesterase with varying activity. Quantitative reduction of pseudocholinesterase occurs in patients who receive organophosphorous compounds like the antineoplastics, cyclophosphamide and thiotepa (N, N′, N″-triethylenethiophosphoramide). Ecothiopate iodide, an anticholinesterase miotic used in the treatment of glaucoma, also reduced pseudocholinesterase levels (McGavie, 1965), and *Trasylol*, a polypeptide inactivator of kallikrein, obtained from animal sources, is also reported to cause prolonged apnoea (Chasapakis and Dimas, 1966).

Prolonged apnoea after suxamethonium is still a serious complication and many authors still report their cases (see Van Dijl, 1968). The treatment of prolonged apnoea depends mostly on good ventilation and maintaining physiological levels of pH, CO_2 and bicarbonate. Administration of whole blood or plasma has been recommended. When suxamethonium is present for a long time, or has been given in large doses, a dual neuromuscular block occurs in which the depolarizing block changes to a non-depolarizing type (i.e. curare-like); in this state edrophonium chloride or neostigmine methylsulphate may be helpful.

The muscle pain that occurs quite frequently after the use of suxamethonium can be so severe as to immobilize the patient and even impair ventilation. Prevention or reduction of this post-operative pain have been the goal of several investigators; their studies and investigations have been reviewed by Van Dijl (1968).

Gallamine, injected (5 mg) just before suxamethonium, reduced the degree and incidence of pain; a prophylactic dose of 3 mg *d*-tubocurarine completely prevented the pain although with this a higher dose of suxamethonium was required to produce muscle relaxation; slow infusion of suxamethonium in place of intermittent injection of doses is claimed to prevent muscle pain, and diazepam reduced the percentage of post-operative muscle pains to a low figure.

CHLOROQUINE NEUROMYOPATHY

Chloroquine has proved to be an effective antimalarial agent. In the treatment of malaria it is used for relatively short periods of time and in the prophylaxis of the disease the dosage is usually low (300 mg chloroquine base). Complications from its antimalarial use are therefore rare; however, chloroquine is an effective anti-inflammatory agent and larger doses extending up to or beyond 600 mg of base daily are used in the treatment of rheumatoid arthritis or discoid lupus erythematosus. It is with these larger doses that toxic side-effects occur [see also CHAPTER 16].

Neuromyopathy due to chloroquine is a rare side-effect although there have been casual references to muscle weakness in the literature. However, a number of clear-cut cases of chloroquine-induced myopathy or neuromyopathy have been described in several papers during more recent years (for example: Loftus, 1963; Whisnant *et al.*, 1963; Begg and Simpson, 1964; *British Medical Journal*, 1964; Bureau *et al.*, 1965; Blom and Lundberg, 1965; Blomberg, 1965; Journe *et al.*, 1965; Lenoir *et al.*, 1965; Renier, 1965; Sanghvi and Mathur, 1965; Bonard, 1966; Eadie and Ferrier, 1966; Millingen and Suerth, 1966; Smith and O'Grady, 1966).

Neuromyopathy usually appeared only in patients receiving 500 mg or more chloroquine daily. Whisnant and colleagues described four patients; in these cases symptoms started with muscular weakness in the lower limbs, usually arising in the proximal muscles and progressing slowly to the upper limbs. Sometimes the trunk, neck and facial muscles were eventually affected. As a rule tendon reflexes were reduced or absent without any sensory disturbances.

In reviewing these and other cases, all patients had clinical similarities, but differed in detail. Most patients were on long-term treatment and symptoms were slow to develop although in one case symptoms were apparent within a few weeks of treatment. Neuropathic and myopathic abnormalities were demonstrated by electromyography and muscle biopsy. Histological studies showed focal necrosis and fibrosis of muscle; some 50 per cent of the sarcoplasmic material was found to have been replaced by vacuoles. Some patients also suffered from blurring of vision due to corneal opacity without retinopathy. Usually a gradual return to normal muscle function followed withdrawal of the chloroquine, although in some cases deep reflexes were still diminished, and in others some muscle weakness still remained. According to some reports, regression of the condition after chloroquine withdrawal is favourably influenced by corticosteroids.

The mechanism of these effects is not clear; individual susceptibility to the pathological reactions seems probable since there is no well established correlation between dose and duration and development of a vacuolar myopathic pattern. The vacuolar changes are accompanied by glycogen accumulation and it has been suggested that chloroquine may act on the muscle by inhibiting enzymes involved in glycogen breakdown in muscle tissue. It has been shown that chloroquine interferes with hexokinase and the flavine adenine nucleotide enzymes; also an increase of the SGO and SGP transaminases has been observed (Schindel, 1968).

Loss of motor units and a rather low speed of motor conduction suggest neurogenic injury. The absence of reflexes even when atrophy and paresis are not very pronounced is also significant although this could be due to muscle damage affecting the small nerve end-plates. The whole clinical picture, however, suggests neuromyopathy rather than pure myopathy. Clinically the condition is rather like that of steroid myopathy but differs clearly from nerve injuries caused by, for example, thalidomide, nitrofurantoin or isoniazid (Schindel, 1968).

An interesting experimental tool has been produced by Smith and O'Grady (1966) who induced chloroquine myopathy in rats and rabbits. Large doses of chloroquine were required, 800–1,050 mg/kg, although only for a short period. Histologically there was necrosis of both cardiac and skeletal muscle fibres. In muscle the main damage was in 'red' fibres and was thought to be due to binding of chloroquine by myohaemoglobin. Histological changes were not observed in the peripheral nervous system although there was damage to spindle muscle fibres. These changes were thought to account for diminished tendon reflexes.

CORTICOSTEROID-INDUCED MYOPATHY

Muscle weakness is described in Cushing's syndrome and muscle weakness and atrophy can occur during systemic corticosteroid treatment; this complication is particularly likely during treatment with 9α-fluorinated steroids such as triamcinolone (16α-hydroxy-9α-fluoroprednisolone) (*Lancet*, 1965).

Dubois (1963) reported on side-effects experienced by 31 patients with systemic lupus erythematosus whilst on paramethasone (6α-fluoro-16α-methylprednisolone). One patient developed muscle weakness and vacuolar degeneration was noted on muscle biopsy in another patient.

Braun *et al.* (1965a) described six patients with rheumatoid arthritis who developed a myopathy whilst on long-term corticosteroid treatment. There was a progressive loss of muscular strength and in all cases the pelvic region was affected; in addition four patients showed affections of the humeral scapular region and one patient had an affected calf muscle. These changes were symmetrical and were not accompanied by pain or cramp. Four cases showed electromyogram changes and muscle biopsy disclosed degenerative changes including granules, hyaline degeneration, vacuolar degeneration and necroses.

Lerique and Chaumont (1965) also described six cases of patients who developed myopathy while on treatment with triamcinolone or methylprednisolone; their EMGs returned to normal 3 or 4 months after the steroid treatment was stopped. Coomes (1965) reported 34 patients on corticosteroids who showed mild signs of hypercortism; EMG reaction was normal, but in the low range. In 17 more severe cases the EMG reaction was well below the normal range.

Other reports of corticosteroid-induced myopathy have been given by Braun *et al.* (1965b); Coste *et al.* (1965a, 1965b); and Raffi *et al.* (1966). Features of the cases are similar; there is a delay in return to normal muscle function after stopping the steroid treatment, and there is no clear relationship between the severity of the myopathy and the duration of treatment. There is a suggestion that the incidence of myopathy is greatest in patients being treated with 9α-fluorinated corticosteroids. Hypokalaemia is a probable contributory cause of this steroid-induced myopathy and, in this respect, it is significant that deoxycorticosterone,

one of the most potent of the mineralocorticoids, also produces muscle weakness associated with hypokalaemia.

EMETINE-INDUCED MYOPATHY

Emetine is highly active against extra-intestinal amoebiasis and against the symptoms of amoebic dysentery. Thus emetine has remained the basis of treatment of the most important forms of amoebic disease in spite of some disadvantages. While the importance of its toxicity may have been exaggerated, it is certainly true that this has precluded its administration in the high doses necessary to treat severe infections and that if it were better tolerated, emetine would be a more acceptable treatment, especially for use in ambulatory patients.

Prolonged administration and large doses of emetine may produce degenerative changes in the heart, skeletal muscles, gastro-intestinal tract, liver and kidneys. Cardiovascular effects are the most important toxic manifestations of emetine treatment and include tachycardia, electrocardiographic abnormalities, pericarditis and hypotension. Excretion and detoxification of emetine is slow and therefore accumulation is a considerable factor in its toxicity.

Reports of muscular weakness and peripheral neuritis are less common than reports of cardiovascular disturbances. Four cases were reported by Keng and Swee (1966). The first, a patient suffering from amoebic hepatitis developed bilateral foot-drop and absent knee and ankle jerks after two emetine injections. Chloroquine therapy was substituted and the patient was discharged 3 months later with normal muscle and reflex function.

The second patient complained of extreme weakness and paraesthesias of both legs after receiving 350 mg of emetine. His ECG records indicated toxic myocarditis as well. Leg movement returned within 9 days and some 6 weeks later the patient was able to walk without support; at the same time the ECG returned to normal.

The third patient received combination therapy of chloroquine, oxytetracycline and a total dose of 780 mg of emetine. The patient had 'head drop', the facial muscles and the sternomastoids were weak, the palate was paralysed and there was pronounced weakness in both limbs. The ECG showed inversion of T-waves.

The fourth case had received a total of 650 mg of emetine together with chloroquine. Eighteen days later this patient experienced aching pain in both thighs, associated with tiredness and weakness of both legs, and at a later time, of the hands also. His ECG showed low voltage, flattening and inversion of the T-waves in all leads. Deltoid muscle biopsy suggested a primary myopathy.

The search for new less toxic amoebicides received a considerable stimulus when work aimed at the elucidation of the chemical structure of natural emetine opened up the way to the synthesis of new emetine derivatives. This work by Brossi et al. (1959) in the Roche Labora-

tories in Switzerland and England led to dehydroemetine (Dehydroemetine) and at about the same time this compound was also synthesized at Glaxo Laboratories (Mebadin).

Experimental chemotherapy and toxicology showed that dehydroemetine possessed equal or slightly superior amoebicidal activity to emetine, that it was eliminated more than twice as rapidly as emetine and that it was half as toxic as natural emetine.

In the clinic, dehydroemetine has been better tolerated than emetine by injection and also by mouth as dehydroemetine resinate. Some patients complained of weakness but this was not severe. Cardiovascular disturbances were evident but treatment with dehydroemetine was far safer than with emetine.

The derivative was effective in both hepatic amoebiasis and amoebic dysentery giving about a 95 per cent cure rate in both conditions (Blanc et al., 1961a, 1961b; Armengaud et al., 1962; Blanc and Nosny, 1962; Powell et al., 1962; Blanc, 1963; Sarin, 1963; Sardesai et al., 1963; Chhabra et al., 1964; Dempsey and Salem, 1966; Shroff and Bodiwala, 1966; Patel and Mehta, 1967).

DRUG-INDUCED NEONATAL MYASTHENIA

Buckley et al. (1968) described a male infant born of a myasthenic patient who was clinically normal until 24 hours after delivery, when he became lethargic, had only a faint cry and had weak sucking and grasping reflexes. Several severe cyanotic and apnoeic attacks occurred and the baby was clinically myasthenic.

A normal electromyogram (EMG) had been obtained at 12 hours after delivery but at 24 hours the EMG pattern was characteristic of myasthenia. The diagnosis was confirmed by the improvement in clinical condition, and by an increase in neuromuscular transmission measured by EMG after an injection of neostigmine (0·1 mg i.m.). The baby was treated for 12 days with intramuscular injection of neostigmine in progressively decreasing dosage, and at the end of this period anticholinesterase therapy was stopped without the reappearance of any myasthenic symptoms.

During pregnancy, EMG tests indicated that the mother was overtreated with pyridostigmine and measurements with ^{14}C-labelled pyridostigmine showed that she excreted this drug more slowly than other myasthenic patients.

The diagnosis of drug-induced neonatal myasthenia due to placental transfer of pyridostigmine was made on the basis of the low level of plasma cholinesterase in maternal and cord blood, the onset of symptoms 24 hours after birth and the decreasing requirement for neostigmine.

PROGRESSIVE CAUDA EQUINA LESIONS INDUCED BY THOROTRAST

Boyd et al. (1968) made a follow-up study on 27 patients who received Thorotrast (232-thorium dioxide) injection into the cerebrospinal fluid in the course of ventriculography or lumbar myelography. Seventeen of these patients died within 5 years of the disease bringing them under investigation. Seven of the remaining ten patients subsequently developed progressive cauda equina lesions, six of which were ultimately fatal. In view of the comparative rarity of this lesion in the population and the high incidence in this treated group, it was concluded that *Thorotrast* was the aetiological factor.

Other iatrogenic effects of *Thorotrast* have been described in CHAPTER 9.

CENTRAL NERVOUS DYSFUNCTION INDUCED BY DRUGS

EXTRAPYRAMIDAL REACTIONS

Phenothiazines

Since the introduction of chlorpromazine in 1951 and the large number of related phenothiazine tranquillizers in the late 1950s, reports have appeared in the literature concerning various neurological disorders resulting from their use: Schwab *et al.* (1956); Kinross-Wright (1959); Orland (1959); Hollister *et al.* (1960); Ayd (1961); McGeer *et al.* (1961); Schiele (1962); Moser (1966).

All members of the three groups of phenothiazine tranquillizers (dimethylaminopropyl side-chain, piperazine side-chain, piperidine side-chain) have been implicated in extrapyramidal reactions to a greater or lesser degree. It is difficult to link frequency of side-effects to chemical structure since there is a considerable variation in patient response, and in this respect it is perhaps significant that in spite of the large number of phenothiazines currently available [FIG. 15.4], chlorpromazine, the earliest member of this family, is still widely prescribed and used with considerable benefit.

The study by Ayd (1961) is one of the most detailed and comprehensive in the literature. He surveyed 3,775 patients treated with phenothiazine tranquillizers of whom 1,472 developed extrapyramidal reactions; 21·2 per cent had acathisia, 15·4 per cent had parkinsonism, and 2·3 per cent dyskinesia. There was correlation between the absolute frequency of these reactions and the chemical structure and milligram potency of the phenothiazine derivative used.

In this series the commonest extrapyramidal reaction to phenothiazines was akinesia. This condition was characterized by weakness and muscular fatigue. It caused the patient to be almost constantly aware of fatigue in a limb used for ordinary, repetitive motor acts such as walking or writing. In advanced form the patients complained of aches and pains in the musculature of the affected limb. Patients were apathetic and were disinclined to initiate or to expend energy to complete a task.

FIG. 15.4. *List of phenothiazine tranquillizers currently available; all have been associated with extrapyramidal side-effects*

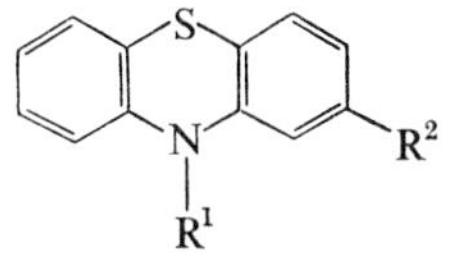

Basic structure of phenothiazine

PREPARATION	STRUCTURE
1. *Dimethylaminopropyl* side-chain	$\left(R^1 = -(CH_2)_3-N\begin{array}{c}CH_3\\CH_3\end{array}\right)$
Chlorpromazine	$R^2 = -Cl$
Promazine	$R^2 = -H$
Acetopromazine (Acetylpromazine) (Acetazine) (Acepromazine)	$R^2 = -COCH_3$
Methotrimeprazine	$R^1 = -CH_2CHCH_2N(CH_3)_2$ (with CH_3 branch)
(Levomepromazine) (Levomeprazine)	$R^2 = -OCH_3$

2. *Piperazine side-chain*

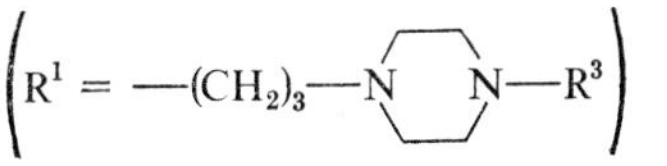

$$\left(R^1 = -(CH_2)_3-N\diagup\diagdown N-R^3\right)$$

Fluphenazine	$R^2 = -CF_3$ $R^3 = -CH_2CH_2OH$
Perphenazine (Chlorpiprazine) (Chlorpiprozine)	$R^2 = -Cl$ $R^3 = -CH_2CH_2OH$
Prochlorperazine (Chlormeprazine) (Prochlorpemazine) (Proclorperazine)	$R^2 = -Cl$ $R^3 = -CH_3$
Thiopropazate	$R^2 = -Cl$ $R^3 = -CH_2CH_2OHOCOCH_3$
Trifluoperazine (Triftazin) (Triphthasine)	$R^2 = -CF_3$ $R^3 = -CH_3$

3. *Piperidine side-chain*

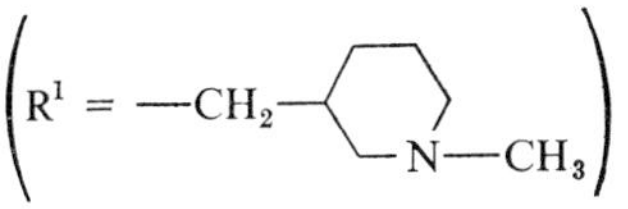

$$\left(R^1 = -CH_2-\bigcirc-N-CH_3\right)$$

Pecazine (Mepazine) (Mepasin)	$R^2 = -H$

Thioridazine

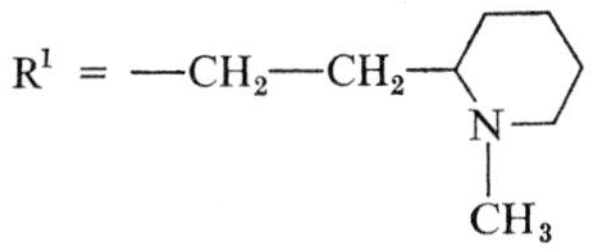

$$R^1 = -CH_2-CH_2-\bigcirc N-CH_3$$

$$R^2 = -SCH_3$$

The acathisia (motor restlessness) of phenothiazine intoxication causes the patient to walk or pace about, when sitting he constantly taps his feet or shifts his legs, if standing the patient may continually rock his body backwards and forwards or side to side. At the same time, there may be chewing movements of the jaw, rolling or smacking of the tongue and twisting of the fingers. In Ayd's series 65 per cent of cases with acathisia were female and 35 per cent were male; the cause of the difference in sex incidence is unexplained.

Dyskinesia or dystonic reactions are characterized by abrupt onset of retrocollis, torticollis, facial grimacing and distortions, dysarthria, laboured breathing and involuntary muscle movements. These may be accompanied by scoliosis, lordosis, opisthotonus, tortipelvis and dystonic gait. Another form of dyskinesia associated with the phenothiazine group is the oculogyric crisis. The attack begins with a fixed stare which is momentary and is followed by rotation of the eyes upwards and to the side and the eyes are then fixed in this position. The patient is unable to move his eyes. At the same time, the head is tilted backwards and laterally, and the mouth is open. Dyskinesia was nearly twice as common in men as in women; again this sex difference is unexplained.

Children under 15 years showed the severest and most bizarre neuromuscular symptoms with phenothiazines. Usually their hyperkinesia was generalized, resulting in a clinical picture resembling advanced cases of dystonia musculorum. The older the patient the more the involvement was restricted to the muscles of the neck, face, tongue and upper limbs. Thus the drug-induced dyskinesia closely resembles the infantile, juvenile and late forms of dystonia. Also, the incidence of drug-induced dyskinesia diminishes with increasing age, as is the case with genuine dystonia.

According to Schwab et al. (1956) genuine parkinsonism begins with tremor (50 per cent), rigidity (30 per cent), impairment of motor activity (10 per cent). By contrast, muscular rigidity, impairment of normal associated movements, and cogwheel phenomena were the initial symptoms of 65 per cent of cases of drug-induced parkinsonism. Tremor, which ultimately appeared in 60 per cent of cases of drug-induced parkinsonism, was the initial symptom in 35 per cent. The age distribution of phenothiazine-induced parkinsonism closely paralleled that of genuine paralysis agitans.

Another difference between drug-induced parkinsonism and genuine parkinsonism was the frequent early manifestation of bulbar symptoms of dysarthria, dysphagia, salivation, and drooling.

With rare exceptions, drug-induced parkinsonism is completely reversible on removal of the offending drug. More rapid reversal may be obtained by treatment with any of a number of antiparkinsonian agents. McGeer and colleagues (1961) postulated that the syndrome was due to interference with the normal functioning of central catecholamines, particularly dopamine, and of central histamine. Extrapyramidal reactions caused by reserpine or phenothiazines were treated with 4–32 grams per day of dopa (dihydroxyphenylalanine), the precursor of the catecholamines, with 0·4 to 0·6 grams per day of the antihistaminic, diphenhydramine or with each drug in turn. Dopa was mildly beneficial in 4 out of 22 patients, whereas diphenhydramine was completely effective in each of 11 cases. Ayd (1961) reported that dystonic reactions could be relieved promptly by parenteral benztropine methanesulphonate or by biperiden in doses of 1–2 mg. The latter two agents, given parenterally, exerted their effect within about 10 minutes with a maximum effect within 30 minutes. In his experience dystonic reactions were not a contraindication to further phenothiazine therapy; a recurrence could be avoided either by giving lower doses of the responsible phenothiazine or by the co-administration of an antiparkinsonian drug. Motor restlessness was also controlled by benztropine or biperiden (2 mg i.m.) or other antiparkinsonian drug by mouth, but acathisia, in Ayd's experience, was the most difficult to manage of the extrapyramidal reactions. Only partial relief was obtained with moderate doses of the antiparkinsonian drugs and larger doses were inadvisable due to their own psychotropic effects. The safest control was moderate dosage of the antiparkinsonian agent together with small doses of a barbiturate.

Rauwolfia Alkaloids

Reserpine and deserpidine are also major tranquillizers and produce much the same spectrum of extrapyramidal signs and symptoms as the phenothiazines. The mechanism by which these extrapyramidal reactions are produced by the phenothiazines and the rauwolfia alkaloids is not known. Much of the available experimental evidence links the mechanism of action of these drugs to interference with the retention in brain tissue of a number of amines, such as 5-hydroxytryptamine (5-HT) and the catecholamines (adrenaline, noradrenaline and hydroxytyramine). The rauwolfia alkaloids, such as reserpine, have been shown to deplete the brain of serotonin and catecholamines by competing for their binding sites. The phenothiazines, on the other hand, do not affect storage of amines but block their action after release. Clinically, the observed results are very similar.

The drugs previously described as effective in the control of phenothiazine-induced extrapyramidal reactions are also effective in those due to reserpine and rauwolfia alkaloids.

DRUG-INDUCED CONVULSIONS

Penicillin

In 1945 Johnson and Walker noted that when 50,000 units of penicillin were injected into the intraventricular system of a 22-year-old man, one hour later the patient lost consciousness and developed clonic spasms. These workers investigated this further (Walker and Johnson, 1945), and showed that application of commercial penicillin to the cerebral cortex of cats, dogs and monkeys and man, gave rise to convulsive manifestations. Since these findings were reported, the association between intracisternal injection of penicillin and convulsions has been established.

Bloomer et al. (1967) have described four cases in which massive doses of penicillin G were given intravenously to four patients in renal failure; this was followed by a reduced level of consciousness, myoclonic jerking and seizures. Weinstein and colleagues (1964) had earlier described similar observations following administration of 40×10^6 units of penicillin G to a uraemic 12-year-old patient, and Oldstone and Nelson (1966) had observed convulsions of a myoclonic type in a 71-year-old woman with renal calculi who had been treated with procaine penicillin for a pyrexia of unknown origin. Bloomer and his associates (1967) have also described a case of loss of consciousness and myoclonic convulsions in a 41-year-old patient treated with sodium cephalothin, 6 grams daily i.v. In this patient renal function was impaired due to glomerulonephritis.

The importance of the concentration of penicillin in the cerebrospinal fluid has been shown by Smith and co-workers (1967), for they found that, even when high doses were given, there was little danger of fits, provided the concentration in the CSF did not exceed 10 units per ml.

Another aspect of this problem has been reported by Seamans et al. (1968). Four patients undergoing open heart surgery with cardiopulmonary bypass at the Royal Victoria Hospital, Montreal, developed status epilepticus and coma in the immediate post-operative period, and three of them died. Each had received large doses of sodium penicillin intravenously over a period of 8 hours before, during, and after the bypass procedure, with the aim of preventing bacterial endocarditis or infection at the site of the valve prosthesis. None of these patients had azotaemia. Penicillin had not been used in this manner in the unit before January 1965 and was not given after March 1965, and there were no previous or subsequent cases. The authors then carried out experiments on dogs and found that, if large amounts of penicillin were given intravenously alone, no fits or electroencephalographic changes were observed, but out of eight animals in which this was combined with a full bypass operation seven developed fits. None of the five animals having full bypass but not receiving penicillin, developed fits. It was suggested that a breakdown, as yet unexplained, of the blood-brain barrier occurs after cardiopulmonary bypass, which does not appear to be related either to changes in the blood pH or to haemolysis, and there has been no convincing evidence of air embolism, particulate embolism or thrombosis of vessels. These authors in another paper do suggest, however, that small aggregates of material such as fat globules may become temporarily trapped in the cerebral capillaries and produce local deficiency in the blood-brain barrier, which may allow passage of abnormal quantities of penicillin.

Whether this is the explanation or not, these cases are another example of the potential neurotoxic effects of penicillin when allowed to come in contact with the brain in high concentration. There is also the possibility that during cardiopulmonary bypass operations other drugs usually given with safety may more readily be able to exert direct influence on the brain and produce unexpected, unfamiliar, and perhaps undesirable effects.

Isoniazid

Adams and White (1965) described a patient with encephalopathy following isoniazid; this was followed by a report of a further eight cases in a Tuberculosis Chemotherapy Centre at Madras (Devadatta, 1965). Six of these eight patients developed convulsions of the grand mal type, the remaining two had symptoms of a toxic psychosis. Of these eight patients, six (five with convulsions and one with psychosis) also developed signs of peripheral neuropathy.

Evans et al. (1960) have suggested that slow inactivators of isoniazid are more prone to develop neurological complications than rapid inactivators. This is well supported by Devadatta's experience of 43 cases of neurotoxicity caused by isoniazid since, of these, 36 patients (83·7 per cent) were classified as slow inactivators (Devadatta, 1965).

This is therefore a further example of a particular type of patient being at peculiar risk in terms of drug toxicity, and once again emphasizes the need to pick out these patients before commencing therapy of this type. In this respect, it is interesting to note that Rao et al. (1970) undertook sulphadimidine acetylation tests for classification of patients as slow or rapid inactivators of isoniazid. A total of 103 patients were studied, 52 of whom had been classified as slow and 51 as rapid inactivators of isoniazid by a standard microbiological assay method. Each patient received sulphadimidine by mouth in a dose of 44 mg/kg body weight, and free and total sulphadimidine were estimated in blood and urine collected at six hours.

The findings of these investigators suggest that patients can be classified as slow inactivators of isoniazid if the proportion of acetylated sulphadimidine (total minus free) is (a) less than 25 per cent in blood or (b) less than 70 per cent in urine. They reported that the sulphadimidine test was easy to perform and that it had the additional advantage that the result could be determined on the same day as the test. Stored samples of urine, kept at room temperature, for over a week, gave satisfactory results.

DRUG-INDUCED C.N.S. DEPRESSION
Corticosteroids
Usually administration of corticosteroids (glucocorticoids) causes euphoria. The intensity of mood change depends on a number of factors including the dosage

administered, the sensitivity of the patient and the underlying personality. However, full-blown psychosis has been described and this mental abnormality may be accompanied by fear, depression or stupor. Patients with chronic adrenal insufficiency are especially sensitive to this effect at the normal dosage required for adequate replacement therapy, as also patients with a previous history of mental disorder.

Curzon and Green (1968), Green and Curzon (1968) and Curzon (1969) have shown that intraperitoneal injection of 5 mg/kg of cortisol into rats caused a fall not only of brain 5-hydroxytryptamine, but also of 5-hydroxyindole acetic acid (a measure of 5-HT turnover), indicating decreased 5-HT synthesis. This seemed to be due to increased pyrrolase activity since firstly, the 5-HT fall was maximal 6–7 hours after injection of cortisol, while the induced increase in pyrrolase activity occurred earlier. Secondly, the pyrrolase inhibitors, allopurinol and yohimbine prevented the 5-HT change and, thirdly, α-methyltryptophan, which induces pyrrolase activity not by affecting adrenal corticoid secretion but by a direct action upon the enzyme, also caused brain 5-HT to fall in both intact and adrenalectomized rats.

Nistico et al. (1969) obtained results in good agreement with those of Curzon. An intramuscular injection of 1 mg/kg of corticosterone caused a 21 per cent fall in brain 5-HT, 12 hours after injection. This effect lasted for 24 hours. Intramuscular betamethasone (5 mg/kg) caused a fall in brain 5-HT of 49 per cent.

The inter-relationship between 5-HT levels and depressive illness and alteration in 5-HT levels by corticoids has been woven into a working hypothesis by Lapin and Oxenkrug (1969) to explain the biochemistry of steroid therapy-induced depression.

Most authors feel that a psychiatric history is a contraindication for therapy with corticosteroids or ACTH. The literature on this has been reviewed by De Lange and Doorenbos (1968).

Oral Contraceptives

Depressive feelings are a not uncommon side-effect of oral contraceptive medication, especially when there is a previous clear-cut history of depression. From 5–30 per cent of women complain of such symptoms as irritability, tension and depression, but many have had premenstrual symptoms before they started on the pill, and in any case those who complain are balanced by the 10–20 per cent who experience relief of premenstrual tension and an increased sense of well-being. High rates of depression appear to be associated with oral contraceptives having a high progestogen content and

depression diminishes with change to a more oestrogenic composition (British Medical Journal, 1969).

Recent work has suggested that prevention of this iatrogenic depression might be possible. Steroids, including cortisol and those in oral contraceptive formulations, appear to influence tryptophan metabolism.

Price and Toseland (1969) have produced evidence of disturbed tryptophan metabolism in 20 women on oral contraceptives. This is based on the finding of increased urinary levels of 3-hydroxyanthranilic acid without prior tryptophan loading. Toseland and Price (1969) and Rose (1966) have shown that these levels can be brought to normal by administration of pyridoxine.

Winston (1969a) suggested that administration of pyridoxine might protect women on oral contraceptives from depression. He bases this on the assumption that dysfunction of tryptophan metabolism is implicated in some forms of depression, and that by activating tryptophan pyrrolase oral contraceptives may create a functional deficiency of pyridoxine along the tryptophan-niacin pathway.

The net effect would seem to be that oestrogen-progestogen combinations create a functional deficiency of pyridoxine (vitamin B_6) which is a co-enzyme in the conversion of tryptophan both to nicotinic acid ribonucleotide and to 5-hydroxytryptamine. It is interesting in this respect to note that there is evidence that premedication with pyridoxine prevents the disturbance of tryptophan metabolism by cortisol (Rose and McGinty, 1968), and some evidence that a very few cases of 'pill'-induced depression have responded to pyridoxine (Winston, 1969b). It is of further interest to learn that an oral contraceptive preparation containing pyridoxine has been marketed in Spain (Otte, 1969).

If it is acceptable, simple withdrawal of oral contraceptive medication is, at the moment, probably the safest and most satisfactory solution to the problem of induced depression. A recent case of one of us (J.P.G.) illustrates this very well and also indirectly demonstrates the problems of drug interaction.

A young asthmatic woman started on oral contraceptives at the time of her marriage. Subsequently she became depressed and the depression was attributed to a bereavement in her family that occurred at about this time. She was started on a MAO inhibitor as a result of which the use of sympathomimetic amines for the treatment of her asthma was contraindicated. Some seven months later she developed a deep vein thrombosis in her right leg and oral contraceptives were stopped. Her emotional state has improved considerably since that time.

RECOMMENDED FURTHER READING

BRITISH MEDICAL JOURNAL (1969) Oral contraception and depression, leading article, *Brit. med. J.*, **4**, 380–1.

DALLY, P. (1967) Current Therapeutics CCXXXVIII. The current status of psychotropic drugs, *Practitioner*, **199**, 553–63.

GLICK, I. D. (1967) Mood and behavioural changes associated with the use of the oral contraceptive agents, *Psychopharmacologia (Berl.)*, **10**, 363–74.

HINTON, J. (1968) Psychotropic drugs, *Postgrad. med. J.*, **44**, 286–96.

LEAR, E. (1966) *Chemistry and Applied Pharmacology of Tranquillizers*, Springfield, Illinois.

MURRAY, M. J. (1968) Pulmonary reactions to nitrofurantoin, in *Drug-Induced Diseases*, Vol. 3, eds. Meyler, L., and Peck, H. M., Excerpta Medica Foundation, Amsterdam, pp. 157–60.

PLATE, W. P. (1968) Ovarian changes after long-term oral contraception, in *Drug-Induced Diseases*, Vol. 3, eds. Meyler, L., and Peck, H. M., Excerpta Medica Foundation, Amsterdam, pp. 235–8.

ROSE, D. P. (1970) Effect of ovarian hormones and oral contraceptives on tryptophan metabolism, *J. clin. Path.*, **23**, Suppl. (Ass. Clin. Path.), **3**, 37–42.

RUBENSTEIN, C. J. (1968) Peripheral polyneuropathy caused by nitrofurantoin, in *Drug-Induced Diseases*, Vol. 3, eds. Meyler, L., and Peck, H. M., Excerpta Medica Foundation, Amsterdam, pp. 161–4.

REFERENCES

ADAMS, P., and WHITE, C. (1965) Isoniazid induced encephalopathy, *Lancet*, **i**, 680–2.

ALLOT, E. N., and THOMPSON, J. C. (1956) The familial incidence of low pseudocholinesterase level, *Lancet*, **ii**, 517.

ARMENGAUD, M., BOURGOIN, J. J., and GUÉRIN, M. (1962) L'amibiase aiguë de l'Africain en milieu hospitalier (à propos de 153 observations), *Bull. Soc. méd. Afr. noire Langue franc.*, **7**, 783–93.

AYD, F. J., JR. (1961) A survey of drug-induced extrapyramidal reactions, *J. Amer. med. Ass.*, **175**, 1054–60.

BARLOW, M. B., and GROESBEEK, A. (1966) Apparent potentiation of neuromuscular block by antibiotics, *S. Afr. med. J.*, **40**, 135–6.

BARON, F., JOINVILLE, R., PIQUET, R., DEJOUR, B., and PRESSARD, P. (1967) Accidents due à la colistine, *Ouest méd.*, **20**, 148.

BEGG, T. B., and SIMPSON, J. A. (1964) Chloroquine neuromyopathy, *Brit. med. J.*, **1**, 770.

BEHAR, A., RACHMILEWITZ, E., RAHAMIMOFF, R., and DENMAN, M. (1965) Experimental nitrofurantoin polyneuropathy in rats; early histological and electrophysiological alterations in peripheral nerves, *Arch. Neurol. (Chic.)*, **13**, 160–3.

BEVERUNGEN, W., FRITZ, K. W., and ROSS, J. (1965) Polyneuritis nach Behandlung mit Nitrofurantoin bei einem Niereninsuffizienz-Kranken, *Münch. med. Wschr.*, **107**, 953–5.

BLANC, F. (1963) Réflexions sur l'amibiase colique et son traitement, *Rev. Prat. (France)*, **13**, 2861–70.

BLANC, F., and NOSNY, Y. (1962) Un amoebicide synthétique diffusible: La 2-déhydro-émétine, *Marseille-med.*, **99**, 153–60.

BLANC, F., NOSNY, Y., ARMENGAUD, M., SANKALÉ, M., MARTIN, M., and CHARMOT, G. (1961a) Un amoebicide synthétique susceptible de remplacer l'émétine: La 2-déhydro-émétine, *Presse méd.*, **69**, 1548–50.

BLANC, F., NOSNY, Y., ARMENGAUD, M., SANKALÉ, M., MARTIN, M., CHARMOT, G., and NOSNY, P. (1961b) La 2-déhydro-émétine dans le traitement de l'amibiase, *Bull. Soc. Path. exot.*, **54**, 29–39.

BLOM, S., and LUNDBERG, P. O. (1965) Reversible myopathy in chloroquine treatment, *Acta med. scand.*, **177**, 685–8.

BLOMBERG, L. H. (1965) Dystrophia myotonica probably caused by chloroquine, *Acta neurol. scand.*, **41**, Suppl. 13, 647–51.

BLOOMER, H. A., BARTON, L. J., and MADDOCK, R. K., JR. (1967) Penicillin-induced encephalopathy in uremic patients, *J. Amer. med. Ass.*, **200**, 121–3.

BONARD, E. C. (1966) Neuropathie due à la chloroquine, *Schweiz. med. Wschr.*, **96**, 1103–5.

BOURNE, J. G., COLLIER, H. O. J., and SOMERS, G. F. (1952) Succinylcholine (succinoylcholine) muscle-relaxant of short action, *Lancet*, **i**, 1225–9.

BOYD, J. L., LANGLANDS, A. O., and MACCABE, J. J. (1968) Long-term hazards of Thorotrast, *Brit. med. J.*, **2**, 517–21.

BRAUN, S., AUREL, M., COSTE, F., and DELBARRE, F. (1965a) La myopathie des corticoïdes, *Sem. Hôp. Paris*, **41**, 1717–35.

BRAUN, S., COSTE, F., and AUREL, M. (1965b) Les myopathies iatrogènes, II. La myopathie des corticoïdes, *Rev. Rhum.*, **32**, 561–5.

BRIAND, P., and TYGSTRUP, I. (1959) Polyneuritis following nitrofurantoin (Furadantin) treatment, *Ugeskr. Laegr.*, **121**, 664–6.

BRITISH MEDICAL JOURNAL (1964) Chloroquine neuromyopathy, leading article, *Brit. med. J.*, **1**, 452.

BRITISH MEDICAL JOURNAL (1969) Oral contraception and depression, leading article, *Brit. med. J.*, **4**, 380–1.

BROSER, F. (1962) Polyneuritiden und funikulare Myelosen nach Conterfan-Gerbrauch, *Med. Klin.*, **57**, 53–7.

BROSSI, A., BAUMANN, M., CHOPPARD-DIT-JEAN, L. H., WÜRSCH, J., SCHNEIDER, F., and SCHNIDER, O. (1959) Syntheseversuche in der Emetin-Reihe, 4. Mitt: Racemisches 2-Dehydroemetin, *Helv. chim. Acta*, **42**, 772–8.

BROWN, J. A. (1961) Neuropathy after thalidomide ('Distaval'), *Brit. med. J.*, **2**, 1359–60.

BUCKLEY, G. A., ROBERTS, D. V., ROBERTS, J. B., THOMAS, B. H., and WILSON, A. (1968) Drug-induced neonatal myasthenia, *Brit. J. Pharmacol.*, **34**, 203P–204P.

BUREAU, Y., BARRIÈRE, H., LITOUX, P., and BUREAU, M. (1965) Les accidents neuromusculaires de la chloroquine, *J. méd. Nantes*, **5**, 107.

BURLEY, D. (1961) Is thalidomide to blame? *Brit. med. J.*, **1**, 130.

BUZARD, J. A., and CONKLIN, J. D. (1964) Placental transfer of nitrofurantoin and furaltadone, *Amer. J. Physiol.*, **206**, 189–92.

CAHILL, P. K. (1961) Neuropathy after thalidomide ('Distaval'), *Brit. med. J.*, **2**, 1223.

CHASAPAKIS, G., and DIMAS, C. (1966) Possible interaction between muscle relaxants and the kallikrein-trypsin inactivator 'Trasylol', *Brit. J. Anaesth.*, **38**, 838–9.

CHHABRA, R. H., BAMJI, D. D., and DESAI, M. M. (1964) Clinical trials of injection of dehydroemetine in amoebiasis, *Curr. med. Pract.*, **8**, 114–16.

CHURCHILL-DAVIDSON, H. C. (1955) Abnormal response to muscle relaxants, *Proc. roy. Soc. Med.*, **48**, 621–4.

COLLIER, G., and MARTIN, A. (1960) Side effects of Tofranil. General review apropos of three cases of polyneuritis of the lower extremities, *Ann. med.-psychol.*, **118**, 719–38.

COLLINGS, H. (1960) Polyneuropathy associated with nitrofurantoin therapy, *Arch. Neurol. (Chic.)*, **3**, 656–60.

CONNELL, P. H. (1968) Central nervous system stimulant and antidepressant drugs, in *Side Effects of Drugs*, Vol. VI, eds. Meyler, L., and Herxheimer, A., Excerpta Medica Foundation, Amsterdam, pp. 1–50.

COOMES, E. N. (1965) Corticosteroid myopathy, *Ann. rheum. Dis.*, **24**, 465–72.

COSTE, F., DELBARRE, F., BRAUN, S., RONDEAU, P., BEDORSEAU, P., and AUREL, M. (1965a) La myopathie des corticoïdes, *Presse méd.*, **73**, 2636.

COSTE, F., DELBARRE, F., BRAUN, S., RONDEAU, P., BEDORSEAU, P., and AUREL, M. (1956b) La myopathie des corticoïdes, *Lyon méd.*, **214**, 91.

CURZON, G. (1969) Metabolic changes in depression, *Lancet*, **i**, 257.

CURZON, G., and GREEN, A. R. (1968) Effect of hydrocortisone on rat brain 5-hydroxytryptamine, *Life Sci.* **7**, 657–63.

DE LANGE, W. E., and DOORENBOS, H. (1968) Hormones and synthetic substitutes, in *Side Effects of Drugs*, Vol. VI, eds. Meyler, L., and Herxheimer, A., Excerpta Medica Foundation, Amsterdam, p. 388.

DEMPSEY, J. J., and SALEM, H. H. (1966) An enzymatic electrocardiographic study on toxicity of dehydroemetine, *Brit. Heart. J.*, **28**, 505–11.

DEVADATTA, S. (1965) Isoniazid-induced encephalopathy, *Lancet*, **ii**, 440.

DUBOIS, E. L. (1963) Paramethasone in the treatment of systemic lupus erythematosus. Analysis of results in 51 patients with emphasis on single daily oral doses, *J. Amer. med. Ass.*, **184**, 463–9.

EADIE, M. J., and FERRIER, T. M. (1966) Chloroquine myopathy, *J. Neurol. Neurosurg. Psychiat.*, **29**, 331–7.

ELLIS, F. G. (1962) Acute polyneuritis after nitrofurantoin therapy, *Lancet*, **ii**, 1136–8.

ENGEL, H. L., and DENSON, J. S. (1957) Respiratory depression due to neomycin, *Surgery*, **42**, 862–4.

EVANS, D. A. P., MANLEY, K. A., and McKUSICK, V. A. (1960) Genetic control of isoniazid metabolism in man, *Brit. med. J.*, **2**, 485–91.

EVANS, F. T., GRAY, P. W. S., LEHMANN, H., and SILK, E. (1952) Sensitivity to succinylcholine in relation to serum-cholinesterase, *Lancet*, **i**, 1229–30.

EVANS, F. T., GRAY, P. W. S., LEHMANN, H., and SILK, E. (1953) Effects of pseudo-cholinesterase level on action of succinylcholine in man, *Brit. med. J.*, **1**, 136–8.

EVERED, D. F., and RANDALL, H. G. (1963) Thalidomide and B vitamins, *Brit. med. J.*, **1**, 610.

FALK, G., REIS, G. VON, and VEERSTEEGH-LIND, A. (1957) Polyneurit vid furadantin-behandling, *Opusc. med. (Stockh.)*, **2**, 130–4.

FLORENCE, A. L. (1960) Is thalidomide to blame? *Brit. med. J.*, **2**, 1954.

FORD-ROBERTSON, W. (1962) Thalidomide ('Distaval') and vitamin-B deficiency, *Brit. med. J.*, **1**, 792–3.

FREYHAN, F. A. (1959) Clinical effectiveness of Tofranil in the treatment of depressive psychoses, *Canad. psychiat. Ass. J.*, **4**, Suppl., S86–S99.

FULLERTON, P. M., and KREMER, M. (1961) Neuropathy after thalidomide ('Distaval'), *Brit. med. J.*, **2**, 855–8.

GILES, H. Mc C. (1963) Imipramine poisoning in childhood, *Brit. med. J.*, **2**, 844–6.

GOLD, G. N., and RICHARDSON, A. P. (1965) Myasthenic reaction to colistimethate, *J. Amer. med. Ass.*, **194**, 1151–2.

GOLD, G. N., and RICHARDSON, A. P. (1966) An unusual case of neuromuscular blockade seen with therapeutic blood levels of colistin methanesulphonate (Coly-mycin), *Amer. J. Med.*, **41**, 316–21.

GREEN, A. R., and CURZON, G. (1968) Decrease of 5-hydroxytryptamine in the brain provoked by hydrocortisone and its prevention by allopurinol, *Nature (Lond.)*, **220**, 1095–7.

HAFSTROM, T. (1959) Prognosen vid furadantin-polyneurit, *Opusc. med. (Stokh.)*, **4**, 17–23.

HARLEY, J. D., FARRAR, J. F., GRAY, J. B., and DUNLOP, I. C. (1964) Aromatic drugs and congenital cataracts, *Lancet*, **i**, 472–3.

HART, S. M., and MITCHELL, J. V. (1962) Suxamethonium in the absence of pseudocholinisterase, *Brit. J. Anaesth.*, **34**, 207–9.

HEATHFIELD, K. W. G. (1961) Neuropathy after thalidomide ('Distaval'), *Brit. med. J.*, **2**, 1084.

HEFFELFINGER, J. C., and ALLEN, R. J. (1964) Neurotoxicity with nitrofurantoin. A case report, *J. Pediat.*, **65**, 611–12.

HERNDON, R. F., and FOX, G. E. (1966) Polyneuropathy due to nitrofurantoin, *Illinois med. J.*, **129**, 164–6.

HOKKANEN, E. (1964) The aggravating effect of some antibiotics on the neuromuscular blockage in myasthenia gravis, *Acta neurol. scand.*, **40**, 346–52.

HOLLISTER, L. E., CAFFEY, E. M., JR., and KLETT, C. J. (1960) Abnormal symptoms, signs and laboratory tests during treatment with phenothiazine derivatives, *Clin. Pharmacol. Ther.*, **1**, 284–93.

HUBMANN, R., and BREMER, G. (1965) Die Ausscheidung von Furadantin bei manifester Niereninsuffizienz, *Med. Welt. (Stuttg.)*, **19**, 1039–49.

ISAACS, A. D., and CARLISH, S. (1963) Peripheral neuropathy after amitriptyline, *Brit. med. J.*, **1**, 1739.

JOHNSON, H. C., and WALKER, A. E. (1945) Intraventricular penicillin: Note of warning, *J. Amer. med. Ass.*, **127**, 217–19.

JOURNE, P., LENOIR, P., MOREL, H., TURPIN, J., DUPONT, B., and BOUREL, M. (1965) Une observation de myopathie vacuolaire au cours d'un traitement par la chloroquine, *Ouest méd.*, **18**, 990.

KALOW, W. (1956) Familial incidence of low pseudocholinesterase level, *Lancet*, **ii**, 576–7.

KALOW, W. (1959) *Ciba Foundation Symposium on the Biochemistry of Human Genetics*, eds. Wolstenholme, G. E., and O'Connor, M. C., London, p. 39.

KALOW, W., and GENEST, K. (1957) A method for the detection of atypical forms of human serum cholinesterase; determination of dibucaine numbers, *Canad. J. Biochem.*, **35**, 339–46.

KALOW, W., and STARON, N. (1957) On distribution of atypical forms of human serum cholinesterase, as indicated by dibucaine numbers, *Canad. J. Biochem.*, **35**, 1305–20.

KAUFMAN, L., LEHMANN, H., and SILK, E. (1960) Suxamethonium apnoea in an infant: Expression of familial pseudocholinesterase deficiency in three generations, *Brit. med. J.*, **1**, 166–7.

KENG, C. B., and SWEE, Y. O. (1966) Neuromuscular manifestations of emetine toxicity, *Singapore med. J.*, **7**, 156–63.

KINROSS-WRIGHT, J. (1959) Newer phenothiazine drugs in treatment of nervous disorders, *J. Amer. med. Ass.*, **170**, 1283–8.

KUENSSBERG, E. V., SIMPSON, J. A., and STANTON, J. B. (1961) Is thalidomide to blame? *Brit. med. J.*, **1**, 291.

LANCET (1965) Corticosteroid myopathy, annotation, *Lancet*, **ii**, 1118.

LAPIN, I. P., and OXENKRUG, G. F. (1969) Intensification of the central serotoninergic processes as a possible determinant of the thymoleptic effect, *Lancet*, **i**, 132–6.

LARSEN, H. W., and BERTELSEN, S. (1956) Neurologic symptoms during treatment with furadantins, *Ugeskr. Laeg.*, **118**, 751–3.

LAURENCE, D. R. (1963) *Clinical Pharmacology*, 2nd ed., London, p. 73.

LEALOCK, A. M., CAMPBELL, D. J., and McINTYRE, J. W. R. (1966) A clinical and biochemical approach to cholinesterase problems in anaesthesia, *Canad. Anaesth. Soc. J.*, **13**, 550–6.

LEHMANN, H., and LIDDELL, J. (1962) *Modern Trends in Anaesthesia*, Series II, London.

LEHMANN, H., and RYAN, E. (1956) Familial incidence of low pseudocholinesterase level, *Lancet*, **ii**, 124.

LEHMANN, H., and SIMMONS, P. H. (1958) Sensitivity to suxamethonium: Apnoea in two brothers, *Lancet*, **ii**, 981–2.

LENOIR, P., JOURNE, P., URVOY, M., and BOUREL, M. (1965) Les complications musculaires et oculaires des traitements par la chloroquine, *Méd. et. Hyg. (Genève)*, **714**, 1223–5.

LERIQUE, J., and CHAUMONT, P. (1965) Exploration électrolytique au cours des syndromes cortisoniques, *Rev. neurol.*, **112**, 342.

LOFTUS, L. R. (1963) Peripheral neuropathy following chloroquine therapy, *Canad. med. Ass. J.*, **80**, 407–12.

LOUGHBRIDGE, L. W. (1962) Peripheral neuropathy due to nitrofurantoin, *Lancet*, **ii**, 1133–5.

MANTEN, A. (1968) Antibiotic drugs, in *Side Effects of Drugs*, Vol. VI, eds. Meyler, L., and Herxheimer, A., Excerpta Medica Foundation, Amsterdam, pp. 263–314.

MARTIN, W. J., CORBIN, K. B., and UTZ, D. C. (1962) Paraesthesias during treatment with nitrofurantoin: Report of case, *Proc. Mayo Clin.*, **37**, 288–92.

McGAVIE, D. D. M. (1965) Depressed levels of serumpseudocholinesterase with ecothiopate-iodide eyedrops, *Lancet*, **ii**, 272–3.

McGEER, P. L., BOULDING, J. E., GIBSON, W. C., and FOULKES, R. G. (1961) Drug-induced extrapyramidal reactions, *J. Amer. med. Ass.*, **177**, 665–70.

MILLER, M. (1963) Neuropathy, agranulocytosis and hepatotoxicity following imipramine therapy, *Amer. J. Psychiat.*, **120**, 185–6.

MILLINGEN, K. S., and SUERTH, E. (1966) Peripheral neuromyopathy following chloroquine therapy, *Med. J. Aust.*, **1**, 840–1.

MONE, J. G., and MATHIE, W. E. (1967) Qualitative and quantitative defects of pseudocholinesterase activity, *Anaesthesia*, **22**, 55–68.

MORRIS, J. S. (1966) Nitrofurantoin and peripheral neuropathy with megaloblastic anaemia, *J. Neurol. Neurosurg. Psychiat.*, **29**, 224–8.

MOSER, R. H. (1966) Reactions to phenothiazine and related drugs, *Clin. Pharmacol. Ther.*, **7**, 683–97.

NISTICÒ, G., SCAPAGNINI, V., and PREZIOSI, P. (1969) Metabolic changes in depression, *Lancet*, **ii**, 159.

OLDSTONE, M. B. A., and NELSON, E. (1966) Central nervous system manifestations of penicillin toxicity in man, *Neurology*, **16**, 693–700.

OLIVARIUS, B. DE F. (1956) Polyneuropathy during treatment with nitrofurantoin, *Ugeskr. Laeg.*, **118**, 753–5.

ORLAND, F. (1959) Use and overuse of tranquillizers, *J. Amer. med. Ass.*, **171**, 633–6.

OTTE, J. (1969) Oral contraceptives and depression, *Lancet*, **ii**, 498.

PALMLOV, A., and TUNEVALL, G. (1956) Furadantin as a urinary tract antiseptic, *Svenska Läk. Tidn.*, **53**, 2864–75.

PARBROOK, G. D., and PIERCE, G. F. M. (1960) Comparison of post-operative pain and stiffness after the use of suxamethonium and suxethonium compounds, *Brit. med. J.*, **2**, 579–80.

PATEL, J. C., and MEHTA, A. B. (1967) Oral dehydroemetine in intestinal and extra-intestinal amoebiasis, *Indian. J. med. Sci.*, **21**, 1–5.

PIRRIE, I. (1961) Neuropathy after thalidomide ('Distaval'), *Brit. med. J.*, **2**, 1498.

PITTINGER, C. B., and LONG, J. P. (1958) Neuromuscular blocking action of neomycin sulphate, *Antibiot. and Chemother.*, **8**, 198–203.

PITTINGER, C. B., LONG, J. P., and MILLER, J. R. (1958) The neuromuscular blocking action of neomycin: A concern of the anesthesiologist, *Curr. Res. Anesth.*, **37**, 276–82.

POHLMANN, G. (1966) Respiratory arrest associated with intravenous administration of polymyxin B sulphate, *J. Amer. med. Ass.*, **196**, 181–3.

POWELL, S. J., McLOED, I. N., WILMOT, A. J., and ELSDON-DEW, R. (1962) Dehydroemetine in amebic dysentery and amebic liver abscess, *Amer. J. trop. Med. Hyg.*, **11**, 607–9.

POWELL-TUCK, G. A. (1961) Neuropathy after thalidomide ('Distaval') *Brit. med. J.*, **2**, 1151.

PRICE, S. A., and TOSELAND, P. A. (1969) Oral contraceptives and depression, *Lancet*, **ii**, 158–9.

PRIDGEN, J. E. (1956) Respiratory arrest thought to be due to intraperitoneal neomycin, *Surgery*, **40**, 571–4.

RAO, K. V. N., MITCHISON, D. A., NAIR, N. G. K., PREMA, K., and TRIPATHY, S. P. (1970) Sulphadimidine acetylation test for classification of patients as slow or rapid inactivators of isoniazid, *Brit. med. J.*, **3**, 495–7.

RAFFI, A., OPPERMAN, H., PAGEAUT, G., PEQUENGOT, J., and LONGCHAMP, D. (1966) Trois cas de myopathie stéroidienne, *Pédiatrie*, **21**, 608–10.

RENIER, J. CL. (1965) Une observation de neuromyopathie due a l'hydroxychloroquine, *Rev. Rhum.*, **32**, 681–2.

ROELSEN, E. (1964) Polyneuritis after nitrofurantoin therapy. A survey and report of two new cases, *Acta med. scand.*, **175**, 145–54.

ROSE, D. P. (1966) The influence of oestrogens on tryptophan metabolism in man, *Clin. Sci.*, **31**, 265–72.

ROSE, D. P., and McGINTY, F. (1968) The influence of adrenocortical hormones and vitamins upon tryptophan metabolism in man, *Clin. Sci.*, **35**, 1–19.

RUBINSTEIN, C. J. (1964) Peripheral polyneuropathy caused by nitrofurantoin, *J. Amer. med. Ass.*, **187**, 647–9.

SAAVEDRA, A., MARIATEGUI, J., and BOGIANO, L. (1960) La imipramima en los estados depresivos, *Rev. Neuro-psiquiat.*, **23**, 195–228.

SANGHVI, L. M., and MATHUR, B. B. (1965) Electrocardiogram after chloroquine and emetine, *Circulation*, **32**, 281–9.

SARDESAI, H. V., SULE, C. R., and GAVANKAR, S. S. (1963) Clinical trials with dehydroemetine (Ro 1-9334) in acute amoebiasis, *Indian J. med. Sci.*, **17**, 334–5.

SARIN, B. P. (1963) Dehydroemetine in the treatment of intestinal amoebiasis in paediatric practice, *Burma med. J.*, **11**, 233–5.

SCHEID, W., WEICK, H. H., STAMMLER, A., KLADETZKY, A., and GIBBELS, E. (1961) Polyneuritische syndrome nach langerer Thalidomid-Medikation, *Dtsch. med. Wschr.*, **86**, 935–40.

SCHIELE, B. C. (1962) Newer drugs for mental illness, *J. Amer. med. Ass.*, **181**, 126–33.

SCHINDEL, L. (1968) Antiprotozoal drugs, in *Side Effects of Drugs*, Vol. VI, eds. Meyler, L., and Herxheimer, A., Excerpta Medica Foundation, Amsterdam, pp. 320–34.

SCHWAB, R. S., DOSHAY, L. J., GARLAND, H., BRADSHAW, P., GARVEY, E., and CRAWFORD, B. (1956) Shift to older age distribution in Parkinsonism: Report on 1000 patients covering past decade from three centres, *Neurology*, **6**, 783–90.

SEAMANS, K. B., GLOOR, P., DOBELL, R. A. R., and WYANT, J. D. (1968) Penicillin-induced seizures during cardiopulmonary bypass. A clinical and electroencephalographic study, *New Engl. J. Med.*, **278**, 861–8.

SHARP, W. L. (1960) Convulsions associated with antidepressant drugs, *Amer. J. Psychiat.*, **117**, 458–9.

SHROFF, K. R., and BODIWALA, N. K. (1966) Clinical trial of dehydroemetine in amoebiasis, *Curr. med. Pract.*, **10**, 233–8.

SIMPSON, J. A. (1961) Neuropathy after thalidomide ('Distaval'), *Brit. med. J.*, **2**, 1287.

SMITH, H., LERNER, P. I., and WEINSTEIN, L. (1967) Neurotoxicity and 'massive' intravenous therapy with penicillin. A study of possible predisposing factors, *Arch. intern. Med.*, **120**, 47–53.

SMITH, B., and O'GRADY, F. (1966) Experimental chloroquine myopathy, *J. Neurol. Neurosurg. Psychiat.*, **29**, 255–8.

TELFER, A. B. M., MACDONALD, D. J. F., and DINWOODIE, A. J. (1964) Familial sensitivity to suxamethonium due to atypical pseudocholinesterase, *Brit. med. J.*, **1**, 153–6.

TIMMERMAN, J. C., LONG, J. P., and PITTINGER, C. B. (1959) Neuromuscular blocking properties of various antibiotic agents, *Toxicol. appl. Pharmacol.*, **1**, 299–304.

TOSELAND, P. A., and PRICE, S. A. (1969) Tryptophan and oral contraceptives, *Brit. med. J.*, **1**, 777.

UESU, C. T. (1962) Peripheral neuropathy due to nitrofurantoin, *Ohio St. med. J.*, **58**, 53–6.

VAN DER GRIENT, A. J. (1968) Antibacterial drugs, in *Side Effects of Drugs*, Vol. VI, eds. Meyler, L., and Herxheimer, A., Excepta Medica Foundation, Amsterdam, pp. 241–62.

VAN DIJL, W. (1968) Muscle relaxant drugs, in *Side Effects of Drugs*, Vol. VI, eds. Meyler, L., and Herxheimer, A., Excerpta Medica Foundation, Amsterdam, pp. 156–61.

VICKERS, F. N. (1965) Peripheral neuropathy due to nitrofurantoin, *J. Ky med. Ass.*, **63**, 38–40.

VOSS, R. (1961) Nil nocere! Contergan-Polyneuritis, *Münch. med. Wschr.*, **103**, 1431–2.

WALKER, A. E., and JOHNSON, H. C. (1945) Convulsive factor in commercial penicillin, *Arch. Surg.*, **50**, 69–73.

WEINSTEIN, L., LERNER, P. I., and CHEW, W. R. (1964) Clinical and bacteriological studies of the effect of 'massive' doses of penicillin G on infections caused by Gram-negative bacilli, *New Engl. J. Med.*, **271**, 525–33.

WHISNANT, J. P., ESPINOSA, R. E., KIERLAND, R. R., and LAMBERT, E. H. (1963) Chloroquine neuromyopathy, *Proc. Mayo Clin.*, **38**, 501–13.

WILLETT, R. W. (1963) Peripheral neuropathy due to nitrofurantoin, *Neurology (Minneap.)*, **13**, 344–5.

WINSTON, F. (1969a) Oral contraceptives and depression, *Lancet*, i, 1209.

WINSTON, F. (1969b) Oral contraceptives and depression, *Lancet*, ii, 377.

WYLIE, W. D., and CHURCHILL-DAVIDSON, H. C. (1960) *A Practice of Anaesthesia*, London, p. 587.

YORKE, R. A., SUTTON, W. S., KILSHAW, D., and TAYLOR, W. H. (1962) Neuropathy, hypoglycaemia and adrenal dysfunction during treatment with thalidomide, *Brit. med. J.*, **2**, 306–7.

16

DISORDERS OF THE EYE

Ocular structures may exhibit the earliest evidence of toxicity of drugs used in general medicine (Perkins, 1968). It is vital to detect toxic changes early since at that stage the observed changes may be reversible. That routine examination of the eyes is essential in all new drug toxicity studies in animals is beyond question and this need has been emphasized by the publication of an excellent and informative symposium *Evaluation of Drug Effects on the Eye* published by the Association of Medical Advisers in the Pharmaceutical Industry (1968). Locally or systemically administered drugs can produce undesirable effects on ocular tissues and ocular function. This knowledge is by no means new since in 1785 Withering noted that 'foxglove when given in large and quickly repeated doses occasions sickness, vomiting, giddiness, confused vision, objects appearing green or yellow'. Today many more drugs are known to be implicated in toxic effects on the eye although it is not possible to relate chemical structure to toxic phenomena since undesirable ocular effects, reversible or irreversible may be produced by almost all categories of systemically administered drugs including cardiovascular agents, diuretics, antibiotics, CNS stimulants and depressants, drugs with a target action on the autonomic effector cells and those which act on the blood or blood forming organs. Local application of preparations to the eye may produce toxic symptoms and these may be due to active principle or to a component of the formulation [see PLATE 2F].

Many factors can influence a selective toxic effect of a drug on the eye; the ability of the drug to penetrate into the ocular structure depends on differential solubility in water and lipids, the polarity, and the ionic charge. Lipid-soluble substances pass freely into the eye whether applied locally or administered systemically; indeed the blood-eye barrier resembles the hypothetical blood-brain barrier in many ways. The physiological state of the eye may itself influence the penetration of such agents. Inflammation of the ocular structure is known to lower the resistance to drug penetration.

All ocular structures are potentially vulnerable to drug toxicity; however, the most frequently affected structures are the conjunctiva, cornea, sclera, lens, retina, optic nerve and extraocular muscles. Drugs can produce functional disturbance of accommodation and intraocular pressure and sometimes damage to the retina and optic nerve which is irreversible and may progress even after withdrawal of the implicated agent, as in chloroquine retinopathy. The drugs specifically implicated in the majority of reports of eye toxicity are the phenothiazine tranquillizers, the corticosteroids, the anti-inflammatory-antimalarial drugs, notably chloroquine, and other drugs which can only be grouped under a miscellaneous category.

PHENOTHIAZINE TRANQUILLIZERS

Ocular effects in patients treated with an experimental phenothiazine derivative (N.P. 207) were first reported by Verrey (1956) and also by Kinross-Wright (1956); these workers found pigmentary retinal changes, and the compound was not marketed. A closely related compound, thioridazine in large doses also produced pigmental retinal changes (May *et al.*, 1960).

Chlorpromazine was introduced into the clinic in 1953 and since that time it and its numerous derivatives have been widely used in general medicine and in psychiatry, especially in the long-term intensive treatment of the chronic schizophrenic. Several ocular effects caused by their use have been reported for these phenothiazines; they include: diplopia due to paresis of extra-ocular muscles (Crews, 1962), transient myopia due to promethazine (Bard, 1964), allergic conditions of conjunctiva or lids (Dencker and Enoksson, 1966; Mathalone, 1967; McClanahan *et al.*, 1966), and optic atrophy with both chlorpromazine (Rab *et al.*, 1969) and with perphenazine combined with large doses of thioridazine (Bonaccorsi, 1967).

Oculogyric crises have occasionally been observed as a part of the parkinsonian syndrome which is sometimes produced (Ayd, 1961) and blurred vision, due to an atropine-like action causing a temporary paralysis of accommodation, has been reported (Sinha and Mitra, 1955; Giacobini and Lassenius, 1954). Jonas (1959) has reported a chlorpromazine-induced miosis and Bock and Swain (1963) observed two cases of raised intra-ocular pressure. There is therefore, little doubt that chlorpromazine and its related phenothiazine tranquillizers have a multifarious range of toxic effects on the eye. It is, however, only since the report of Greiner and Berry (1964) that the long-term effects of phenothiazine therapy on the eye have been fully appreciated relative especially to pigmentation and lenticular and corneal changes and, more recently, to retinopathy.

Greiner and Berry (1964) reported lenticular opacity and cutaneous pigmentation in 70 women, of a series of many thousand patients undergoing prolonged and intensive chlorpromazine therapy. In the following year Margolis and Goble (1965) found lenticular opacities in eight of 31 schizophrenic patients who had received phenothiazine therapy for between 3 and 5 years. Trifluoperazine was implicated as the cause of these opacities. Barsa *et al.* (1965) performed slit-lamp examinations on 658 women under treatment for psychiatric disorders; all except seven were receiving phenothiazine therapy. Characteristic opacities of both lens and cornea were found in 33 patients and lens opacity alone in 145 patients. In all 178 patients (27 per cent) were affected with lens opacities. These opacities were characteristic and could easily be distinguished from the varying degrees of senile cataract found in 175 patients.

In the series of cases reported by Barsa *et al.* (1965) chlorpromazine had been given to all but two of the patients showing lens changes.

In 1967, Mathalone reported on an ocular examination of 462 patients in seven mental hospitals in England. Of those patients receiving more than 300 mg of chlorpromazine daily for 3 years or longer, 36 per cent showed lens changes and 17 per cent had corneal changes.

The typical findings in the lens and cornea in patients with opacities due to phenothiazines are as follows: The sites of the lesions are the anterior part of the lens and the back of the cornea, and this leads, as De Long *et al.* (1965), have suggested, to the strong implication that the drug or some metabolite accumulates in the anterior chamber and is responsible for these changes.

The corneal stroma contains a diffuse, yellow, granular pigmentation; the pigment does not accumulate on the cornea shielded by the upper eye lid. On the lens the opacities are situated just under the anterior capsule of the lens and are confined to the central pupillary zone. These opacities consist of fine, yellow, granular clusters. Photosensitivity would therefore appear to play a part in the development of these opacities.

The toxic effect of phenothiazines on the eye is not only confined to the lens and cornea; indeed Cant (1969) has written that 'prolonged administration of all phenothiazines must be considered as liable to lead to retinopathy'. Phenothiazines accumulate in the pigment cells, particularly within the melanin fraction (Potts, 1962) and pigmentary retinal changes have been reported following the use of chlorpromazine and prochlorperazine (Weekley *et al.*, 1960), piperdichlorphenothiazine, and thioridazine (Leopold, 1968).

The retinal effects superficially resemble retinitis pigmentosa in that night blindness occurs and the retinal arteries show diffuse narrowing. Central vision is affected early. However, unlike typical retinitis pigmentosa, the pigment usually aggregates in large clumps rather than in bone corpuscle configuration.

High and continued dosage of thioridazine is required before ocular damage is observed (e.g. above 200 mg daily for many months), and most instances of reported complications were in patients who had received 600–800 mg of thioridazine hydrochloride daily. Pigmentary retinopathy has occurred when thioridazine was administered for as little as 3 weeks. Applebaum (1963) failed to find characteristic changes at smaller dosage.

CORTICOSTEROIDS

Raised Intraocular Pressure

Elevation of intraocular pressure is a well-documented side-effect of both local and systemic administration of corticosteroids. The onset is usually in a matter of weeks after local, and months after systemic, therapy (David and Berkowitz, 1969). This occurs in about 30 per cent of patients receiving local therapy and in a lower percentage when the steroid is given systemically. Severe increases resembling those of acute glaucoma have been reported, and cupping of the optic disc and visual field defects produced by the raised pressure are similar to those of open-angle glaucoma. The changes are usually reversible providing treatment is withdrawn, although an irreversible increase in intraocular pressure has been reported in one patient on topical dexamethasone. The fact that some individuals have a rise in intraocular pressure in response to corticosteroids does not necessarily indicate that they are in a preglaucoma state, and although the tendency to this response is probably hereditary, the exact manner of inheritance is uncertain. Since increased intraocular tension is more likely to develop in patients with simple open-angle glaucoma and their offspring, a simple Mendelian autosomal recessive pattern of inheritance has been postulated. According to this hypothesis, the patients with the greatest degree of elevation of intraocular pressure after topical corticosteroids are homozygotes for primary open-angle glaucoma. However, later work seems to indicate that glaucoma is transmitted by a polygenic mode of inheritance, and that the development of increased tension secondary to corticosteroid therapy does not predict the development of glaucoma.

Levene and Schwartz (1968) found little difference between the pressure rise induced by topical steroids in 'normal' patients and in those thought to have glaucoma. It cannot be concluded, however, that subjects showing only a slight rise of pressure with topical corticosteroids have no tendency to develop glaucoma.

Raised intraocular pressure after topical corticosteroids is common in diabetics without proliferative retinopathy and in patients susceptible to steroid-induced carbohydrate abnormality, but the distribution of intraocular-pressure response to corticosteroids is normal in the diabetic population with proliferative retinopathy. Diabetics who tend to develop a corticosteroid-induced rise in intraocular pressure may be resistant to the development of proliferative retinopathy, since the raised intraocular pressure may prevent extravasation from the retinal capillaries.

Topical corticosteroids have produced an increased incidence of intraocular-pressure elevations in myopic patients with no family history of glaucoma. A correlation between myopia and corticosteroid elevation of intraocular pressure has also been found in twin pairs, possibly due to shared genetic factors. The mechanism of steroid-induced ocular hypertension may involve increased aqueous production, but an increase in resistance to the outflow tract seems to be the most important contributing factor. The trabecular meshwork, which separates the anterior chamber from the canal of Schlemm, contains collagen strands and a single layer of endothelial cells. Corticosteroids may cause swelling of the collagen strands by increasing viscosity and water-binding capacity of the mucopolysaccharides. This would block the outflow tract and increase resistance. The incidence of ocular hypertension may be correlated with the anti-inflammatory effect of the topical steroid used. In glaucomatous eyes there may be a greater accumulation of mucopolysaccharides in the degenerated trabecular meshwork, thus causing heightened susceptibility to the increased outflow resistance induced by corticosteroids. Other effects of topical corticosteroids that could raise outflow resistance include increased vasoconstriction and pupil dilatation, both being a potentiation of the normal sympathetic tone of the eye.

Perkins (1965) has suggested that the normal diurnal variation in intraocular pressure is associated with the diurnal variation in circulating corticosteroid levels. These pressure variations may be related to changes in the rate of formation of aqueous humor rather than to changes in outflow resistance. Patients with Cushing's disease and patients with adrenal insufficiency maintained on corticosteroids lose the diurnal variation in intraocular pressure. Patients with Cushing's disease often have abnormally high intraocular pressures, fundus changes, and positive water-loading tests for glaucoma. After adrenalectomy these abnormalities return to normal. The serum-levels of 17-hydroxycorticosteroids are normal in patients with glaucoma but those who exhibit increased intraocular pressure in response to topical steroids show a slight fall in plasma-cortisol after oral dexamethasone, analogous to patients with Cushing's disease.

Posterior Subcapsular Cataracts

Black and his co-workers in 1960 first described posterior subcapsular cataracts (PSC) in rheumatoid arthritis patients on long-term corticosteroid therapy; since then there have been numerous articles in the literature reporting varying incidences of the association of posterior subcapsular cataracts and long-term corticosteroid therapy in adults (for example Spencer and Andelman, 1965; Fürst et al., 1966) and in children (for example Havre, 1965; Braver et al., 1966, 1967).

However, the relationship of posterior subcapsular cataracts to corticosteroid therapy needs further clarification. There have been only a few reports of lens changes related to local corticosteroid therapy as opposed to the frequent reports of steroid cataract associated with systemic therapy.

Spencer and Andelman (1965) have surveyed the literature for the incidence of PSC formation in patients receiving long-term steroid therapy for various diseases (e.g. asthma, rheumatoid and non-rheumatoid arthritis,

systemic lupus erythematosus and nephrotic syndrome). This varies from 0 to 42 per cent. In the control studies reported in the literature on patients with rheumatoid arthritis who were not treated with corticosteroids the incidence of PSC formation varied from 0 to 3 per cent.

In a specific study on 58 rheumatoid arthritis patients who had previously received intramuscular injections of triamcinolone acetonide, Spencer and Andelman (1965) reported an overall incidence of 60 per cent PSC formation. Generally the greater the total amount of drug received, the higher the incidence of PSC formation. For example there was PSC formation in 33 per cent of patients receiving between 500 and 1,000 mg of steroid and this incidence rose to 100 per cent in patients who received more than 2,000 mg of the drug.

In a related study on 113 patients comprising 56 children with Still's disease and 57 adults with classical rheumatoid arthritis, receiving maintenance therapy, Fürst et al. (1966) found seven adults and six children to have posterior subcapsular lens opacities. The duration of therapy with the steroid (prednisone) seemed to be less important than the average daily dose; while this tended to be higher in the patients developing cataract, particularly among the juveniles, eight of the 13 cataracts occurred in patients whose daily dose of prednisone was 10 mg or less.

In specific studies on children, Braver et al. (1966, 1967) confirmed that in children, as in adults, PSC is associated with prolonged corticosteroid therapy and is not associated with a particular disease. No children on therapy for less than 2 years developed PSC and the authors reported that when PSC did occur in three children there was no regression of the PSC 3 months after stopping corticosteroids, suggesting that if regression did occur it would be very slow.

There is some evidence to suggest that PSC complications of systemic corticosteroids are more common in children (Braver et al., 1967) with lower dosage and with shorter periods of therapy (Fürst et al., 1966). The incidence of cataracts with systemic corticosteroids is felt to depend predominantly upon the dose and duration of drug therapy rather than the underlying disease (Braver et al., 1967; Giles et al., 1962) and in this respect it is of interest to note that the use of intermittent steroid therapy is thought to explain the fact that patients with asthma develop cataracts less frequently than those with rheumatoid arthritis, who generally receive continuous steroid therapy (Giles et al., 1962).

With regard to the aetiology of the disease, steroid-induced cataract is almost always bilateral; the lesion usually occupies the polar region of the posterior cortex, just within the posterior lens capsule; it extends forward into the cortex irregularly but its borders are sharply defined (Oglesby et al., 1961). Vision is not usually impaired early in the development of a steroid-induced cataract, and slit-lamp examination is necessary for early detection and such investigations should certainly be done at least twice each year on any patient on long-term corticosteroid therapy. There is some contention as to whether steroid-induced cataract can be distinguished from cataracts associated with intraocular disease and from cataracts which occasionally develop in adult rheumatoid arthritic patients. There is agreement, however, that the steroid-induced cataract can usually be distinguished from the senile cataract which tends to spread peripherally, is associated with other cortical changes, and tends to cause early loss of vision. David and Berkowitz (1969) have reviewed the literature on this topic. Similar cataracts have been reported following oral contraceptive medication [see PLATE 3B].

Exophthalmos

It has been known for some time that corticosteroids will induce exophthalmos in experimental animals (Williams, 1953, 1955; Aterman and Greenberg, 1954). However, the mechanism of production is controversial and it has been reported only in young growing animals.

Cortisone and corticotrophin have been advocated in the treatment of exophthalmos and some favourable reports have appeared (Kinsell et al., 1953; Rubin and Billet, 1954; MRC Panel, 1955). However, there is now evidence in man that the long-term use of corticosteroids at high dosage can induce exophthalmos.

Slansky et al. (1967) reported four cases of exophthalmos associated with high doses of prednisone of 3 to 12 years' duration. Prior to steroid therapy, these patients exhibited no signs of exophthalmos, and during steroid therapy they were euthyroid with normal thyroid function. In one case there was a reduction in exophthalmos when the prednisone dosage was reduced from 25 mg to 5 mg per day. In these patients the exophthalmos accompanied other known complications of prolonged corticosteroid therapy including hyperglycaemia, posterior subcapsular cataract and elevated intraocular tension.

Although Slansky et al. (1967) were the first to report exophthalmos associated with long-term steroid therapy, there have been previous reports in the literature of exophthalmos being found in 6–8 per cent of patients with Cushing's disease with elevated steroid production (Plotz et al., 1952). In 1958, Morgan and Mason reported a case of Cushing's disease in which the initial manifestation was exophthalmos, while in 1962 Schwarz et al. reported a further five cases of exophthalmos in Cushing's disease and demonstrated an exophthalmic-producing factor in those patients.

All these findings suggest that the long-term use of corticosteroids, in high dosage, can induce exophthalmos and that such therapy should be carefully monitored with this complication in view.

CHLOROQUINE AND OTHER SYNTHETIC ANTIMALARIALS

Apart from their obvious use in the prophylaxis and treatment of malaria, the synthetic antimalarial drugs are widely used in relatively high dosage in the long-term treatment of various skin diseases, collagen diseases and arthritis. This later usage is related to their anti-inflammatory properties. Continued high dosage causes ocular damage of varying severity and reports in the literature have implicated all the commonly used synthetic 4-aminoquinolines: chloroquine, hydroxychloroquine, amodiaquine, and the earlier and now largely superseded aminoacridine, mepacrine (quinacrine), (Kersley and Palin, 1959; Hobbs et al., 1961; Grant, 1962; Merwin and Winkelmann, 1962). It must be emphasized that ocular damage does not occur with the lower dosage used in the prophylaxis and treatment of malaria; there is a danger of damage only at the prolonged and high dosage required for the non-malaria treatments when the drugs are being used for their anti-inflammatory or anti-arthritic properties.

Chloroquine and its near relative hydroxychloroquine are the two synthetic compounds of this group most commonly implicated in ocular damage, largely because they have greater use in their non-malaria role than any of the other synthetic antimalarials. Chloroquine and hydroxychloroquine are known to produce a number of ocular complications such as whitening of the lashes, extraocular muscle palsy, subepithelial corneal deposits, decreased corneal sensitivity and retinal damage. Retinal damage is the most serious of these complications [see PLATE 3C and D] and it may progress to a severe retinal degeneration even after cessation of therapy (Journal of the American Medical Association, 1966).

Henkind and Rothfield (1963) examined 56 clinic patients suffering from either rheumatoid arthritis or systemic or chronic discoid lupus erythematosus who were undergoing long-term medication with chloroquine (250–750 mg per day) or hydroxychloroquine (200–400 mg per day) or mepacrine (100 mg per day). Treatment had continued for a number of years. There was a high incidence of ocular involvement with corneal deposits (68 per cent), retinopathy (18 per cent) and decreased corneal sensitivity in 50 per cent of the patients, all of which appeared to be directly related to the medication. Lens opacities in the posterior subcapsular region were present in 37 per cent of patients, but could not be attributed to the medication. A factor of major importance revealed by this study was that retinopathy was present in asymptomatic patients and that, in the asymptomatic stage, could be reversed by discontinuing therapy. The objective demonstration of retinopathy before symptoms were present emphasized the importance of periodic ophthalmic examination of patients on such a treatment regimen.

The mechanism of retinal damage by antimalarial drugs is unknown; several workers have proposed that damage is initially produced by vascular spasm, although vascular spasm has not been noted in all cases (Hobbs et al., 1961; Smith, 1962). Others have suggested that chloroquine may be a retinal enzyme inhibitor (Schmidt and Mueller-Limmroth, 1962). Chloroquine has local anaesthetic properties (Mandel, 1960) and the reduction in corneal sensitivity experienced by patients may be attributable to this property (Henkind and Rothfield, 1963). The presence of corneal deposits appears to depend on a time-dose relationship and they disappear after cessation of therapy without causing permanent ocular damage. Corneal opacities have been reported in the literature as occurring with all the commonly used 4-aminoquinolines even at low dosage when given over prolonged periods of time. Henkind and Rothfield (1963) have reviewed and summarized the progress of such corneal pigmentation.

Leopold (1968) in his comprehensive review on the ocular complications of drugs has cited an incidence of about 4 per cent retinopathy in patients with collagen disease who were receiving long-term chloroquine therapy, and in common with other authors has emphasized the importance of periodically examining the ocular functions of such patients. Earnshaw et al. (1966) have studied methods of screening patients at risk, to determine which test or combination of tests were most useful. They concluded that no single test was suitable to detect early chloroquine retinopathy but that a combination of tests of colour-vision, elicitation of recent symptoms, especially photophobia, and ophthalmoscopy was reliable. The electro-oculogram was unsatisfactory as a screening test.

MISCELLANEOUS DRUGS (ANTI-CHOLINESTERASES, CHLORAMPHENICOL, ETC.)

Anticholinesterase Drugs and Cataracts

In 1960 Harrison published the first documented evidence of lens opacities produced by a miotic. A 13-year-old girl with esotropia had been treated with 0·025 per cent dyflos (di-isopropyl fluorophosphate) eye drops for 3 months when rosette-like anterior capsular lens opacities were noted. They did not interfere with vision and slowly disappeared after treatment was stopped.

In 1963 Axelsson and Holmberg (1966) commenced a carefully documented study of 3 years' duration in which they planned to compare the relative efficiency of the long-acting cholinesterase inhibitor phospholine iodide with pilocarpine in the treatment of glaucoma. Within a year these workers had become impressed by the increased incidence of cataracts in the phospholine-treated cases and so altered the direction of their study to compare the frequency of cataract formation in the two treatment groups. A total of 181 eyes was included in the study; of 103 eyes treated with pilocarpine (2–4 per cent solution, 2–4 times a day) for a mean period of 22 months, 10 eyes (about 10 per cent) developed or had an increase in lens opacities. Seventy-eight eyes were treated with phospholine iodide (0·06–0·25 per cent solution twice daily) for a mean period of 12 months; of these eyes, 39, or 50 per cent, had an increase in lens opacities. Of the 87 eyes with clear lenses when therapy was started three out of 47 were listed as positive

after the pilocarpine treatment and 16 out of 40 after phospholine treatment. An increase in the duration or strength of the anti-cholinesterase therapy significantly added to the cataractogenicity.

In later studies Holmberg (1966) reported that similar lens changes were seen with other long-acting anti-cholinesterase drugs, including dyflos and demecarium bromide, and De Roetth (1966) described 19 cases of anterior subcapsular lens changes in patients treated for 7 to 17 months with phospholine iodide. Shaffer and Hetherington (1966) have reviewed the literature to that date and in addition have published the results of their own studies which were largely aimed at determining whether the findings of Axelsson and Holmberg (1966) in Sweden were comparable with results in California. They also found that anticholinesterase agents (dyflos, demecarium bromide, and phospholine iodide) could initiate cataract formation and cited a 38 per cent incidence in their anti-cholinesterase-treated patients. There was a 6 per cent incidence in the pilocarpine-treated glaucoma cases. The lenses of patients over 60 years of age seemed more vulnerable to cataractous changes than those of younger patients and few lens opacities were seen in patients under 60 years of age.

Shaffer and Hetherington (1966) have concluded that in spite of the established cataractogenic effect of the long-acting anti-cholinesterases they have a useful and definite role in therapy especially since with surgery there is also a risk of cataract formation. Anticholinesterases should not be used, however, in those cases where tension can be controlled by parasympathomimetic agents, combined with adrenaline (epinephrine) and possibly carbonic anhydrase inhibitors. If used, the patient's pupils should be dilated at least every 6 months and the lenses examined for the characteristic vacuoles.

Chloramphenicol and Optic Neuritis

In 1951, Gewin and Friou reported the history of a patient with staphylococcal endocarditis who was treated with 247·5 grams of chlortetracycline, and 190·5 grams of chloramphenicol. Three days after medication was stopped, the patient complained of blurred vision. Ophthalmoscopy revealed blurred nerve heads. Since then there have been other reports of optic neuritis associated with chloramphenicol therapy in adults and children. (For example: Wallenstein and Snyder, 1952; Lasky et al., 1953; Dinning et al., 1963; Keith, 1964; Huang et al., 1966; Chang et al., 1966; Cocke et al., 1966.) In children with cystic fibrosis, the lesions appear to differ from the ocular changes frequently seen in those patients with cystic fibrosis who are not receiving chloramphenicol.

In all patients with associated optic neuritis, large total doses of chloramphenicol were given and therapy was prolonged. The changes have always been bilateral and central scotomata have been present; withdrawal of the antibiotic does not ensure a complete return of vision. The mechanism by which the optic neuritis develops is not known, it may be related to the neurological and hypersensitivity reactions occasionally reported with this agent.

Drug-induced Myopia and Scotomata

Drug-induced transient myopia is a rare phenomenon; it has been noted following therapy with organoarsenicals, acetazolamide, sulphonamides, phenothiazines and prochlorperazine. The transient myopia has a characteristic clinical course. There is a rapidly progressive blurring of distance-vision caused by a myopic shift in refractive error of 1 to 5 diopters superimposed on the patient's normal refractive index. The pupils remain normal in size and reactivity. Cycloplegia usually has little or no effect on the induced myopia. The myopia begins to disappear 24 to 48 hours after treatment has been withdrawn, and has totally gone in 3 to 5 days. Bard (1964) has reviewed the literature on this drug-induced disorder and has discussed the possible mechanisms involving this effect including an allergic origin.

Drug-induced scotomata is also uncommon although Robertson *et al.* (1966) have described three cases of blurred vision with central scotomata associated with digitalis intoxication. The only other compound that has been reported in the literature as causing scotomata is clomiphene citrate, a non-steroidal synthetic oestrogen (Roch *et al.*, 1967). Chlorpropamide, a member of the sulphonylurea group of oral hypoglycaemics, has also been implicated, although not proven, in central scotomata (Givner, 1961; George, 1963). The reaction has been observed only rarely, and it is not certain on the basis of present evidence that chlorpropamide alone is responsible for this complication in the diabetic patient.

The total incidence of ocular manifestations in patients with digitalis toxicity has been estimated to be as high as 25 per cent (Leopold, 1968), and in approximately 10 per cent of patients with digitalis toxicity the ocular complications may occur prior to other symptoms of toxicity although with the majority of patients adverse ocular effects appear simultaneously with, or after, signs of cardiac toxicity. The most common of these are blurred and disturbed colour vision (xanthopsia), photophobia, 'snowy vision', flickerings, flashes, sparks and scintillating scotomata. Disturbances of visual acuity are common and both transient and permanent amblyopias accompanied by central scotomata have been described. Central scotomata may be secondary to retrobulbar neuritis or to toxic effects of digitalis on the retinal receptor cell.

RECOMMENDED FURTHER READING

CANT, J. S. (1969) Iatrogenic eye disease, *Practitioner*, **202**, 787–95.

GRANT, W. M. (1969) Ocular complications of drugs: Glaucoma, *J. Amer. med. Ass.*, **207**, 2089–91.

GREEN, H., and SPENCER, J. (1969) *Drugs with Possible Ocular Side-Effects*, The British Optical Association, London.

LEOPOLD, I. H. (1968) Ocular complications of drugs: Visual changes, *J. Amer. med. Ass.*, **205**, 631–3.

MARZULLI, F. N. (1968) Ocular side effects of drugs, *Food Cosmet. Toxicol.*, **6**, 221–34.

PIGOTT, P. V., ed. (1968) *Evaluation of Drug Effects on the Eye*, Association of Medical Advisers in the Pharmaceutical Industry, London.

REFERENCES

ATERMAN, K., and GREENBERG, S. M. (1954) Experimental exophthalmos produced by cortisone, *Arch. Ophthal.*, **51**, 822–31.

APPLEBAUM, A. (1963) Ophthalmoscopic study of patients under treatment with thioridazine, *Arch. Ophthal.*, **69**, 578–80.

AXELSSON, U., and HOLMBERG, A. (1966) The frequency of cataract after miotic therapy, *Acta ophthal. (Kbh.)*, **44**, 421–9.

AYD, F. J. (1961) A survey of drug-induced extra pyramidal reactions, *J. Amer. med. Ass.*, **175**, 1054–60.

BARD, L. A. (1964) Transient myopia associated with promethazine (Phenergan) therapy, *Amer. J. Ophthal.*, **58**, 682–6.

BARSA, J. A., NEWTON, J. C., and SAUNDERS, J. C. (1965) Lenticular and corneal opacities during phenothiazine therapy, *J. Amer. med. Ass.*, **193**, 10–12.

BLACK, R. L., OGLESBY, R. B., VON SALLMANN, L., and BUNIM, J. J. (1960) Posterior subcapsular cataracts induced by corticosteroids in patients with rheumatoid arthritis, *J. Amer. med. Ass.*, **174**, 166–71.

BOCK, R., and SWAIN, J. (1963) Ophthalmological findings in patients on long-term chlorpromazine therapy, *Amer. J. Ophthal.*, **56**, 808–10.

BONACCORSI, M. T. (1967) Atrophie optique et atteinte systémique: Deux cas de réactions secondaires aux phénothiazines chez des enfants, *Laval méd.*, **38**, 84–8.

BRAVER, D. A., RICHARDS, R. D., and GOOD, T. A. (1966) Posterior subcapsular cataracts in corticosteroid-treated children, *J. Pediat.*, **69**, 735–8.

BRAVER, D. A., RICHARDS, R. D., and GOOD, T. A. (1967) Posterior subcapsular cataracts in steroid-treated children, *Arch. Ophthal.*, **77**, 161–2.

CANT, J. S. (1969) Iatrogenic eye disease, *Practitioner*, **202**, 787–95.

CHANG, N., GILES, C. L., and GREGG, R. H. (1966) Optic neuritis and chloramphenicol, *Amer. J. Dis. Child.*, **112**, 46–8.

COCKE, J. G., JR., BROWN, R. E., and GEPPERT, L. J. (1966) Optic neuritis with prolonged use of chloramphenicol. Case report and relationship to fundus changes in cystic fibrosis, *J. Pediat.*, **68**, 27–31.

CREWS, S. J. (1962) Toxic effects on the eye and visual apparatus resulting from the systemic absorption of newly introduced chemical agents, *Trans. ophthal. Soc. U.K.*, **82**, 387–406.

DAVID, D. S., and BERKOWITZ, J. S. (1969) Ocular effects of topical and systemic corticosteroids, *Lancet*, **ii**, 149–51.

DELONG, S., POLLEY, B. J., and McFARLANE, J. R. (1965) Ocular changes associated with long-term chlorpromazine therapy, *Arch. Ophthal.*, **73**, 611–17.

DENCKER, S. J., and ENOKSSON, P. (1966) Ocular changes produced by chlorpromazine, *Acta ophthal. (Kbh.)*, **44**, 397–403.

DE ROETTH, A., JR. (1966) Lenticular opacities in glaucoma patients receiving echothiophate iodide therapy, *J. Amer. med. Ass.*, **195**, 664–6.

DINNING, C. R., BRUCE, G. M., and SPALTER, H. F. (1963) Optic neuritis in chloramphenicol-treated patients with cystic fibrosis, *J. Pediat.*, **63**, 878.

EARNSHAW, E. R., MILES, D. W., and STEWART, T. W. (1966) Screening for chloroquine retinopathy, *Brit. J. Derm.*, **78**, 669–74.

FÜRST, C., SMILEY, W. K., and ANSELL, B. M. (1966) Steroid cataract, *Ann. rheum. Dis.*, **25**, 364–7.

GEORGE, C. W. (1963) Central scotomata due to chlorpropamide (Diabenese), *Arch. Ophthal.*, **69**, 773.

GEWIN, H. M., and FRIOU, G. J. (1951) Manifestations of vitamin deficiency during Aureomycin and chloramphenicol therapy of endocarditis due to *Staphylococcus aureus*: Report of a case, *Yale J. Biol. Med.*, **23**, 332–8.

GIACOBINI, E., and LASSENIUS, B. (1954) Chlorpromazine therapy in psychiatric practice; secondary effects and complications, *Nord. Med.*, **52**, 1693–9.

GILES, C. L., MASON, G. L., DUFF, I. F., and McLEAN, J. A. (1962) The association of cataract formation and systemic corticosteroid therapy, *J. Amer. med. Ass.*, **182**, 719–22.

GIVNER, I. (1961) Centrocecal scotomatas due to chlorpropamide, *Arch. Ophthal.*, **66**, 64.

GRANT, W. M. (1962) *Toxicology of the Eye*, Springfield, Illinois, pp. 39, 40, 130–3, 274, 450–6.

GREINER, A. C., and BERRY, K. (1964) Skin pigmentation and corneal and lens opacities with prolonged chlorpromazine therapy, *Canad. med. Ass. J.*, **90**, 663–5.

HARRISON, R. (1960) Bilateral lens opacities associated with the use of di-isopropylfluorophosphate eyedrops, *Amer. J. Ophthal.*, **50**, 153–4.

HAVRE, D. C. (1965) Cataracts in children on long-term corticosteroid therapy, *Arch. Ophthal.*, **73**, 818–21.

HENKIND, P., and ROTHFIELD, N. F. (1963) Ocular abnormalities in patients treated with synthetic antimalarial drugs, *New Engl. J. Med.*, **269**, 433–9.

HOBBS, H. E., EADIE, S. P., and SOMERVILLE, F. (1961) Ocular lesions after treatment with chloroquine, *Brit. J. Ophthal.*, **45**, 284–97.

HOLMBERG, A. (1966) cited by Shaffer and Hetherington (1966).

HUANG, N. N., HARLEY, R. D., PROMADHATTAVEDI, V., and SPROUL, A. (1966) Visual disturbances in cystic fibrosis following chloramphenicol administration, *J. Pediat.*, **68**, 32–44.

JONAS, S. (1959) Miosis following administration of chlorpromazine, *Amer. J. Psychiat.*, **115**, 817–18.

JOURNAL OF THE AMERICAN MEDICAL ASSOCIATION (1966) Chloroquine retinopathy, editorial, *J. Amer. med. Ass.*, **195**, 774.

KEITH, C. G. (1964) Optic atrophy induced by chloramphenicol, *Brit. J. Ophthal.*, **48**, 567–70.

KERSLEY, G. D., and PALIN, A. G. (1959) Amodiaquine and hydroxychloroquine in rheumatoid arthritis, *Lancet*, **ii**, 886–8.

KINROSS-WRIGHT, V. (1956) in An evaluation of the newer psychopharmacologic agents and their role in current psychiatric practice, *Psychiat. Res. Rep. Amer. psychiat. Ass.*, **4**, 89–94.

KINSELL, L. W., PARTRIDGE, J. W., and FOREMAN, N. (1953) The use of ACTH and cortisone in the treatment and in the differential diagnosis of malignant exophthalmos: A preliminary report, *Ann. intern. Med.*, **38**, 913–17.

LASKY, M. A., PINCUS, M. H., and KATLAN, N. R. (1953) Bilateral optic neuritis following chloromphenicol therapy, *J. Amer. med. Ass.*, **151**, 1403–4.

LEOPOLD, I. H. (1968) Ocular complications of drugs, *J. Amer. med. Ass.*, **205**, 631–3.

LEVENE, R. Z., and SCHWARTZ, B. (1968) Depression of plasma cortisol and the steroid ocular pressure response, *Arch. Ophthal.*, **80**, 461–6.

MANDEL, E. H. (1960) New local anaesthetic with anticoagulant properties, chloroquine (Aralen) dihydrochloride, *Arch. Derm.*, **81**, 260–3.

MARGOLIS, L. H., and GOBLE, J. L. (1965) Lenticular opacities with prolonged phenothiazine therapy, *J. Amer. med. Ass.*, **193**, 7–9.

MATHALONE, M. B. R. (1967) Eye and skin changes in psychiatric patients treated with chlorpromazine, *Brit. J. Ophthal.*, **51**, 86–93.

MAY, R. H., SELYMES, P., WEEKLEY, R. D., and POTTS, A. M. (1960) Thioridazine therapy; results and complications, *J. nerv. ment. Dis.*, **130**, 230–4.

McCLANAHAN, W. S., HARRIS, J. E., KNOBLOCH, W. H., TREDICI, L. M., and UDASCO, R. L. (1966) Ocular manifestations of chronic phenothiazine derivative administration, *Arch. Ophthal.*, **75**, 319–25.

MERWIN, C. F., and WINKELMANN, R. K. (1962) Antimalarial drugs in therapy of lupus erythematosus, *Proc. Mayo Clin.*, **37**, 253–68.

MORGAN, D. C., and MASON, A. S. (1958) Exophthalmos in Cushing's syndrome, *Brit. med. J.*, **2**, 481–3.

OGLESBY, R. B., BLACK, R. L., VON SALLMANN, L., and BUNIM, J. J. (1961) Cataracts in rheumatoid arthritis patients treated with corticosteroids, *Arch. Ophthal.*, **66**, 519–23.

PANEL APPOINTED BY THE MEDICAL RESEARCH COUNCIL (1955) Cortisone in exophthalmos, *Lancet*, **i**, 6–9.

PERKINS, E. S. (1965) Steroid-induced glaucoma, *Proc. roy. Soc., Med.*, **58**, 531–3.

PLOTZ, C. M., KNOWLTON, A. I., and RAGAN, C. (1952) The natural history of Cushing's syndrome, *Amer. J. Med.*, **13**, 597–614.

POTTS, A. M. (1962) Concentration of phenothiazines in the eye of experimental animals, *Invest. Ophthal.*, **1**, 522–30.

RAB, S. M., ALAM, M. N., and SADEQUZZAMAN, M. D. (1969) Optic atrophy during chlorpromazine therapy, *Brit. J. Ophthal.*, **53**, 208–9.

ROBERTSON, D. M., HOLLENHORST, R. W., and CALLAHAN, J. A. (1966) Ocular manifestations of digitalis toxicity, *Arch. Ophthal.*, **76**, 640–5.

ROCH, L. M., GORDON, D. L., BARR, A. B., and PAULSEN, L. A. (1967) Visual changes associated with clomiphene citrate therapy, *Arch. Ophthal.*, **77**, 14–17.

RUBIN, I. L., and BILLET, E. W. (1954) Treatment of malignant exophthalmos with ACTH and cortisone, *N.Y. Med J.*, **54**, 2991–2.

SCHMIDT, B., and MUELLER-LIMMROTH, W. (1962) Electroretinographic examinations following application of chloroquine, *Acta ophthal. (Kbh.)*, **70**, Suppl., 245–51.

SCHWARZ, F., DER KINDEREN, P. J., and HOUTSTRALANZ, M. (1962) Exophthalmos-producing activity in the serum and in the pituitary of patients with Cushing's syndrome and acromegaly, *J. clin. Endocr.*, **22**, 718–25.

SHAFFER, R. N., and HETHERINGTON, J., JR. (1966) Anti-cholinesterase drugs and cataracts, *Amer. J. Ophthal.*, **62**, 613–18.

SINHA, G. B., and MITRA, S. K. (1955) Case of acute chlor-promazine hydrochloride poisoning, *J. Indian med. Ass.*, **24**, 557–8.

SLANSKY, H. H., KOLBERT, G., and GARTNER, S. (1967) Exophthalmos induced by steroids, *Arch. Ophthal.*, **77**, 579–81.

SMITH, J. L. (1962) Chloroquine macular degeneration, *Arch. Ophthal.*, **68**, 186–90.

SPENCER, R. W., and ANDELMAN, S. Y. (1965) Steroid cataracts: posterior subcapsular cataract formation in rheumatoid arthritis patients on long-term steroid therapy, *Arch. Ophthal.*, **74**, 38–41.

VERREY, F. (1956) Dégénérescence pigmentaire de la rétine d'origine medicamenteuse, *Ophthalmologica (Basel)*, **131**, 296–303.

WAGNER, P. (1956) Untersuchungen über die Wirkung von Phenothiazinderivaten auf den Augenhintergrund des Tieres, *Klin. Mbl. Augenheilk.*, **129**, 772–81.

WALLENSTEIN, L., and SNYDER, J. (1952) Neurotoxic reactions to chloromycetin, *Ann. intern. Med.*, **36**, 1526–8.

WEEKLEY, R. D., POTTS, A. M., REBOTON, J., and MAY, R. H. (1960) Pigmentary retinopathy in patients receiving high doses of new phenothiazine, *Arch. Ophthal.*, **64**, 65–76.

WILLIAMS, A. W. (1953) Exophthalmos in cortisone-treated experimental animals, *Brit. J. exp. Path.*, **34**, 621–4.

WILLIAMS, A. W. (1955) Pathogenesis of cortisone-induced exophthalmos in guinea pigs, *Brit. J. exp. Path.*, **36**, 245–7.

WITHERING, W. (1785) cited by White, P. D. (1965) Important toxic effect of digitalis overdosage on vision, *New Engl. J. Med.*, **272**, 904–5.

17

DISORDERS OF THE EAR

The ototoxic effects of a number of drugs are well established, yet to date the participation of experimental animal studies in the elucidation of drug-induced ototoxicity has been virtually nil. There are no tests used routinely to screen new molecules for absence of ototoxicity and it has been the patient who has provided the first indication of vestibular or auditory damage.

It is commonplace now to screen all new molecules, and even re-examine some older compounds, for absence of general toxicity and absence of terato-genicity. Indeed, these are statutory requirements common to all drug-registration authorities. More recently, many laboratories have introduced tests to screen drugs for absence of ocular toxicity. It is time that tests were also devised to screen compounds for absence of toxic effects on the vestibular apparatus and for absence of auditory disturbance. There are a number of drugs with known ototoxic actions well suited as reference standards and there are sufficient indications in the literature to suggest that meaningful and comparable toxicity tests would be possible. Perhaps the required catalyst would be more interest in this aspect of toxicity on the part of some of the drug-registration authorities.

Among agents known at the present time to produce vestibular and/or auditory damage are specific antibiotics produced by *Streptomyces* species; these amino-glycoside antibodies could be much more freely used but for their peculiar capacity to damage the eighth cranial nerve. Streptomycin and gentamicin attack mainly the vestibular branch and neomycin and kanamycin the auditory. It is fairly well recognized that any of these antibiotics should be used with caution, especially in patients with poor renal function, though, in the past, vestibular damage in such patients from streptomycin has unfortunately been far from uncommon (*British Medical Journal*, 1969).

The diuretic, ethacrynic acid, and the much abused family of salicylates are also ototoxic drugs. Quinine should also be added to this list, although with the advent of the synthetic antimalarials, many fewer patients now suffer from a vertigo, tinnitus and deafness that this agent was wont to cause. In view of its present usage, confined perhaps to emergency intravenous treatment in severe *Plasmodium falciparum* malaria, its ototoxicity will not be discussed here. In passing, however, it is of interest to speculate why with the close structural relationship between quinine and some of the synthetic antimalarials, the latter do not share in the ototoxicity of quinine especially when they are used in high dosage for their anti-inflammatory effects.

STREPTOMYCIN AND DIHYDROSTREPTOMYCIN

Soon after the introduction of streptomycin, damage to the eighth cranial nerve, vestibular and auditory fibres, was recognized (Hinshaw and Feldman, 1945). In order to find a drug as efficacious but less toxic, dihydro-streptomycin was introduced, but was found to be toxic to the cochlea (Hobson *et al.*, 1948) and caused a high incidence of ototoxicity. Deafness occurred without preliminary warnings of disturbed vestibular function and occurred even after treatment had stopped. Hobson (1953) suggested that a combination of equal parts of streptomycin and dihydrostreptomycin might reduce the toxic effects of both components; however, this was unsuccessful and this combination product, strepto-duocin, is little used.

Streptomycin continues to be used as a 'first-line' drug in antitubercular therapy either alone or in combination with other agents; there is, however, no rationale for the use of dihydrostreptomycin alone and this agent has virtually disappeared from use. The most frequent toxic effect of streptomycin is disturbance of vestibular function (Glorig and Fowler, 1947; Northington, 1950) and the commonest symptom is giddiness in the upright position, sometimes associated with nausea and vomiting. This state is replaced in a few days by a chronic condition of uncertainty of balance in which only sudden movements produce vertigo. In time this difficulty is overcome and the eyes become of great importance in maintaining balance. The danger of developing vestibular disturbance increases with age and the drug should not be given to patients with renal impairment, as shown by a raised blood urea, otherwise high blood levels may be produced by normal therapeutic doses and result in severe damage to the vestibular nerve. Deafness, except in patients with tuberculous meningitis, is an extremely rare complication of streptomycin therapy. It seems likely that in these patients, streptomycin which usually appears in the cerebrospinal fluid in low concentration, reaches the CNS in higher concentration, either because it was given intrathecally or because, after intramuscular injection, the inflamed meninges permit more of the streptomycin to enter the cerebrospinal fluid.

Rasmussen (1969) examined the ototoxic effects of streptomycin and dihydrostreptomycin on the foetus and showed that the dangers of ototoxic damage to the foetus during maternal treatment was slight. Thirty-six children aged 2 to 15 years, whose mothers had received streptomycin, dihydrostreptomycin, or both during pregnancy were examined. Slight unilateral sensory-neural high-tone hearing loss was found in one child but all children were found to have normal vestibular function. In eight of 33 mothers there was impaired hearing attributable to dihydrostreptomycin therapy and in one mother there was reduced vestibular function. Similar results to these findings were reported by earlier investigators (for example Heilman *et al.*, 1945; Sakula, 1954; Kreibich, 1954).

Riskaer *et al.* (1952) conducted experiments in streptomycin and dihydrostreptomycin-treated pregnant guinea-pigs and found normal hearing among the siblings. In these studies, however, only small amounts of antibiotic (8·65 per cent) passed the placenta. In man the antibiotic concentrations in the foetus are equal or higher than in the mother (Jakobsen, 1953).

There have been other interesting studies in animals which may also indicate the route towards definitive screening tests. Streptomycin reduced the cochlea microphonic potential in cats after a few days' treatment at 200 mg/kg although there was no adverse effect when 100 mg/kg was given for as long as 60 days. Dihydrostreptomycin had an opposite effect in the cat in that it enhanced the cochlea microphonic potential, whilst depressing the action potentials of the auditory nerve. Histological studies have also been interesting; peripheral end organ lesions in the crista ampulloris have been described in streptomycin-treated mice (Causse *et al.*, 1948) and cats (Berg, 1949; Hawkins and Lurie, 1952) and evidence of a central lesion in the cochlea system was described by Winston *et al.* (1948) in the streptomycin-treated cat. Microscopic sections of the temporal bones from dihydrostreptomycin-treated cats showed degeneration of the neuroepithelium of the vestibular end organs and of the external hair cells of the organ of Corti.

Data from human pathology is scarce, since few patients come to autopsy, but Stevenson *et al.* (1947) described pathological changes in five patients who had vestibular damage from streptomycin. In these patients there were lesions in the ventral cochlea nuclei, but not in the dorsal cochlea nuclei.

NEOMYCIN

Absorption of neomycin from the alimentary tract is slight although it can be enhanced by ulceration. However, when large doses are given for long periods, as for example in the prevention of hepatic coma, and if the patient also has diminished renal function, the amounts absorbed are sufficient to produce ototoxic effects.

The risk of ototoxicity from administering neomycin is much greater than that of streptomycin, both because deafness is a more severe handicap than vestibular dysfunction and because a smaller total dose may produce it. Since kanamycin, with very similar therapeutic effects, is less ototoxic, the parenteral administration of neomycin has been almost entirely abandoned (*British Medical Journal*, 1969). Neomycin still continues, however, to be used in topical preparations, in inhalent solutions, in tablets swallowed for their effect

on bowel flora, and is also used to treat infection of the peritoneal cavity and the bladder. Recent evidence has suggested that absorption from these local sites is not insignificant and ototoxic effects have been reported.

Neomycin affects the basal coil of the cochlea first. This has been demonstrated by the loss of high-frequency tones during life, and by post-mortem histopathology of the temporal bones (Hawkins and Lurie, 1953). Profound loss of hearing after the intravenous or intramuscular use of neomycin was reported shortly after the clinical introduction of the antibiotic (Waisbren and Spink, 1950) and later reports drew attention to impairment of hearing caused by prolonged oral administration or colonic irrigation with neomycin (Halpern and Heller, 1961; Fields, 1964; Gibson, 1967).

Inhalation of neomycin in the treatment of bronchiectasis is also not without risk of ototoxicity. Lorian (1962) showed that the aminoglycosides are particularly well absorbed after intrabronchial administration, and the inhalation of an aerosol of neomycin several times a day has been reported to cause hearing loss in children (Fuller, 1960).

Recently Kelly *et al.* (1969) reported a case of deafness after irrigation of a granulating wound with a topical solution of neomycin (0·5 per cent) and polymyxin (0·1 per cent). Hearing impairment progressed in the patient after treatment was stopped and 10 months later there was an 89 per cent loss of hearing in the left ear and a 100 per cent loss in the right. Caloric examination was within normal limits indicating that the vestibular system was intact.

The case cited by Kelly *et al.* (1969), apart from indicating a new route for the absorption and subsequent ototoxic action of neomycin, has illustrated some of the features of neomycin ototoxicity that need to be given emphasis. Firstly, hearing loss can occur and progressively deteriorate days, weeks or even months after cessation of the drug (Kohonen, 1965) and may progress to involve the entire auditory frequency range. Secondly, the vestibular labyrinth is usually unaffected, and accordingly, vertigo is rarely a symptom. Thirdly, ototoxicity is enhanced by renal impairment since the antibiotic is normally excreted by the kidneys; this may be complicated by the additional nephrotoxic action of neomycin. Fourthly, although nephrotoxicity is often reversed with cessation of the drug, neomycin ototoxicity is not, and finally, local treatment is not free from dangers of ototoxicity. If local treatment with neomycin is adopted, it is a sensible precaution to limit the daily amount to that considered safe by injection—certainly not more than 1 gram—and the treatment should not continue for more than 7 days. The same considerations should apply to all forms of local application, including the treatment of skin infections and burns and instillations into serous and other cavities (Trimble, 1969).

KANAMYCIN AND VIOMYCIN

Like neomycin both of these antibiotics are related chemically to streptomycin; they are aminoglycosides produced by species of *Streptomyces*. Kanamycin and viomycin have vestibular toxicity, cochlea toxicity and nephrotoxicity. Both antibiotics are 'second-line' antitubercular agents whose main usage is when drug-resistant organisms emerge to the first-line drugs or when patients develop hypersensitivity to them. The usefulness of both the antibiotics is greatly limited by their range of toxicity and their potential ototoxicity increases in the presence of renal dysfunction.

A comparative assessment of the ototoxicity and renal toxocity of this whole group of aminoglycoside antibiotics is shown in TABLE 17.1; toxicity ratings are shown by the number of pluses.

TABLE 17.1

TOXICITY RATINGS FOR STREPTOMYCIN AND
OTHER AMINOGLYCOSIDE ANTIBIOTICS

	VESTIBULAR TOXICITY	AUDITORY TOXICITY	RENAL TOXICITY
Streptomycin	+++	+	−
Dihydrostreptomycin	+	++	−
Viomycin	+	+++	++
Neomycin	+	++++	++++
Kanamycin	+	+++	++

With kanamycin, ototoxicity is related to the total dosage administered; damage to the inner ear is to be expected after total doses of 40–60 grams when the daily dose is 1 gram, or 30 grams total dose, when the daily dose is 2 grams. There is, however, considerable variation in the level of reported ototoxic dosage and an 18-year-old girl with septicaemia suffered deafness and loss of vestibular function after a total dose of 14 grams of kanamycin administered over 8 days.

Some authorities have stated that the total dose should not exceed 80 grams whereas others have adopted wider margins of safety and have advocated maximum total doses of 40 or 50 grams. The reasons for this variation in opinions are almost certainly related to the fact that elderly patients are especially at risk from the ototoxicity of kanamycin, and also at special risk are those patients with impaired renal function and those with existing auditory disturbances such as might well have been caused by prior streptomycin or dihydrostreptomycin treatment. Intermittent administration of the antibiotic lessens the risk of ototoxicity, possibly by a three-fold margin.

Since kanamycin causes late auditory damage, similar to that produced by dihydrostreptomycin, medication must be discontinued as soon as the first audiological changes are noted. Regular audiological examination is therefore imperative. Although the ototoxic effect of kanamycin must be regarded as serious there is no doubt that nephrotoxicity is a more serious hazard associated with the use of kanamycin. The occurrence of hearing damage and impaired renal function, especially in the presence of already diseased kidneys, has greatly limited the usefulness of kanamycin.

Meyler (1963, 1966) has produced a comprehensive survey of literature on the toxicity of kanamycin.

ETHACRYNIC ACID

Ethacrynic acid, a desulphamyl compound, is an effective diuretic of novel chemical structure; however, since its introduction numerous adverse effects have been reported (Brest *et al.*, 1965; Cannon *et al.*, 1965; Hagedorn, 1965; Maher and Schreiner, 1965) including development of acute transient deafness in patients with marked impairment of renal function (Maher and Schreiner, 1965; Schneider and Becker, 1966; Schmidt and Friedman, 1967).

Recently Pillay *et al.* (1969) and Hanzelik and Peppercorn (1969) have re-emphasized the need for caution in the use of ethacrynic acid in uraemic patients; Pillay *et al.* (1969) presented case histories of five uraemic patients in whom deafness followed ethacrynic acid treatment; in three the deafness was permanent, this being the first report of permanent deafness occurring. In one case intravenous injection of 200 mg ethacrynic acid was followed, 90 minutes later, by deafness which persisted; in another case 800 mg of intravenous ethacrynic acid daily produced hearing impairment within 2 days, which persisted while dosage was continued but cleared soon after it was stopped. Oral ethacrynic acid (300–600 mg per day) produced deafness within 2 days of commencement of treatment. Hanzelik and Peppercorn (1969) reported the history of one patient in chronic renal failure who was given 100 mg of ethacrynic acid intravenously. Within 5 minutes the patient complained of diminished hearing with tinnitus but without vertigo or nausea. Ten minutes after the dosage, examination revealed bilateral nerve deafness. Over the next few hours, hearing gradually returned to normal and was fully restored by 8 hours. Further administration of ethacrynic acid did not result in impairment of hearing.

Mathog and Klein (1969) have reported moderate to severe permanent hearing loss in three uraemic patients after administration of ethacrynic acid and small amounts of aminoglycoside antibiotics (streptomycin alone or combined with kanamycin plus colonic irrigation with neomycin). The authors suggested that the combined effect of diuretic and aminoglycosides might be toxic to hair cells or damage them through an alteration in supporting cells and composition of cochlear fluids since, although differing in chemical structures, both ethacrynic acid and the aminoglycoside antibiotics have separately been shown to produce deterioration of outer hair cells and depression of cochlear microphonic potentials (Hawkins, 1959; Matz *et al.*, 1965; Kunin, 1966; Matz and Naunton, 1968).

Other investigators have also discussed the possible mode of the ototoxic action of ethacrynic acid. Schneider and Becker (1966) suggested that it could be related to an alteration in the formation of perilymph in the cochlea, although they discounted their own theory in view of the lack of vertigo and nausea in their patients. However, the theory is perhaps tenable since in the series reported by Pillay *et al.* (1969) one patient had nausea and severe vertigo, and another experienced dizziness in association with hearing loss.

In animal studies, Schneider and Becker (1966) found that 20–30 per cent of ethacrynic acid recovered in the urine resembled the cysteine derivative of ethacrynic acid—a substance which was withdrawn from clinical trial because of the high incidence of transient hearing loss. Retention of this substance in patients with renal insufficiency, if the route of metabolism in man is the same as in the animal study, could be the cause of the hearing loss.

Others have suggested that ethacrynic acid is directly toxic to the auditory nerves and certainly the speed with which impaired hearing followed the intravenous injection of the diuretic, in the patients described by Pillay *et al.* (1969) and Hanzelik and Peppercorn (1969) would add considerable weight to this opinion.

Mathog and Klein (1969) seemed reluctant to ascribe ototoxicity solely to ethacrynic acid in their studies with combined diuretic and aminoglycoside antibiotics, and advocated a combined effect as the cause of deafness in their patients. This view is not in accordance with the mass of evidence that is accumulating on the ototoxicity of ethacrynic acid itself, some of which has been summarized in this review. Ethacrynic acid is ototoxic and the uraemic patient is at special risk. If renal function is impaired the blood concentration of ethacrynic acid (or a metabolite) is raised and a direct ototoxic effect results related to the raised concentration of the drug. If diuresis results the blood concentration of drug or metabolite falls and the risk of ototoxicity is reduced.

It would be prudent to use other diuretics initially in uraemic patients and to reserve ethacrynic acid for those cases which are resistant to other therapy. Even then, it would be wise to monitor the patient carefully for evidence of hearing loss, preferably with serial audiograms. Treatment with ethacrynic acid should be stopped at the first sign of impaired hearing and, even if hearing loss is transient, ethacrynic acid treatment should not be re-introduced for fear of inducing permanent deafness. There is some evidence, and indeed it would be logical to expect, that therapy with combinations of known ototoxic agents (e.g. ethacrynic acid plus aminoglycoside antibiotics) is liable to produce deafness at relatively low doses of each component; this is, presumably, mutual potentiation of ototoxicity.

FRUSEMIDE (FUROSEMIDE, FURSEMIDE)

Frusemide, a compound unrelated to ethacrynic acid, is a diuretic that has achieved wide use because of its great potency as a saluretic agent and its low order of toxicity. However, Schwartz *et al.* (1970) have recently described transient ototoxic effects of high-dose intravenous frusemide therapy in five patients with diminished renal function.

All reactions occurred immediately after rapid intravenous administration and the individual doses ranged from 800–2,000 mg. In four of the five cases large doses of frusemide had been given previously and the remaining case had a potentially ototoxic drug (colistin 100 mg) administered as well. In three of the five cases the diuretic effect was poor.

The ototoxic effect consisted of hearing loss in four patients, vertigo in two, and tinnitus in two. In all cases the effect was transient and recovery was apparently complete within 5 hours.

The authors concluded that frusemide is a potentially ototoxic agent when given in large intravenous doses to patients with impaired renal function. Without conjecturing whether patients prone to ototoxicity with ethacrynic acid therapy are the most likely to sustain frusemide-induced hearing loss, these authors cautioned against the arbitrary substitution of frusemide for ethacrynic acid in such cases.

SALICYLATES

Tinnitus is a recognized side-effect of salicylate treatment in acute rheumatic fever and rheumatoid and osteo-arthritis, largely due to the high level of dosage required. However, Jager and Alway (1946) reported both tinnitus and moderate reduction in hearing in 34 of 38 patients being treated for acute rheumatic fever with large doses of salicylates. These effects disappeared 2 or 3 days after treatment was stopped.

Waltner (1955) described tinnitus and deafness in a woman who had taken 200 aspirin tablets in 6 days. The patient had severe bilateral sensorineural loss with recruitment. This hearing loss was completely reversible in 7 days.

In more recent studies McCabe and Dey (1965) and Myers and Bernstein (1965) investigated the effects of aspirin upon auditory sensitivity. The former workers found that salicylates caused tinnitus and reduction in pure tone sensitivity in five women who previously had normal hearing; with pure tone sensitivity the higher frequencies were more severely impaired than the lower. Audiometric studies indicated that the locus of aspirin ototoxicity was intracochlear. Myers and Bernstein (1965) undertook a clinical study using 25 arthritic patients as subjects. Twenty-one patients were actually intoxicated with aspirin and developed a bilateral symmetrical elevation of pure tone thresholds. The magnitude of hearing loss was dependent on the plasma salicylate level and was quickly reversible after aspirin treatment was stopped. Patients who had experienced tinnitus and hearing loss when on aspirin dosage lost the tinnitus and reverted to normal hearing when the drug was withdrawn. Audiometric studies indicated that the cochlear was the probable site of the ototoxicity. An experimental study on squirrel monkeys was made using behavioural conditioning methods to plot the audiograms. Reversible hearing loss was produced and this could be correlated with plasma salicylate levels. However, subsequent light and electron microscopic examination of the cochlea failed to show any morphological change.

In general terms, ototoxicity with the salicylates is not serious provided the drug is withdrawn when ototoxic symptoms first occur. The real danger, however, is that salicylate-containing 'over-the-counter' preparations are readily available and excessive self-medication may induce ototoxic effects without the subject correlating tinnitus or hearing impairment with the remedy that is being taken. It is also worthy of mention in this context that other side-effects of salicylates notably renal damage and gastro-intestinal bleeding are of equal if not greater potential danger to the patient.

Rheumatoid arthritis is often quoted as a condition in which patients are treated with large quantities of salicylates over long periods of time without developing renal damage. This view is in conflict with the evidence which shows a high incidence of serious renal damage (including papillary necrosis) in patients with rheumatoid arthritis treated in this way (Kincaid-Smith, 1970).

With regard to gastro-intestinal bleeding, Croft (1970) has reported that in south-east England 56 per cent of all patients admitted to hospital with haematemesis and melaena have taken aspirin during the previous few days, compared with only 32 per cent of those who are admitted for other reasons. This suggests that at least a quarter of all clinically serious upper gastro-intestinal tract bleeds are caused by aspirin. Aspirin causes an even higher proportion of radiologically negative bleeds from gastric erosion.

The trilogy of ototoxicity, renal damage and gastro-intestinal bleeding together with the common usage and ready availability of aspirin in particular, and salicylates in general, make this class of drug a prime contributor to iatrogenic disease when used in high and continuous dosage by the patient with or without the benefit of medical advice.

RECOMMENDED FURTHER READING

MANTEN, A. (1968) Antibiotic drugs, in *Side Effects of Drugs*, Vol. VI, eds. Meyler, L., and Herxheimer, A., Excerpta Medica Foundation, Amsterdam, pp. 291–302.

PRESCOTT, L. F. (1968) Antipyretic analgesic drugs, in *Side Effects of Drugs*, Vol. VI, eds. Meyler, L., and Herxheimer, A., Excerpta Medica Foundation, Amsterdam, pp. 101–9.

REFERENCES

BERG, K. (1949) The toxic effect of streptomycin on the eighth cranial nerve, *Ann. Otol. (St. Louis)*, **58**, 448–56.

BREST, A. N., ONESTI, G., SELLER, R., RAMIREZ, O., HEIDER, C., and MOYER, J. H. (1965) Pharmacodynamic effects of a new diuretic drug, ethacrynic acid, *Amer. J. Cardiol.*, **16**, 99–105.

BRITISH MEDICAL JOURNAL (1969) Deafness after topical neomycin, leading article, *Brit. med. J.*, **2**, 181–2.

CANNON, P. J., HEINEMANN, H. O., STASON, W. B., and LARAGH, J. H. (1965) Ethacrynic acid. Effectiveness and mode of diuretic action in man, *Circulation*, **31**, 5–18.

CAUSSÉ, R., GONDET, I., and VALLANCIEN, B. (1948) Action vestibulaire de la streptomycine chez la souris, *C.R. Soc. Biol. (Paris)*, **142**, 747–9.

CROFT, D. N. (1970) Gastric bleeding due to drugs, *Prescribers' J.*, **10**, 14–19.

FIELDS, R. L. (1964) Neomycin ototoxicity: Report of case due to rectal and colonic irrigations, *Arch. Otolaryng.*, **79**, 67–70.

FULLER, A. (1960) Ototoxicity of neomycin aerosol, *Lancet*, **i**, 1026.

GIBSON, S. W., JR. (1967) Deafness due to orally administered neomycin, *Arch. Otolaryng.*, **86**, 163–5.

GLORIG, A., and FOWLER, E. P., JR. (1947) Tests for labyrinth function following streptomycin therapy, *Ann. Otol. (St. Louis)*, **56**, 379–94.

HAGEDORN, C. W., KAPLAN, A. A., and HULET, W. H. (1965) Prolonged administration of ethacrynic acid in patients with chronic renal disease, *New Engl. J. Med.*, **272**, 1152–5.

HALPERN, E. B., and HELLER, M. F. (1961) Ototoxicity of orally administered neomycin: Report of a case, *Arch. Otolaryng.*, **73**, 675–7.

HANZELIK, E., and PEPPERCORN, M.) (1969 Deafness after ethacrynic acid, *Lancet*, **i**, 416.

HAWKINS, J. E., JR. (1959) Antibiotics and inner ear, *Trans. Amer. Acad. Ophthal.*, **63**, 206–18.

HAWKINS, J. E., JR., and LURIE, M. H. (1952) The ototoxicity of streptomycin, *Ann. Otol. (St. Louis)*, **61**, 789–809.

HAWKINS, J. E., JR., and LURIE, M. H. (1953) The ototoxicity of dihydrostreptomycin and neomycin in the cat, *Ann. Otol. (St. Louis)*, **62**, 1128–48.

HEILMAN, D. H., HEILMAN, F. R., HINSHAW, H. C., NICHOLS, D. R., and HERRELL, W. E. (1945) Streptomycin: Absorption diffusion, excretion and toxicity, *Amer. J. med. Sci.*, **210**, 576–84.

HINSHAW, H. C., and FELDMAN, W. H. (1945) Streptomycin in treatment of clinical tuberculosis: A preliminary report, *Proc. Mayo Clin.*, **20**, 313–18.

HOBSON, L. B. (1953) cited by Heck, W. E., Lynch, W. J., and Graves, H. L. (1953) Controlled comparison on eighth nerve toxicity of streptomycin and dihydrostreptomycin, *Ann. Otol. (St. Louis)*, **62**, 101–6.

HOBSON, L. B., TOMPSETT, R., MUSCHENHEIM, C., and McDERMOTT, W. (1948) Laboratory and clinical investigation of dihydrostreptomycin, *Amer. Rev. Tuberc.*, **58**, 501–24.

JAGER, B. V., and ALWAY, R. (1946) The treatment of acute rheumatic fever with large doses of sodium salicylate with special reference to dose management and toxic manifestations, *Amer. J. med. Sci.*, **211**, 273–85.

JAKOBSEN, B. E. (1953) Streptomycinets overgang fra moder til foster, *Ugeskr. Laeg.*, **115**, 1181–3.

KELLY, D. R., NILO, E. R., and BERGGREN, R. B. (1969) Deafness after topical neomycin wound irrigation, *New Engl. J. Med.*, **280**, 1338–9.

KINCAID-SMITH, P. (1970) Analgesic nephropathy, *Prescribers' J.*, **10**, 8–13.

KOHONEN, A. (1965) Effect of some ototoxic drugs upon the pattern and innervation of cochlear sensory cells in the guinea pig, *Acta oto-laryng (Stockh.)*, **208**, Suppl., 1–70.

KREIBICH, H. (1954) Sind nach einer Streptomycinbehandlung tuberkulöser Schwangerer Schädigungen des Kindes zu erwarten?, *Dtsch. Gesundh.-Wes.*, **9**, 177–81.

KUNIN, C. M. (1966) Absorption, distribution, excretion and fate of kanamycin, *Ann. N.Y. Acad. Sci.*, **132**, 811–18.

LORIAN, V. (1962) Experimental intrabronchial administration of antibiotics in man and animals, *Acta tuberc. pneumol. belg.*, **42**, 149–57.

MAHER, J. E., and SCHREINER, G. E. (1965) Studies on ethacrynic acid in patients with refractory edema, *Ann. intern. Med.*, **62**, 15–29.

MATHOG, R. H., and KLEIN, W. J., JR. (1969) Ototoxicity of ethacrynic acid and aminoglycoside antibiotics in uremia, *New Engl. J. Med.*, **280**, 1223–4.

MATZ, G. J., and NAUNTON, R. F. (1968) Ototoxic drugs and poor renal function, *J. Amer. med. Ass.*, **206**, 2119.

MATZ, G. J., WALLACE, T. H., and WARD, P. H. (1965) Ototoxicity of kanamycin: Comparative histological study, *Laryngoscope (St. Louis)*, **75**, 1680–98.

McCABE, P. A., and DEY, F. L. (1965) The effect of Aspirin upon auditory sensitivity, *Ann. Otol. (St. Louis)*, **74**, 312–25.

MEYLER, L., ed. (1963) *Side Effects of Drugs*, 4th ed., Excerpta Medica Foundation, Amsterdam, pp. 189–91.

MEYLER, L., ed. (1966) *Side Effects of Drugs*, Vol. V, Excerpta Medica Foundation, Amsterdam, pp. 319–20.

MYERS, E. N., and BERNSTEIN, J. M. (1965) Salicylate ototoxicity. A clinical and experimental study, *Arch. Otolaryng.*, **82**, 483–93.

NORTHINGTON, P. (1950) Syndrome of bilateral vestibular paralysis and its occurrence from streptomycin therapy, *Arch. Otolaryng.*, **52**, 380–96.

PILLAY, V. K. G., SCHWARTZ, F. D., AIMI, K., and KARK, R. M. (1969) Transient and permanent deafness following treatment with ethacrynic acid in renal failure, *Lancet*, i, 77–9.

RASMUSSEN, F. (1969) The oto-toxic effect of streptomycin and dihydrostreptomycin on the foetus, *Scand. J. resp. Dis.*, **50**, 61–7.

RISKAER, N., CHRISTENSEN, E., and HERTZ, H. (1952) The toxic effects of streptomycin and dihydrostreptomycin in pregnancy illustrated experimentally, *Acta tuberc. scand.*, **27**, 211–16.

SAKULA, A. (1954) Streptomycin and the foetus, *Brit. J. Tuberc.*, **48**, 69–72.

SCHMIDT, P., and FRIEDMAN, I. S. (1967) Adverse effects of ethacrynic acid, *N.Y. St. J. Med.*, **67**, 1438–42.

SCHNEIDER, W. J., and BECKER, E. L. (1966) Acute transient hearing loss after ethacrynic acid therapy, *Arch. intern. Med.*, **177**, 715–17.

SCHWARTZ, G. H., DAVID, D. S., RIGGIO, R. R., STENZEL, K. H., and RUBIN, A. L. (1970) Ototoxicity induced by furosemide, *New Engl. J. Med.*, **282**, 1413–14.

STEVENSON, L. D., ALVORD, E. C., JR., and CORRELL, J. W. (1947) Degeneration and necrosis in eighth cranial nuclei caused by streptomycin, *Proc. Soc. exp. Biol. N.Y.*, **65**, 86–8.

TRIMBLE, G. X. (1969) Neomycin ototoxicity: Dossier and doses, *New Engl. J. Med.*, **281**, 219.

WAISBREN, B. A., and SPINK, W. W. (1950) Clinical appraisal of neomycin, *Ann. intern. Med.*, **33**, 1099–1119.

WALTNER, J. (1955) The effect of salicylates on the inner ear, *Ann. Otol. (St. Louis)*, **64**, 617–22.

WINSTON, J., LEWEY, F. H., PARENTEAU, A., MARDEN, P. A., and CRAMER, F. B. (1948) An experimental study of the toxic effects of streptomycin on the vestibular apparatus of the cat, Part 1. The central nervous system, *Ann. Otol. (St. Louis)*, **57**, 738–53.

18

DRUG-INDUCED OR AGGRAVATED INFECTIVE CONDITIONS

A separate chapter on these comparatively rare complications of therapy has been deemed necessary in view of the potential hazard and severity of many of these conditions. The major drugs involved are the oral contraceptives, corticosteroids, the tetracyclines, and immunosuppressive and antineoplastic agents.

ORAL CONTRACEPTIVES

INTRACTABLE VAGINAL CANDIDIASIS

Several reports of severe candidiasis in women taking oral contraceptives have appeared. In many of these women, local antifungal therapy has been ineffective until oral contraceptives have been stopped (Yaffee and Grots, 1965). Pregnant women are at a higher risk of contracting vaginal candidiasis than non-pregnant women; diabetics also have a higher risk of vaginal candidiasis than normal women. Since oral contraceptives induce a pseudo-pregnancy state and have a diabetogenic action it is not surprising that they increase the risk of vaginal candidiasis. With all these conditions, pregnancy, diabetes, and oral contraceptive therapy, there is an increase in epithelial cell glycogen, a rise of pH and a fall in the Döderlein's bacillus population.

PYELONEPHRITIS

During contraceptive regimes as in ordinary pregnancy there is a tendency for non-striated muscle of various organs to relax. In the case of the ureters this has led to an increased incidence of pyelonephritis (Marshall et al., 1966).

CORTICOSTEROIDS

Like many other drugs now at our disposal, the corticosteroids constitute a two-edged weapon; they exert both beneficial and detrimental effects on infectious disease. With regard to beneficial effects, it is common knowledge that the Addisonian patient is highly sensitive to infection and intoxication and that replacement therapy with corticoids in proper amounts restores the resistance of these patients to a normal level. Moreover as first observed by Kass et al. (1950) cortisone exerts a favourable influence on the toxaemia associated with severe infectious diseases.

In the early days of corticosteroid research, it was repeatedly demonstrated that corticotrophin and corticoids, when injected in large doses, would interfere with the host defence mechanism against bacterial infections (Foley et al., 1957a). It was suggested that the steroids interfered both with antibody formation and with the development of tissue immunity (Foley et al., 1957a, 1957b). In addition, other investigators showed that cortisone would lower the resistance of laboratory animals to a wide range of bacterial, viral, protozoal and fungal infections (Kass and Finland, 1953).

Early reviewers (Robinson, 1956; James, 1957; Romansky, 1959; Shubin et al., 1959) were cautious about the exact status of steroids in the collateral management of infections, as indeed they had every right to be. Corticosteroids produced beneficial effects in the hands of some, less beneficial with others. All, however, had common ground in their recognition of the realities of harmful effects. It is to the latter that this section refers.

BACTERIAL INFECTIONS

Tuberculosis is the major bacterial infection of concern associated with corticosteroid treatment and it is with this infection that this section will deal. An excellent review entitled 'Corticosteroids in the treatment of infectious diseases' by Romansky (1960), summarizes evidence for and against the use of steroids in infective conditions and it is to this review that readers are referred for information about other bacterial infections.

D'Arcy Hart and Rees (1950) were the first to show that the severity of a tuberculous infection in mice could be increased by concurrent administration of massive doses of cortisone. Other investigators found similar results in other animal species. It is now universally recognized that in man manifestations of tuberculous infection, or aggravation of existing tuberculosis as well as reactivation of completely quiet tuberculosis, can occur during treatment with corticosteroids (Espersen, 1963). The course is often severe owing to a decreased reaction around the lesion and can continue undiagnosed due to the masking effect of the corticosteroid (Veuthey, 1962).

Mayfield (1962) has discussed tuberculosis occurring in association with corticosteroid treatment and has assembled some revealing statistics on the extent of the danger. In 1959, of a total of 7,785 patients treated with corticosteroids for asthma, rheumatoid arthritis, eczema and leukaemia, 13 developed tuberculosis during or within six months of the end of therapy. In 1960, there were 21 such patients out of a total of 6,584. In an earlier study Shubin et al. (1959) reported that during

1958 they had seen 58 patients in whom active tuberculosis developed during or after steroid therapy without antituberculosis drugs.

Although most cases of steroid-induced or steroid-aggravated tuberculosis can be related to continuous long-term use of corticosteroids at virtually pharmacological dosage levels, this is not always so. Tobias (1964) has reported the development of active tuberculosis after intra-articular use of cortisone in one patient and after the use of steroid-containing suppositories in another.

It is worth bearing in mind that the anterior pituitary gland secretes about 1 unit of ACTH daily, while the average daily output of cortisol from the adrenal cortex varies between 12 and 20 mg (Kern, 1957). Most steroid therapy is therefore used in doses far in excess of normal intrinsic secretion (i.e. pharmacological rather than physiological dose levels). The potential dangers are obviously apparent and cannot be, nor should they be, minimized. Investigation of the presence of tuberculosis by skin tests and by radiographs of the chest should always be done before starting long-term corticosteroid therapy and at suitable intervals thereafter. When steroids have to be used in patients at risk from tuberculosis, antitubercular chemotherapy will tend to safeguard against tuberculosis reactivation.

VIRAL INFECTIONS

Increased susceptibility to all kinds of viral infection has been noted and viral infections may run a very severe course in patients on corticosteroid treatment. Even in the early days of cortisone-availability it was known from animal studies that corticosteroids and ACTH permitted a more rapid multiplication of such viruses as poliomyelitis, Rift Valley fever, Coxsackie and encephalomyocarditis in host tissues (Findlay and Howard, 1952).

Infections with herpes virus seem especially dangerous; dissemination of herpes zoster has been reported (Irons, 1964; Merselis et al., 1964), and ocular herpes simplex may be exacerbated by corticosteroids (Crompton, 1965).

Haemorrhagic varicella with pneumopathy has been described in an adult patient on prednisone treatment for acute leukaemia (Domart et al., 1964) and a number of cases of interstitial pneumonitis has been described in children on corticosteroid treatment (Goetz and Ohrt, 1964).

Children would especially seem to be at risk from exacerbation of viral infection whilst on corticosteroids. Meyler (1963) has reviewed some of the literature and commented that chickenpox is not uncommonly a fatal disease in children on steroid treatment. There is also a greater susceptibility to poliomyelitis virus and simple respiratory infections may progress to fatal illness in these children, especially if resistant staphylococci are present. Thirteen cases of interstitial plasma-cell pneumonia in children were cited; most of the

cases were receiving corticosteroids. This complication did not occur until corticosteroids or ACTH had been administered for at least 50 days. Damage to the lymphatic system was suggested. Nine of the 13 children died from this complication.

Gerbeaux et al. (1963) have produced some revealing statistical data which emphasize the true nature of this problem; 194 cases of infectious disease were reported in 154 children on long-term corticosteroid treatment for various complications of tuberculosis. Viral, fungal, and bacterial diseases are included in the list which is summarized as follows:

Chickenpox	102 cases
Pyogenic infections	17 cases
Poliomyelitis	3 cases
Measles	16 cases
Ocular herpes	2 cases
Whooping cough	11 cases
Mumps	28 cases
Lymphocytic meningitis	1 case
Moniliasis	3 cases
German measles	6 cases
Herpes zoster	4 cases
Undetermined (fatal)	1 case

PROTOZOAL INFECTIONS

There are relatively few reports of parasitic protozoal infection in man being enhanced by corticosteroids, although early work in experimental animals showed that this was likely to occur (Kass and Finland, 1953). Meyler (1963) has reviewed the literature on amoebiasis and corticosteroids and comments that colitis with ulceration due to amoebiasis under the influence of steroid therapy has been reported although aggravation of a latent amoebiasis is rather a rare complication. A case described was observed in a young soldier treated with corticosteroids for severe arthritic complaints associated with Reiter's disease.

Mody (1959) reported two cases of corticosteroid treatment unmasking latent infection of the bowel with Entamoeba histolytica. The first case was diagnosed as non-specific ulcerative colitis and treatment by retention enemas of hydrocortisone hemisuccinate was given. Subsequent examination of stools and scrapings from the ulcers revealed swarms of E. histolytica trophozoites and cysts to an abnormal degree. In the second case, initial diagnosis was non-specific proctocolitis; amoebiasis had been excluded by careful examination. Prenisolone suppositories (5 mg) were used twice daily for over a month. On examination a most profuse infection with E. histolytica trophozoites was found in the stools. The ulcers on scraping yielded copious evidence of amoebic infection. The author suggested that corticosteroids might alter the environmental or nutritive condition of E. histolytica in a like manner to that known to occur with cholesterol which acts as a growth factor for the organism (Sharma, 1959).

FUNGAL INFECTIONS

Fungal infections may run a more severe course in corticosteroid-treated patients and such patients frequently have a greater susceptibility to them. Nabarro (1960) reviewed the uses of ACTH and adrenal steroids in general medicine and mentioned under the dangers of steroid therapy that death due to pulmonary aspergillosis occurred in a patient on prolonged steroid therapy for pemphigus. Boyd and Chappell (1961) reported a case of a 17-year-old girl who had recurrent acute rheumatic fever. A fatal mycetosis occurred due to *Candida albicans* which was associated with long-continued corticosteroid therapy and intensive antibiotic therapy. The therapy given was designed to counteract complications, including agranulocytosis, anaemia, and a severe staphylococcal infection, but it proved ineffective.

Jacobs (1963) has reported a case of a 64-year-old woman with postnecrotic liver cirrhosis treated with prednisone 20 mg daily. The woman died three years later of sepsis caused by *Cryptococcus neoformans*. Bennington *et al.* (1964) reported a case of fatal cryptococcal meningitis in an 84-year-old man who had received steroid treatment for over one year for his asthma. Other cases of fungal infection after steroid therapy have been reviewed by Meyler (1966) and include cryptococcal osteitis in one scapula followed by fatal cryptococcal meningitis in a 33-year-old man given prednisone for Boeck's sarcoid, and a primary cutaneous cryptococcosis which developed after long-term corticosteroid treatment for arthropathy associated with psoriasis in a 41-year-old man.

Apart from systemic fungal infections, the topical infections due to yeasts are also a hazard during long-term corticosteroid treatment. Hayes (1965) has reported two cases of oesophageal moniliasis whilst Lehner (1964) found oral thrush in a group of 44 patients who had been given corticosteroids in association with antibiotics or cytotoxic agents. Dennis and Itkin (1964) reported monilial infection after the use of an aerosol containing dexamethasone in asthmatic patients. Five of the 25 patients developed infection of the oropharynx and two infection of the larynx with *Candida albicans*.

The topical application of corticosteroids may also promote fungal infection especially if occlusive dressings are used (Gill *et al.*, 1963). Grant Peterkin and Khan (1969) in discussing iatrogenic skin disease, remarked that not only did topical corticosteroids increase the incidence of fungal infections but also they rendered them atypical. Ive and Marks (1968) reported 14 cases in which unusual clinical pictures resulted from the use of such treatment. The usual eczematous reaction produced by the fungus was suppressed and fungal growth continued uninhibited. There was, in addition, an apparent enhancement of virulence by suppression of the local immune response. Clinical appearance was so modified that the disease was almost unrecognizable. Several patients presented with patches of atrophy and telangiectasia. Two who were infected with *Epidermophyton floccosum* had lesions in the flexures resembling moniliasis, one patient had a facial eruption resembling rosacea and another had an area of marginated hypopigmentation on the face. The suppression of the immune response led to unusually widespread lesions, and in one instance infection with *Trichophyton rubrum* produced a kerion. This fungus has only rarely been implicated in kerion formation.

TETRACYCLINE-INDUCED GASTRO-INTESTINAL INFECTION

Although of low toxicity, when given orally, the tetracyclines cause gastro-intestinal upsets, flatulence, nausea, vomiting and diarrhoea, the most troublesome general adverse effect.

Tetracyclines are only partially absorbed from the alimentary tract and enough remains in the intestine to produce a local irritant action and to suppress the normal flora and replace it by resistant pathogenic species.

Superinfection in the bowel following alteration of the flora may be with *Candida albicans*, which can give rise to soreness and redness of the mouth (thrush), diarrhoea due to monilial enteritis and troublesome pruritus of the anus and genitalia. A case of melanotrichia linguae has also been reported.

Staphylococcal enteritis has been reported after treatment with tetracyclines, as with the use of other antibiotics. Tetracycline, however, has been mentioned as the commonest cause of staphylococcal enterocolitis. Sudden loss of appetite, abdominal pain or discomfort and distention are usually the first signs of this serious condition which has been reported by Spaulding (1962) to carry a mortality rate of 40–60 per cent.

Superinfection may occur even when the antibiotics are given intravenously since tetracycline is excreted in appreciable amounts in the bile. When superinfection occurs tetracycline or any other incriminated antibiotic should be stopped. The stool should be cultured and rectal swabs taken to identify the organisms involved. In the case of *Candida albicans*, nystatin may be given although it is doubtful whether its routine incorporation into oral tetracycline tablets (e.g. *Lederstatin*, demethylchlortetracycline plus nystatin; *Mysteclin*, tetracycline plus nystatin and amphotericin B) is useful, especially as it can cause diarrhoea. Spontaneous recovery is usual after withdrawal of the drug; alternatively, lactobacillus (cream cheese) can be given in large amounts to displace the offending superinfecting organism (Laurence, 1966). There is some evidence that administration of vitamin B preparations may prevent or arrest alimentary tract symptoms. It is probably justifiable to give these vitamins routinely if prolonged tetracycline therapy is envisaged; some preparations contain combinations of tetracycline and vitamins (e.g. *Terramycin S.F.*, *Tetracyn S.F.*).

IMMUNOSUPPRESSIVE AND ANTINEOPLASTIC AGENTS

AZOTHIOPRINE AND CORTICO-STEROIDS

Opportunistic infection is a common complication of renal transplantation and an important factor in most deaths. This complication is largely due to the use of immunosuppressive drugs which reduce the rejection process. The combination of drugs most frequently used is azothioprine and prednisone or prednisolone.

Infections frequently reported as the cause of death following renal transplantation have usually been bacterial and fungal. Infections with viruses of the herpes group (herpes zoster, herpes simplex, varicella and cytomegalic virus) have been described, but recently Montgomerie et al. (1969) have described four cases in which normally benign infections of herpes simplex have proved fatal. In one patient, the herpes infection involved the face, mouth, oesophagus, ileum and anogenital areas.

All four of Montgomerie's patients also showed evidence of infection with cytomegalic virus. There were two cases with candidiasis, two patients with cysts in the lungs typical of *Pneumocystis carinii* infection and one patient had a post-operative staphylococcal septicaemia. Two of the patients described above also developed reticulum cell sarcoma, a recognized complication of azothioprine therapy.

The prolonged use of potent synthetic glucocorticoids, alone or in combination with immunosuppressive agents, has re-emphasized the fact that infectious illness ranks as a major cause of death in patients receiving high-dose steroid therapy for extended periods.

In a large series of patients receiving renal homotransplants, late (non-surgical) deaths were due to intractable infection in 39 of 44 patients (Hill *et al.*,

1967). Since the use of antimetabolites was markedly restricted in these patients, steroid therapy could be incriminated directly. The infecting organisms were generally ubiquitous non-pathogens or pathogenic organisms that under normal circumstances rarely penetrate the host's defensive mechanisms. Previously non-pathogenic organisms became pathogenic and normally localized infections became systemic.

These points are particularly pertinent when immunosuppressive agents are used in conditions other than transplants. There are widening indications for the use of these agents in common conditions such as rheumatoid arthritis, indeed much of the current research into new non-steroidal anti-inflammatory agents is closely linked with the search for new immunosuppressive compounds. Many new compounds have both properties to a greater or lesser degree and if these are eventually to be used in rheumatoid conditions then certainly their potential induction or aggravation of infective conditions must be a constant source of reflection.

CYCLOPHOSPHAMIDE

Meadow and colleagues (1969) described the case of a 4-year-old boy who had a relapsing nephrotic syndrome treated with cyclophosphamide. He developed measles and died of giant cell pneumonia. Before treatment he had been immunologically competent, but in his terminal illness measles antibody failed to develop. The findings suggested that the defective immunological response may have been due to cyclophosphamide therapy.

Cyclophosphamide is a useful drug in the treatment of childhood nephrotic syndrome and its use is increasing, therefore it might be wise to consider the possibility of measles immunization before cyclophosphamide treatment is commenced in the hope that immunization may give these children some protection.

RECOMMENDED FURTHER READING

BEISEL, W. R., and RAPOPORT, M. I. (1969) Inter-relations between adrenocortical functions and infectious illness, *New Engl. J. Med.*, **280**, 541–6.

REFERENCES

BENNINGTON, J. L., HABER, S. L., and MORGENSTERN, N. L. (1964) Increased susceptibility to cryptococcosis following steroid therapy, *Dis. Chest*, **45**, 262–3.

BOYD, J. F., and CHAPPELL, A. G. (1961) Fatal mycetosis due to *Candida albicans* after combined steroid and antibiotic therapy, *Lancet*, **ii**, 19–22.

CROMPTON, D. O. (1965) Corticosteroids exacerbate ocular herpes simplex, *Med. J. Aust.*, **1**, 487.

D'ARCY HART, P., and REES, R. J. W. (1950) Enhancing effect of cortisone on tuberculosis in mouse, *Lancet*, **ii**, 391–5.

DENNIS, M., and ITKIN, I. H. (1964) Effectiveness and complications of aerosol dexamethasone phosphate in severe asthma, *J. Allergy*, **35**, 70–6.

DOMART, A., HAZARD, J., LABRAM, C., HUSSON, R., and

PORTOS, J. L. (1964) Varicelle hémorrhagique avec pneumopathie chez un adult traité par la delta-cortisone pour leucose aiguë, *Presse méd.*, **72**, 235–8.

ESPERSEN, E. (1963) Corticosteroids and pulmonary tuberculosis. Activation of four cases, *Acta tuberc. pneumol. belg.*, **43**, 1–8.

FINDLAY, G. M., and HOWARD, E. M. (1952) The effects of cortisone and adrenocorticotrophic hormone on poliomyelitis and on other virus infections, *J. Pharm. Pharmacol.*, **4**, 37–42.

FOLEY, E. J., MORGAN, W. A., and GRECO, G. (1957a) Effect of prednisone and prednisolone on streptococcus infections in mice treated with chlortetracycline, *Antibiot. and Chemother.*, **7**, 65–9.

FOLEY, E. J., MORGAN, W. A., and GRECO, G. (1957b) Effect of prednisone and prednisolone on antibody formation in mice, *Antibiot. and Chemother.*, **7**, 70–4.

GERBEAUX, J., COUVREUR, J., BACULARD-BEAUCHEF, A., and JOLY, J. B. (1963) Maladies infectieuses sous corticothérapie au long cours (194 observations dont 102 varicelles), *Sem. Hôp. Paris*, **39**, 61–75.

GILL, K. A., JR., KATZ, H. I., and BAXTER, D. L. (1963) Fungus infections occurring under occlusive dressings, *Arch. Derm.*, **88**, 348–9.

GOETZ, O., and OHRT, B. (1964) Cortison-Langzeitbehandlung und interstitelle Pneumonie, *Mschr. Kinderheilk.*, **112**, 163–4.

GRANT PETERKIN, G. A., and KHAN, S. A. (1969) Iatrogenic skin disease, *Practitioner*, **202**, 117–26.

HAYES, M. (1965) Esophageal moniliasis, *Amer. J. Gastroent.*, **43**, 143–9.

HILL, R. B., JR., DAHRLING, B. E., STARZI, T. E., and RIFKIND, D. (1967) Death after transplantation: Analysis of sixty cases, *Amer. J. Med.*, **42**, 327–34.

IRONS, G. V. (1964) Steroids and herpes zoster, *J. Amer. med. Ass.*, **189**, 649.

IVE, F. A., and MARKS, R. (1968) Tinea incognito, *Brit. med. J.*, **3**, 149–52.

JACOBS, H. W. (1963) Unusual fatal infectious complications of steroid-treated liver disease, *Gastroenterology*, **44**, 519–26.

JAMES, D. G. (1957) The use of corticosteroids in the management of infections, *Practitioner*, **179**, 176–80.

KASS, E. H., and FINLAND, M. (1953) Adrenocortical hormones in infection and immunity, *Ann. Rev. Microbiol.*, **7**, 361–88.

KASS, E. H., INGBAR, S. H., and FINLAND, M. (1950) Effects of adreno-corticotrophic hormone in pneumonia: Clinical, *Ann. intern. Med.*, **33**, 1081–98.

KERN, R. (1957) cited by Shubin, H., Lambert, R. E., Heiken, C. A., Sokmensuer, A., and Glaskin, A. (1959) *J. Amer. med. Ass.*, **170**, 1885–90.

LAURENCE, D. R. (1963) *Clinical Pharmacology*, 2nd ed., London, pp. 53–5.

LEHNER, T. (1964) Oral thrush, or acute pseudomembranous candidiasis. A clinicopathologic study of forty-four cases, *Oral. Surg.*, **18**, 27–37.

MARSHALL, S., LYON, R. P., and MINKLER, D. (1966) Ureteral dilatation following use of oral contraceptives, *J. Amer. med. Ass.*, **198**, 782–3.

MAYFIELD, R. B. (1962) Tuberculosis occurring in association with corticosteroid treatment, *Tubercle (Edinb.)*, **43**, 55–60.

MEADOW, S. R., WELLER, R. O., and ARCHIBALD, R. W. (1969) Fatal systemic measles in a child receiving cyclophosphamide for nephrotic syndrome, *Lancet*, **ii**, 876–8.

MERSELIS, J. G., KAYE, D., and HOOK, E. W. (1964) Disseminated herpes zoster. A report of 17 cases, *Arch. intern. Med.*, **113**, 679–86.

MEYLER, L., ed. (1963) *Side Effects of Drugs*, 4th ed., Excerpta Medica Foundation, Amsterdam, p. 236.

MEYLER, L., ed. (1966) *Side Effects of Drugs*, Vol. V, Excerpta Medica Foundation, Amsterdam, pp. 415–16.

MODY, V. R. (1959) Corticosteroids in latent amoebiasis, *Brit. med. J.*, **2**, 1399.

MONTGOMERIE, J. Z., BECROFT, D. M. O., CROXSON, M. C., DOAK, P. B., and NORTH, J. D. K. (1969) Herpes simplex infection after renal transplantation, *Lancet*, **ii**, 867–71.

NABARRO, J. D. N. (1960) The pituitary and adrenal cortex in general medicine, *Brit. med. J.*, **2**, 553–88, 625–33.

ROBINSON, H. J. (1956) Adrenal cortical hormones and infection, *Pediatrics*, **17**, 770–80.

ROMANSKY, M. J. (1959) Steroid therapy in systemic infections, *J. Amer. med. Ass.*, **179**, 1179–83.

ROMANSKY, M. J. (1960) Corticosteroids in the treatment of infectious diseases, *Antibiot. et Chemother. (Basel)*, **8**, 313–24.

SHARMA, R. (1959) Effect of cholesterol on the growth and virulence of *Entamoeba histolytica*, *Trans. roy. Soc. trop. Med. Hyg.*, **53**, 278–81.

SHUBIN, H., LAMBERT, R. E., HEIKEN, C. A., SOKMENSUER, A., and GLASKIN, A. (1959) Steroid therapy and tuberculosis, *J. Amer. med. Ass.*, **170**, 1885–90.

SPAULDING, W. B. (1962) Dangers in the use of some potent drugs, *Canad. med. Ass. J.*, **87**, 1275–81.

TOBIAS, J. M. (1964) The dangers of administering steroids to patients suffering from incipient, latent or inactive tuberculosis, *S. Afr. med. J.*, **38**, 91–2.

VEUTHEY, J. (1962) Tuberculose aiguë au cours de traitements par la cortisone. A propos de cinq observations, *Praxis*, **51**, 403–6.

YAFFEE, H. S., and GROTS, I. (1965) Moniliasis due to Norethynodrel with Mestranol, *New Engl. J. Med.*, **272**, 647.

19

DRUG-INDUCED NEOPLASIA

Reports of drug-induced neoplasia are rare. This is probably due to difficulty in establishing a cause and effect relationship between a drug and its possible carcinogenic action, rather than to an actual rarity of occurrence, since clinical manifestations of neoplasia usually occur many years after completion of the implicated course of therapy. Examples of these long latencies are the 20 or more years before the appearance of haemangioendothelioma of the liver after *Thorotrast* (232-thorium dioxide) and periods of up to 30 years before the manifestations of arsenic-induced neoplasia of skin, bronchus, or genito-urinary tract.

A number of broadly based generalizations can be made about drug-induced neoplasia. Firstly, such neoplasms tend to develop at sites where there is maximum concentration of the drug. Thus carcinogenic drugs which are excreted via the kidneys reach their maximum concentration in the genito-urinary tract, and it is at this site that neoplasms are likely to develop. For example, *Thorotrast* has been reported as causing renal carcinoma and chlornaphazine (chlornaphazin) has been implicated in bladder cancer. Also Bengtsson *et al.* (1968) have described transitional cell tumours of the renal pelvis and bladder in patients taking excessive doses of phenacetin-containing analgesics.

Similarly, carcinogenic drugs which are metabolized and excreted by the liver tend to affect predominantly the development of neoplasia in the liver, for example *Thorotrast*-induced haemangioendothelioma (Da Silva Horta *et al.*, 1965).

Drugs may also be deposited in specific organs and may attain high local concentration. Thus, arsenic deposited in the skin may ultimately lead to the development of basal cell carcinoma (Fierz, 1965).

If the drug is a carcinogen then there is a strong possibility that there will be a dose-effect relationship between the amount of drug administered and the incidence of neoplasia. This has been shown, for example, in respect of chlornaphazine-induced bladder tumour (Laursen, 1970).

The second mechanism by which drugs may induce neoplasia is by their interference with the patient's immune mechanisms. For example, azothioprine (azathioprine, *Imuran*) and prednisone in combined therapy are commonly used in renal transplantation to prevent graft rejection. Such treatment has been implicated in reticulum cell sarcoma (Doak *et al.*, 1968).

Such generalizations as have been mentioned are as yet based only on sparse evidence. They do, however, serve to pin-point those drugs which currently can be regarded as having potential carcinogenic hazard. It is

obvious that with such agents their metabolism and distribution within the tissues are directly related to the site of their possible carcinogenic action.

THOROTRAST-INDUCED NEOPLASIA

Thorotrast-induced haemangioendothelioma of the liver has already been discussed in CHAPTER 9, but it is important to note that *Thorotrast* has also been reported to cause renal carcinoma (Krückemeyer *et al.*, 1960).

PHENACETIN-INDUCED GENITO-URINARY TUMOURS

Phenacetin-induced tumours of the renal pelvis and bladder have been described by Bengtsson *et al.* (1968) in patients taking excessive amounts of phenacetin-containing analgesics. This has been fully discussed in CHAPTER 14.

ARSENICAL CARCINOGENESIS

The first suggestion that the therapeutic administration of arsenic could lead to cancer was made by Hutchinson in 1887 who described five cases of skin cancer following the medicinal use of arsenic. It is now generally accepted that arsenic given by mouth can cause cancer of the skin, which is usually preceded by arsenical pigmentation, keratosis and dermatosis. Fierz (1965) found that, in a series of 262 patients treated with Fowler's solution for from 6 to 26 years, carcinoma of the skin developed in 21 patients (8 per cent). The type of cancer most frequently encountered was a basal cell carcinoma, and in 16 of these patients there were multiple basal cell carcinomata.

Sommers and McManus (1953) described a series of 27 cases of arsenical skin cancer and drew attention to the fact that 10 of these patients also had other primary sites of neoplastic change. Two cases had bronchial carcinoma and three had primary carcinomata arising in the genito-urinary tract. This association of arsenic with visceral carcinogenesis was further elaborated by Robson and Jelliffe (1963) who described six cases (four female and two male) who all developed bronchial carcinoma with an average latent period of 32 years after receiving arsenic therapy. Arsenic had been prescribed to these patients for psoriasis, rheumatic fever, 'convulsions', or as a 'tonic'. Each of these patients had the dermatological stigmata of arsenic ingestion.

The major importance of discussing arsenic-induced cancers at this current time is that owing to the long latent period of onset of clinical neoplasia such patients may still present themselves for treatment. It should also be borne in mind that although there are no indications today for using arsenic, the organo-arsenicals have been used in chemotherapy, and tryparsamide, which contains about 25 per cent of penta-valent arsenic in organic combination, is still used in the treatment of African trypanosomiasis.

ISONIAZID: IS IT A CARCINOGEN?

The observation that isoniazid caused pulmonary tumours in experimental animals (Biancifiori and Severi, 1966) has suggested the need to re-examine the lung cancer mortality of tuberculous patients and to determine whether this was increased by ioniazid therapy. Two earlier investigations, one from Australia (Campbell, 1961) and the other from Israel (Steinitz, 1965) had already demonstrated that patients with tuberculosis had an excess mortality from lung cancer.

Campbell and Guilfoyle (1970) examined a group of 3,064 tuberculous ex-Servicemen and compared them with a control population of 14,241 ex-Servicemen who had been prisoners of war. All these men had served with the Australian Armed Services during the Second World War. It was found that the tuberculous patients experienced a significant excess mortality from all cancers (92 observed cases compared with 68 expected cases) during a 6-year period of observation. This was largely contributed to by increased mortality from lung cancer (33 observed, 16 expected) and carcinoma of the upper respiratory and digestive tracts (12 observed, 5 expected). Nevertheless the use of isoniazid was not shown conclusively in this small series to affect the higher incidence of lung cancer in patients who had been treated for tuberculosis.

CHLORNAPHAZINE-INDUCED BLADDER CARCINOMA

Three reports of individual cases of chlornaphazine-induced bladder cancer have been cited by Meyler (1966). The first case was a woman of 68 being treated for polycythaemia vera; she had received a total of 156·6 grams of chlornaphazine over a period of 10 years. The second patient, a woman of 45, had received 149·5 grams of the drug over a period of 5 years for the treatment of Hodgkin's disease. The third patient, a man aged 30, had been treated for Hodgkin's disease with chlornaphazine for 6 years.

It would seem from these cases that a high dose of chlornaphazine is associated with neoplastic changes in the bladder epithelium. This is in keeping with the findings of Thiede et al. (1964) who treated 60 patients suffering from polycythaemia rubra vera with chlornaphazine. Only 20 of these patients received over 100 grams of chlornaphazine, and, of these, seven patients developed bladder carcinoma. However, in a recent paper Laursen (1970) reported two patients treated for Hodgkin's disease with chlornaphazine who developed cancer of the bladder 5 and 6 years after the drug had been stopped. In these cases the total doses were only 78 and 85 grams respectively.

AZOTHIOPRINE AND PREDNISONE THERAPY

Burnet (1959) postulated that the immune system plays an important role in preventing and restricting the growth of neoplastic cells, and Swanson and Schwartz (1967) carried this concept a stage further when they suggested that neoplasia might occur as a complication of treatment with immunosuppressive agents.

Unfortunately this concept has been shown to be true and Doak and colleagues (1968) reported two such cases in which prednisone and azothioprine had been used to suppress the immunological mechanisms after renal transplantation. Both of these patients developed reticulum cell sarcoma; the first patient a 34-year-old man with chronic renal failure due to glomerulonephritis had a cadaver kidney transplanted. The other patient, a 46-year-old woman, had been similarly treated by renal transplant because she had renal failure due to pyelonephritis. Both patients developed infections with *Candida albicans*, and the woman also developed labial herpes simplex and a systemic staphylococcal infection.

NEOPLASTIC EFFECTS OF RADIATION

In human experience the best documented carcinogen is ionizing radiation which for practical purposes means X-rays as applied in the course of diagnosis and therapy. In the early days of the use of X-rays it was commonplace to find that the radiologists suffered from multiple skin carcinomata of the hands. One hundred radiologists were said to have died of malignant disease induced by radiation prior to 1922.

Fortunately in recent years much more attention has been paid to the increasing incidence of leukaemia attributable to ionizing radiation from the medical use of X-rays. Data concerning this incidence can be summarized as follows:

1. Patients heavily irradiated for the treatment of ankylosing spondylitis showed a significant incidence of myeloid leukaemia (Court-Brown and Doll, 1957).
2. Children irradiated *in utero* have a greater risk of developing leukaemia in the first decade of life (Stewart *et al.*, 1956).
3. There is a considerably higher death rate from leukaemia amongst radiologists than amongst other members of the medical profession.

In all cases there is evidence that there is a quantitative relationship between dose of irradiation and the risk of developing leukaemia. A latent period of 3–4 years after a single heavy dose of radiation is common.

Other neoplastic conditions have also been reported following X-irradiation; these have been classified by Bailey and Love (1959) as follows:

1. Skin: rodent ulcers and squamous cell carcinoma.
2. Soft tissue and bone sarcoma: sarcoma may arise in the mesenchyme.

3. Thyroid carcinoma: this may follow irradiation of the thymus gland in infancy, or repeated irradiation of tuberculous lymph nodes sufficient to produce skin damage in adolescents.

4. Myelogenous leukaemia.

In this context it is interesting that Sypkens Smit and Meyler (1970) described a case of myeloid leukaemia induced by cyclophosphamide which had been used for the treatment of bilateral papilliferous ovarian cyst adenomas in a woman of 44 years. They drew attention to the fact that the activity of alkylating agents such as thiotepa (triethylene thiophosphoramide) and cyclophosphamide in many respects resembled that of ionizing radiation.

RECOMMENDED FURTHER READING

ROBB, G. H. (1970) Arsenic, *Hosp. Med.*, **4**, 200–2.

REFERENCES

BAILEY, H., and LOVE, MCN. (1959) *A Short Practice of Surgery*, London, p. 1347.

BENGTSSON, U., ANGERVALL, L., EKMAN, H., and LEHMANN, L. (1968) Transitional cell tumours of the renal pelvis in analgesic abusers, *Scand. J. Urol. Nephrol.*, **2**, 145–50.

BIANCIFIORI, C., and SEVERI, L. (1966) The relation of isoniazid (INH) and allied compounds to carcinogenesis in some species of small laboratory animals, *Brit. J. Cancer*, **20** 528–38.

BURNET, F. M. (1959) *The Clonal Selection Theory of Acquired Immunity*, Cambridge.

CAMPBELL, A. H. (1961) The association of lung cancer and tuberculosis, *Aust. Ann. Med.*, **10**, 129–36.

CAMPBELL, A. H., and GUILFOYLE, P. (1970) Pulmonary tuberculosis, isoniazid, and cancer, *Brit. J. Dis. Chest*, **64**, 141–9.

COURT-BROWN, W. M., and DOLL, R. (1957) Leukaemia and aplastic anaemia in patients irradiated for ankylosing spondylitis, *Medical Research Council Special Report Series*, No. 295, London, H.M.S.O.

DA SILVA HORTA, J., DA MOTTA, L. C., ABBATT, J. D., and RORIZ, M. L. (1965) Malignancy and other latent effects following administration of Thorotrast, *Lancet*, **ii**, 201–5.

DOAK, P. B., MONTGOMERIE, J. Z., NORTH, J. D. K., and SMITH, F. (1968) Reticulum cell sarcoma after renal homotransplantation and azothioprine and prednisone therapy, *Brit. med. J.*, **4**, 746–8.

FIERZ, U. (1965) Katamnestiche Untersuchungen uber die Nebenwirkungen der Therapie von HautKrankheiten mit an organischem Arsen bei HautKrankheit, *Dermatologica (Basel)*, **131**, 41–58.

HUTCHINSON, J. (1887) Arsenic cancer, *Brit. med. J.*, **2**, 1280–1.

KRÜCKEMEYER, K., LESSMANN, H. D., and PUDWITZ, K. R. (1960) Nierenkarzinom als Thorotrastschaden, *Fortschr. Röntgenstr.*, **93**, 313–21.

LAURSEN, B. (1970) Cancer of the bladder in patients treated with chlornaphazine, *Brit. med. J.*, **3**, 684–5.

MEYLER, L., ed. (1966) *Side Effects of Drugs*, Vol. V, Excerpta Medica Foundation, Amsterdam, pp. 475–6.

ROBSON, A. O., and JELLIFFE, A. M. (1963) Medicinal arsenic poisoning and lung cancer, *Brit. med. J.*, **2**, 207–9.

SOMMERS, S. C., and MCMANUS, R. G. (1953) Arsenical tumours of the skin and viscera, *Cancer (Philad.)*, **6**, 347–59.

STEINITZ, R. (1965) Pulmonary tuberculosis and carcinoma of the lung, *Amer. Rev. resp. Dis.*, **92**, 758–66.

STEWART, A., WEBB, J., GILES, D., and HEWITT, D. (1956) Malignant disease in childhood and diagnostic irradiation in utero, *Lancet*, **ii**, 447.

SWANSON, H. A., and SCHWARTZ, R. S. (1967) Immunosuppressive therapy, *New Engl. J. Med.*, **277**, 163–70.

SYPKENS SMIT, G. C., and MEYLER, L. (1970) Acute myeloid leukaemia after treatment with cytostatic agents, *Lancet*, **ii**, 671–2.

THIEDE, T., CHIEVITZ, E., and CHRISTENSEN, B.CH. (1964) Chlornaphazine as a bladder carcinogen, *Acta med. scand.*, **175**, 721–5.

CROSS-INDEX OF OFFICIAL AND PROPRIETARY NAMES

Where possible the British Pharmacopoeia Commission approved name is given as the official name for each drug.

The proprietary names listed are those in most common use in Great Britain, the United States and on the Continent, the list is not intended to be comprehensive.

The index covers only those drugs mentioned in the text of the book.

PROPRIETARY NAME	OFFICIAL NAME
Acetamox	acetazolamide
Achromycin	tetracycline
ACTH	corticotrophin
Actomol	mebanazine
Adalin	carbromal
Adcortyl	triamcinolone
Adcortyl-A	triamcinolone
Adreson	cortisone
Adroyd	oxymetholone
Aerosporin	polymyxin
Aerotrol	isoprenaline
Aetina	ethionamide
Akineton	biperiden
Aktiran	thiacetazone
Albamycin	novobiocin
Aldactone-A	spironolactone
Aldocorten	aldosterone
Aldomet	methyldopa
Alepsin	phenytoin
Aleudrin	isoprenaline
Aleukon	chlornaphazine
Alficetyn	chloramphenicol
Alflorone	fludrocortisone
Alindor	phenylbutazone
Alkeran	melphalan
Alphadrol	fluprednisolone
Alserin	reserpine
Alupent	orciprenaline
Amargyl	chlorpromazine
Ambramycin	tetracycline
Amechol	methacholine
Amethopterin	methotrexate
Amidofebrin	aminopyrine
Aminoquin	pamaquin
Amphicol	chloramphenicol
Amuno	indomethacin
Anabolex	stanolone
Anacobin	cyanocobalamin
Anafebrina	aminopyrine
Anapolon	oxymetholone
Anaprotin	stanolone
Anastress	meprobamate
Andaxin	meprobamate
Androdiol	methylandrostenediol
Androstalone	mestanolone
Androteston	methyltestosterone
Anectine	suxamethonium chloride
Anodynine	phenazone
Anovlar	{norethisterone / ethinyloestradiol
Ansolysen	pentolinium
Antadol	phenylbutazone
Antilusin	pentamethonium

PROPRIETARY NAME	OFFICIAL NAME
Antistin	antazoline
Anturan	sulphinpyrazone
Apresoline	hydrallazine
Aprinox	bendrofluazide
Apsin VK	phenoxymethylpenicillin
Aquamox	quinethazone
Aralen	chloroquine
Aramine	metaraminol
Arfonad	trimetaphan
Aristocort	triamcinolone
Arlef	flufenamic acid
Artane	benzhexol
Artolon	meprobamate
Artosin	tolbutamide
Aspirin	acetylsalicylic acid
Aspro	acetylsalicylic acid
Asucrol	chlorpropamide
Atebrin	mepacrine
Atebrine	mepacrine
Atensin	mephenesin
Atromid	clofibrate
Aureomycin	chlortetracycline
Auriquin	quinidine sulphate
Avloclor	chloroquine
Avlosulfon	dapsone
Avosyl	mephenesin
Ayfivin	bacitracin
Azaron	tripelennamine
Bactrim	{trimethoprim / sulphamethoxazole
Barbital	barbitone
Bayrena	sulphamethoxydiazine
Benadryl	diphenhydramine
Benemid	probenecid
Berkfurin	nitrofurantoin
Berkomine	imipramine
Berkozide	bendrofluazide
Betnelan	betamethasone
Betnesol	betamethasone
Betnovate	betamethasone
Bidizole	sulphasomizole
Bindan	phenindione
Biogastrone	carbenoxolone
Bioral	carbenoxolone
Biotexin	novobiocin
Bistrium chloride	hexamethonium chloride
Bretylan	bretylium tosylate
Brevidil E	suxethonium
Brevidil M	suxamethonium bromide
Bristab	hydroflumethiazide
Bromural	bromvaletone
Bucrol	carbutamide

PROPRIETARY NAME	OFFICIAL NAME	PROPRIETARY NAME	OFFICIAL NAME
Butadion	phenylbutazone	*Debenal*	sulphadiazine
Butazolidin	phenylbutazone	*Debenal M*	sulphamerazine
Buzon	phenylbutazone	*Decadron*	dexamethasone
BZQ	benzquinamide	*Deca-Durabolin*	nandrolone
		Declinax	debrisoquine
Camoquin	amodiaquine	*Declomycin*	demethylchlortetracycline
Camoquinal	amodiaquine	*DeCortisyl*	prednisone
Cardioquin	quinidine	*Dehistin*	tripelennamine
	polygalacturonate	*Dehydroemetine*	dehydroemetine
Catanil	chlorpropamide	*Delta-Cortef*	prednisolone
Cathomycin	novobiocin	*Delta-Cortelan*	prednisone
Catron	pheniprazine	*Deltacortone*	prednisone
Catroniazid	pheniprazine	*Deltacortril*	prednisolone
Cavodil	pheniprazine	*Delta-Stab*	prednisolone
Cefalotin	cephalothin	*Deprinol*	imipramine
Ceflorin	cephaloridine	*Deracil*	thiouracil
Celbenin	methicillin	*Deronil*	dexamethasone
Centyl	bendrofluazide	*Deseril*	methysergide
Ceporin	cephaloridine	*Desernil*	methysergide
Chemofuran	nitrofurazone	*DexaCortisyl*	dexamethasone
Chlornaftina	chlornaphazine	*Dexamed*	dexamphetamine
Chloromycetin	chloramphenicol	*Dexedrine*	dexamphetamine
Chlor-Trimeton	chlorpheniramine	*Dextelan*	dexamethasone
Chlotride	chlorothiazide	*Dextraven*	dextran
Ciba 1906	thiambutosine	*DFP*	dyflos
Cibazol	sulphathiazole	*Diabechlor*	chlorpropamide
Cidamex	acetazolamide	*Diabetamid*	tolbutamide
Cidomycin	gentamicin	*Diabinese*	chlorpropamide
Clomid	clomiphene	*Diabuton*	tolbutamide
Clotride	chlorothiazide	*Di-Ademil*	hydroflumethiazide
Cobalin	cyanocobalamin	*Di-Adreson*	prednisone
Cobastab	cyanocobalamin	*Di-Adreson-F*	prednisolone
Cobione	cyanocobalamin	*Diagnothorine*	232-thorium dioxide
Codelcortone	prednisolone	*Dianabol*	methandienone
Cogentin	benztropine	*Diamox*	acetazolamide
Colomycin	colistin	*Diazyl*	sulphadiazine
Colomycin	colistin sulphomethate	*Dibencil*	benzathine penicillin
Collothor	232-thorium dioxide	*Dibenyline*	phenoxybenzamine
Comazine	prochlorperazine	*Dibenzyline*	phenoxybenzamine
Compazine	prochlorperazine	*Dichlotride*	hydrochlorothiazide
Conteban	thiacetazone	*Dilantin*	phenytoin
Corlan	hydrocortisone	*Dimerin*	methyprylone
Cortelan	cortisone	*Dimycin*	streptoduocin
Cortistab	cortisone	*Dindeval*	phenindione
Cortisyl	cortisone	*Dindevan*	phenindione
Cortril	hydrocortisone	*Diolandrone*	methylandrostenediol
Cortrophin	corticotrophin	*Diolandrone*	methylandrostenediol
Coslan	mefenamic acid	*Di-paralene*	chlorcyclizine
Crestabolic	methylandrostenediol	*Dipirin*	aminopyrine
Crovaril	oxyphenbutazone	*Direma*	hydrochlorothiazide
Cuprimine	*d*-penicillamine	*Distamine*	*d*-penicillamine
Cylphenicol	chloramphenicol	*Distaquaine V*	phenoxymethylpenicillin
Cytacon	cyanocobalamin	*Distivit oral*	cyanocobalamin (peptide)
Cytamen	cyanocobalamin	*Disulone*	dapsone
Cytoxan	cyclophosphamide	*Diuril*	chlorothiazide
		Doriden	glutethimide
Dagenan	sulphapyridine	*Dormwell*	dichloralphenazone
Danilone	phenindione	*Dosulfin*	sulphaproxyline
Darenthin	bretylium tosylate	*Drazine*	phenoxypropazine
Dartal	thiopropazate	*Dumogran*	methyltestosterone
Dartalan	thiopropazate	*Duo-Autohaler*	{ isoprenaline phenylephrine
Davosin	sulphamethoxypyridazine		
DDT	chlorphenthane	*Duogastrone*	carbenoxolone

PROPRIETARY NAME	OFFICIAL NAME	PROPRIETARY NAME	OFFICIAL NAME
Durabolin	nandrolone	Fulcin	griseofulvin
Durenate	sulphamethoxydiazine	Fungizone	amphotericin B
Dyna-Zina	imipramine	Furacin	nitrofurazone
Dytac	triamterene	Furadantin	nitrofurantoin
Dytransin	ibufenac	Furan	nitrofurantoin
		Furosemide	frusemide
Edecril	ethacrynic acid	Furoxane	furazolidone
Edecrin	ethacrynic acid	Furoxone	furazolidone
Edemox	acetazolamide		
Ef-Cortelan	hydrocortisone	Gammexane	gamma benzene hexachloride
Elavid	amitriptyline	Gantanol	sulphamethoxazole
Electrocortin	aldosterone	Gantrisin	sulphafurazole
Eleudron	sulphathiazole	Garamycin	gentamicin
Elkosin	sulphasomidine	Gardenal	phenobarbitone
Elrodorm	glutethimide	Genticin	gentamicin
Emedan	carbutamide	Giardil	furazolidone
Enavid E	{norethynodrel / mestranol	Grisovin	griseofulvin
		Guethine	guanethidine
Endecril	ethacrynic acid	Gynovlar 21	{norethisterone / ethinyloestradiol
Endoxana	cyclophosphamide		
Enturen	sulphinpyrazone		
Epanutin	phenytoin	Haldol	haloperidol
Epidione	troxidone	Haldrate	paramethasone
Eporal	dapsone	Halotensin	fluoxymesterone
Eptoin	phenytoin	Harmonin	meprobamate
Equanil	meprobamate	Harmonyl	deserpidine
Ercoquin	hydroxychloroquine	Hebanil	chlorpromazine
Erysan	chlornaphazine	Hedulin	phenindione
Erythrocin	erythromycin	Hexameton chloride	hexamethonium chloride
Erythroped	erythromycin	Hexathide	hexamethonium iodide
Esbatal	bethanidine	Hipoftalin	hydrallazine
Esidrex	hydrochlorothiazide	Histantin	chlorcyclizine
Eskacillin V	phenoxymethylpenicillin	Humatin	paromomycin
Eskadiazine	sulphadiazine	Humorsol	demecarium bromide
Eskaserp	reserpine	Hydralazine	hydrallazine
Esmarin	trichlormethiazide	Hydrea	hydroxyurea
Eubasin	sulphapyridine	Hydrenox	hydroflumethiazide
Eulissin	decamethonium	Hydril	hydroflumethiazide
Eurinol	trichlormethiazide	Hydro-Adreson	hydrocortisone
Eustigmin	neostigmine	Hydrocortistab	hydrocortisone
Eutonyl	pargyline	HydroCortisyl	hydrocortisone
Evramycin	triacetyloleandomycin	Hydrocortone	hydrocortisone
		Hydrodiuril	hydrochlorothiazide
Favistan	methimazole	Hydrol	hydroflumethiazide
Fentazin	perphenazine	Hydromedin	ethacrynic acid
Flaxedil	gallamine	Hydrosaluric	hydrochlorothiazide
Flexin	zoxazolamine	Hygroton	chlorthalidone
Flogoril	oxyphenbutazone	Hyperstat	diazoxide
Florinef	fludrocortisone	Hypothalin	hydrallazine
Floropryl	dyflos		
Fludrocortone	fludrocortisone	INH	isoniazid
Fluitran	trichlormethiazide	Icipen V	phenoxymethylpenicillin
Fluothane	halothane	Ilosone	erythromycin estolate
Fluracil	5-fluorouracil	Ilotycin	erythromycin
Fluril	5-fluorouracil	Imperacin	oxytetracycline
Flutra	trichlormethiazide	Imuran	azathioprine
Fortral	pentazocine	Inacid	indomethacin
Fouadin	stibophen	Inderal	propranolol
Fovane	benzthiazide	Indocid	indomethacin
Frabel	oxyphenbutazone	Indomed	indomethacin
Frademicina	lincomycin	Indon	phenindione
5-FU	5-fluorouracil	Insulton	mephenytoin
Fuadin	stibophen	Intradex	dextran

PROPRIETARY NAME	OFFICIAL NAME	PROPRIETARY NAME	OFFICIAL NAME
Inventol	carbutamide	*Mebadin*	dehydroemetine
Inversine	mecamylamine	*Medaron*	furazolidone
Isaverin	dipyrone	*Medihaler-Duo*	⎧isoprenaline ⎩phenylephrine
Ismelin	guanethidine		
Iso-Autohaler	isoprenaline	*Medihaler-Iso*	isoprenaline
Isobarin	guanethidine	*Medihaler-Iso-Forte*	isoprenaline
Isodormid	apronal	*Medinal*	barbitone
Isolevin	isoprenaline	*Medrol*	methylprednisolone
Isomist	isoprenaline	*Medrone*	methylprednisolone
Isovon	isoprenaline	*Megalovel*	cyanocobalamin
Isupren	isoprenaline	*Megaphen*	chlorpromazine
ItCH	gamma benzene hexachloride	*Mekamine*	mecamylamine
		Meladinin	methoxsalen
Kamycin	kanamycin	*Melleretten*	thioridazine
Kannasyn	kanamycin	*Melleril*	thioridazine
Kantrex	kanamycin	*Meloxine*	methoxsalen
Kaoxidin	succinylsulphathiazole	*Mepavlon*	meprobamate
Kapilon soluble	menadoxime	*Mephyton*	phytomenadione
Keflin sodium	cephalothin	*MER-29*	triparanol
Kinidin	quinidine bisulphate	*Mercaleukin*	mercaptopurine
Kiron	sulphamethoxydiazine	*Mercazole*	methimazole
Konakion	phytomenadione	*Mercloran*	chlormerodrin
Kynex	sulphamethoxypyridazine	*Mersalyl*	mersalyl
		Mesontoin	mephenytoin
Lampren	clofazimine	*Mestinon*	pyridostigmine
Lamprene	clofazimine	*Mesulfa*	sulphamerazine
Lapaquin	chloroquine	*Metahydrin*	trichlormethiazide
Largactil	chlorpromazine	*Metalcaptase*	*d*-penicillamine
Laroxyl	amitriptyline	*Metandren*	methyltestosterone
Lasilix	frusemide	*Metastab*	methylprednisolone
Lasix	frusemide	*Meterdos-Iso*	isoprenaline
Ledercort	triamcinolone	*Meterdos-Iso-Forte*	isoprenaline
Lederkyn	sulphamethoxypyridazine	*Methampyrone*	dipyrone
Ledermycin	demethylchlortetracycline	*Methotrexate*	methotrexate
Lederstatin	⎧demethylchlortetracycline ⎩nystatin	*Methoxa-Dome*	methoxsalen
		Metilar	paramethasone
Lehidrome	nalorphine	*Mevasine*	mecamylamine
Lepsiral	primidone	*Mezolin*	indomethacin
Lethidrone	nalorphine	*Miaquin*	amodiaquine
Leukeran	chlorambucil	*Microtin*	cephalothin
Leukerin	mercaptopurine	*Midicel*	sulphamethoxypyridazine
Levophed	noradrenaline	*Millicorten*	dexamethasone
Levoprome	methotrimeprazine	*Miltown*	meprobamate
Librium	chlordiazepoxide	*Minilyn*	⎧ethinyloestradiol ⎩lynoestrenol
Lincocin	lincomycin		
Lindane	gamma benzene hexachloride	*Minovlar*	⎧ethinyloestradiol ⎩norethisterone
Lispamol	iminopromazine		
Lissephen	mephenesin	*Mitosan*	busulphan
Locorten	flumethasone	*Mixtamycin*	streptoduocin
Lomodex	dextran	*Mogadon*	nitrazepam
Lorexane	gamma benzene hexachloride	*Mopazine*	methopromazine
Luminal	phenobarbitone	*Mutabase*	diazoxide
Lyndiol	⎧lynoestrenol ⎩mestranol	*Myambutol*	ethambutol
		Myanesin	mephenesin
Lyovac	ethacrynic acid	*Mybasan*	isoniazid
Lysivane	ethopropazine	*Mycifradin*	neomycin
		Myciguent	neomycin
Macrodex	dextran	*Mycivin*	lincomycin
Madribon	sulphadimethoxine	*Mycostatin*	nystatin
Malloral	thioridazine	*Myeleukon*	busulphan
Marevan	warfarin	*Myelosan*	busulphan
Marplan	isocarboxazid	*Mylepsin*	primidone
Marsilid	iproniazid	*Myleran*	busulphan
Masidol	methylandrostenediol		
M & B 693	sulphapyridine		

PROPRIETARY NAME	OFFICIAL NAME	PROPRIETARY NAME	OFFICIAL NAME
Myocrisin	sodium aurothiomalate	*Nydrazid*	isoniazid
Mysoline	primidone	*Nystan*	nystatin
Mysteclin	tetracycline nystatin amphotericin B	*Octachlor*	chlordan
		Oncovin	vincristine
		Opinsul	sulphamethoxypyridazine
Naclex	hydroflumethiazide	*Orabolin*	ethyloestrenol
Nadisan	carbutamide	*Oradexon*	dexamethasone
Nalline	nalorphine	*Oragulant*	diphenadione
Nardil	phenelzine	*Oranil*	carbutamide
Natrionex	acetazolamide	*Oranabol*	oxymesterone
Natulan	procarbazine	*Orasulin*	carbutamide
Nazinan	laevomepromazine	*Orgametril*	lynoestrenol
Nefrolan	clorexolone	*Orinase*	tolbutamide
Neftin	furazolidone	*Orisulf*	sulphaphenazole
Negram	nalidixic acid	*Orlest 28*	ethinyloestradiol norethisterone
Neoantimosan	stibophen		
Neodrenal	isoprenaline	*Ornid*	bretylium tosylate
Neo-Epinine	isoprenaline	*Orthonovin 1/50*	mestranol norethisterone
Neo-Hombreol	testosterone propionate		
		Otophen	chloramphenicol
Neolin	benzathine penicillin	*Ovulen 50*	mestranol norethisterone
Neo-Mercazole	carbimazole		
Neomin	neomycin	*Oxsoralen*	methoxsalen
Neo-Naclex	bendrofluazide		
Neopenyl	clemizole penicillin	*Pacatal*	pecazine
Neophryn	phenylephrine	*Pacinol*	fluphenazine
Neosteron	methylandrostenediol	*Palacrin*	mepacrine
Neosynephrine	phenylephrine	*Pantestin*	testosterone propionate
Neo-Thyreostat	carbimazole	*Pantestin oral*	methyltestosterone
Neptal	mercuramide theophylline	*Paradione*	paramethadione
		Paralgin	dipyrone
Neumandin	isoniazid	*Paramez*	sulphadimidine
Neuractil	methotrimeprazine	*Paraxin*	chloramphenicol
N-Fur	nitrofurantoin	*Pargonyl*	paromomycin
Niamid	nialamide	*Parke-med*	mefenamic acid
Nicetal	isoniazid	*Parnate*	tranylcypromine
Nifulidone	furazolidone	*Parodyne*	phenazone
Nilevar	norethandrolone	*Paxital*	pecazine
Nirvan	methotrimeprazine	*PBZ*	tripelennamine
Nitrofural	nitrofurazone	*Pelentan*	ethyl biscoumacetate
Nivaquine	chloroquine	*Penavlon-V*	phenoxymethylpenicillin
Nivembin	chloroquine	*Penbritin*	ampicillin
Nivemycin	neomycin	*Penicals*	phenoxymethylpenicillin
Noctan	methyprylone	*Penicillin N*	adicillin
Nogram	nalidixic acid	*Penicillin V*	phenoxymethylpenicillin
Noludar	methyprylone	*Penidural*	benzathine penicillin
Noracid	dipyrone	*Penitracin*	bacitracin
Norinyl-1	mestranol norethisterone	*Penspek*	phenbenicillin
		Penthonium	pentamethonium
Norisodrine	isoprenaline	*Pentilium*	pentolinium
Norlestrin 21	ethinyloestradiol norethisterone	*Pentrium*	chlordiazepoxide
		Perandren	methyltestosterone
Norlutin-A	norethisterone	*Permapen*	benzathine penicillin
Nortestosterone	nandrolone	*Perolysen*	pempidine
Notensil	acepromazine	*Pertofran*	desipramine
Nothiazine	pecazine	*Petidon*	troxidone
Novacid	dipyrone	*Phenantoin*	mephenytoin
Novalgin	dipyrone	*Phenergan*	promethazine
Novarsenobillon	neoarsphenamine	*Phospholine iodide*	ecothiopate iodide
Novocamid	procainamide	*Piriton*	chlorpheniramine
Nozinan	methotrimeprazine	*Planovin*	megestrol ethinyloestradiol

PROPRIETARY NAME	OFFICIAL NAME
Plaquenil	hydroxychloroquine
Plasmochin	pamaquin
Plasmoquine	pamaquin
Plegangrin	mecamylamine
Polybrene	hexadimethrine bromide
Ponstan	mefenamic acid
Ponstel	mefenamic acid
Prazine	promazine
PreCortisyl	prednisolone
Prednelan	prednisolone
Predsol	prednisolone
Prenomiser	isoprenaline
Prenomiser-Forte	isoprenaline
Primobolan	methenolone
Primobolan-Depot	methenolone
Primodos	norethisterone
Primolut N	norethisterone
Procamide	procainamide
Procardyl	procainamide
Procasil	propylthiouracil
Procytox	cyclophosphamide
Pronestyl	procainamide
Propacil	propylthiouracil
Propycil	propylthiouracil
Proserine	neostigmine
Prostigmin	neostigmine
Prothyran	propylthiouracil
Prothromadin	warfarin
Provera	medroxyprogesterone
Provost	{medroxyprogesterone / ethinyloestradiol
Ptimal	troxidone
Puri-nethol	mercaptopurine
Pycazide	isoniazid
Pyradone	aminopyrine
Pyramidon	aminopyrine
Pyriamid	sulphapyridine
Pyribenzamine	tripelennamine
Pyrimal	sulphadiazine
Pyrimal M	sulphamerazine
Pyrodin	hydracetin
Pyrostib	stibophen
Quantril	benzquinamide
Quensyl	hydroxychloroquine
Rastinon	tolbutamide
Redomex	amitriptyline
Resistomycin	kanamycin
Resochin	chloroquine
Resulfon	sulphaguanidine
Reudrox	phenylbutazone
Rheomacrodex	dextran
Rifadin	rifampicin
Rimactane	rifampicin
Rimifon	isoniazid
Ritalin	methylphenindate
Rogitine	phentolamine
Roniacol	nicotinyl alcohol
Ronicol	nicotinyl alcohol
Rontyl	hydroflumethiazide
Ruocid	sulphaguanidine

PROPRIETARY NAME	OFFICIAL NAME
Salazopyrin	sulphasalazine
Salupres	hydrochlorothiazide
Saluric	chlorothiazide
Salurin	trichlormethiazide
Sandoxan	cyclophosphamide
Sandril	reserpine
Sanodin	carbenoxolone
Sansert	methysergide
Sarcoclorin	merphalan
Saroten	amitriptyline
Scoline	suxamethonium chloride
Sedatine	phenazone
Sedor	dichloralphenazone
Sedormid	apronal
Sefacin	cephaloridine
Sendoxan	cyclophosphamide
Septrin	{trimethoprim / sulphamethoxazole
Serenace	haloperidol
Seroden	thiacetazone
Seromycin	cycloserine
Serpasil	reserpine
Sinthrome	nicoumalone
Sintrom	nicoumalone
Siqualon	fluphenazine
Siquil	fluopromazine
S-Mez	sulphadimidine
Sodium antimosan	stibophen
Solu-Cortef	hydrocortisone
Sominat	dichloralphenazone
Soneryl	butobarbitone
Sparine	promazine
Spaznil	dichloralphenazone
Stabilin V-K	phenoxymethylpenicillin
Stanozol	stanozolol
Staphcillin	methicillin
Starazine	promazine
Steclin	tetracycline
Stelazine	trifluoperazine
Stemetil	prochlorperazine
Stenediol	methylandrostenediol
Strepolin	streptomycin
Streptolin	streptomycin
Streptaquaine	streptomycin
Streptomycin	streptomycin
Streptonivicin	novobiocin
Stromba	stanozolol
Sulfabutin	busulphan
Sulfacetin	phthalylsulphathiazole
Sulfamul	sulphathiazole
Sulfasuxidine	succinylsulphathiazole
Sulfidine	sulphapyridine
Sulla	sulphamethoxydiazine
Sulmet	sulphadimidine
Sulphetrone	solapsone
Sulphix	sulphadimidine
Sulzol	sulphathiazole
Synacthen	corticotrophin
Synalar	fluocinolone
Synandrone	fluocinolone
Syncurine	decamethonium
Synkavit	menadiol sodium diphosphate

PROPRIETARY NAME	OFFICIAL NAME	PROPRIETARY NAME	OFFICIAL NAME
Talofen	promazine	Tromexan	ethyl biscoumacetate
Tandearil	oxyphenbutazone	Trophenium	phenactropinium
Tanderil	oxyphenbutazone	Tryptizol	amitriptyline
Taractan	chlorprothixene	Tubomel	isoniazid
Tega-Cetin	chloramphenicol		
Tegretal	carbamazepine	Ultandren	fluoxymesterone
Tegretol	carbamazepine	Ultracortenol	prednisone
Tementil	prochlorperazine	Ultracorten-H	prednisolone
Tenormal	pempidine	Ultralanum	fluocortolone
Tensilon	edrophonium chloride	Ultrapen	propicillin
Terramycin	oxytetracycline	Ultrax	sulphamethoxydiazine
Tetracyn	tetracycline	Unephral	{mercuramide {theophylline
Tespamin	thiotepa		
Tevabolin	stanozolol	Urolucosil	sulphamethizole
Thalazole	phthalylsulphathiazole		
Thiacyl	succinylsulphathiazole	Vazadrine	isoniazid
Thiazamide	sulphathiazole	V-Cil-K	phenoxymethylpenicillin
Thiomerosal	thiomersal	Vegolysen	hexamethonium bromide
Thiomerin	mercaptomerin	Vegolysen T	hexamethonium tartrate
Thiomersalate	thiomersal	Vegolystin	hexamethonium bromide
Thioparamizone	thiacetazone	Velban	vinblastine
Thiosporin	sulphomyxin	Velbe	vinblastine
Thiotepa	thiotepa	Ventolin	salbutamol
Thiozone	thiacetazone	Veractil	methotrimeprazine
Thorazine	chlorpromazine	Veronal	barbitone
Thoriophanin	232-thorium dioxide	Vertolan	sulphadimidine
Thorotrast	232-thorium dioxide	Vespazine	fluphenazine
Thycapsol	methimazole	Vespral	fluopromazine
Tifosyl	thiotepa	Vesprin	fluopromazine
Tintorane	warfarin	Veta-Merazine	sulphamerazine
Tofranil	imipramine	Vetibenzamina	tripelennamine
Tolseram	mephenesin	Vikastab	potassium menaphthosulphate
Tonaril	tripelennamine	Viocin	viomycin
Tordiol	232-thorium dioxide	Vionactane	viomycin
Toriofanina	232-thorium dioxide	Virormone	testosterone propionate
Totazina	colistin	Virormone-Oral	methyltestosterone
Toxichlor	chlordan	Viton	gamma benzene hexachloride
Trecator	ethionamide	Volidan 21	{ethinyloestradiol {megestrol
Trescatyl	ethionamide		
Trescazide	{ethionamide {isoniazid	Welldorm	dichloralphenazone
Trevintix	prothionamide	Winstrol	stanozolol
Triclordiuride	trichlormethiazide	Wintomylon	nalidixic acid
Tridione	troxidone		
Triflumen	trichlormethiazide	Xylocaine	lignocaine
Trilafon	perphenazine	Xyloproct	lignocaine
Trimedal	troxidone	Xylotox	lignocaine
Trimethadione	troxidone		
Trisoralen	trioxsalen	Zinamide	pyrazinamide

OFFICIAL NAME	PROPRIETARY NAME
acenocoumarol	*see* nicoumalone
acepromazine	*Notensil*
acetazolamide	*Acetamox, Cidamex, Diamox, Edemox, Natrionex*
acetopromazine	*see* acepromazine
acetylsalicylic acid	*Aspirin, Aspro*
adicillin	*Penicillin N*
aldosterone	*Aldocorten, Electrocortin*
aminopyrine	*Amidofebrin, Anafebrina, Dipirin, Pyradone, Pyramidon*
amitriptyline	*Elavid, Redomex, Saroten, Tryptizol*
amodiaquine	*Camoquin, Camoquinal, Miaquin*
amphotericin B	*Fungizone*
ampicillin	*Penbritin*
androstanazole	*see* stanozolol
antazoline	*Antistin, Histostab*
apronal	*Isodormid, Sedormid*
azathioprine	*Imuran*
bacitracin	*Ayfivin, Penitracin*
barbitone	*Barbital, Medinal, Veronal*
bendrofluazide	*Aprinox, Berkozide, Centyl, Neo-Naclex*
bendroflumethiazide	*see* bendrofluazide
benzathine penicillin	*Dibencil, Neolin, Penidural, Permapen*
benzhexol	*Artane, Pipanol*
benzquinamide	*BZQ, Quantril*
benzthiazide	*Fovane*
benztropine	*Cogentin*
betamethasone	*Betnelan, Betnesol, Betnovate*
bethanidine	*Esbatal*
biperiden	*Akineton*
bretylium tosylate	*Bretylan, Darenthin, Ornid*
bromvaletone	*Bromural*
busulphan	*Mitosan, Myeleukon, Myelosan, Myleran, Sulfabutin*
butobarbitone	*Soneryl*
carbamazepine	*Tegretal, Tegretol*
carbenoxolone	*Biogastrone, Bioral, Duogastrone, Sanodin*
carbimazole	*Neo-Mercazole, Neo-Thyreostat*
carbromal	*Adalin*
carbutamide	*Bucrol, Emedan, Inventol, Nadisan, Oranil, Orasulin*
cephaloridine	*Ceforin, Ceporin, Sefacin*
cephalothin	*Cefalotin, Keflin sodium, Microtin*
chlorambucil	*Leukeran*
chloramphenicol	*Alficetyn, Amphicol, Chloromycetin, Cylphenicol, Otophen, Paraxin, Tega-Cetin*
chlorcyclizine	*Histantin, Di-Paralene*
chlordan	*Octachlor, Toxichlor*
chlordiazepoxide	*Librium, Pentrium*
chlormerodin	*Mercloran*
chlornaphazine	*Aleukon, Chlornaftina, Erysan.*
chlorophenothane	*DDT*
chloroquine	*Aralen, Avloclor, Lapaquin, Nivaquine, Nivembin, Resochin*
chlorothiazide	*Chlotride, Clotride, Diuril, Saluric*
chlorpheniramine	*Chlor-Trimeton, Piriton*

OFFICIAL NAME	PROPRIETARY NAME
chlorpromazine	*Amargyl, Hebanil, Largactil, Megaphen, Thorazine*
chlorpropamide	*Asucrol, Catanil, Diabechlor, Diabinese*
chlorprothixene	*Taractan*
chlortetracycline	*Aureomycin*
chlorthalidone	*Hygroton*
clemizole penicillin	*Neopenyl*
clofazimine	*Lampren, Lamprene*
clofibrate	*Atromid*
clorexolone	*Nefrolan*
colistin	*Colomycin, Totazina*
colistin sulphomethate	*Colomycin*
corticotrophin	*ACTH, Cortrophin, Synacthen*
cortisone	*Adreson, Cortelan, Cortistab, Cortisyl*
cyanocobalamin	*Anacobin, Cobalin, Cobastab, Cobione, Cytacon, Cytamen, Distivit Oral, Megalovel*
cyclophosphamide	*Cytoxan, Endoxana, Procytox, Sandoxan, Sendoxan*
cycloserine	*Seromycin*
dapsone	*Avlosulfon, Disulone, Eporal*
debrisoquine	*Declinax*
decamethonium	*Eulissin, Syncurine*
dehydroemetine	*Dehydroemetine, Mebadin*
demecarium bromide	*Humorsol, Tosmilen*
demethylchlortetracycline	*Declomycin, Ledermycin*
demethylchlortetracycline nystatin	} *Lederstatin*
deserpidine	*Harmonyl*
desipramine	*Pertofran*
dexamethasone	*Decadron, Deronil, Dexa Cortisyl, Dextelan, Millicorten, Oradexon*
dexamphetamine	*Dexamed, Dexedrine*
dextran	*Dextraven, Intradex, Lomodex, Macrodex, Rheomacrodex*
diazoxide	*Hyperstat, Mutabase*
dichloralphenazone	*Sedor, Sominat, Spaznil, Welldorm*
diphenadione	*Oragulant*
diphenhydramine	*Benadryl*
dipyrone	*Isaverin, Methampyrone, Noracid, Novacid, Novalgin, Paralgin*
dyflos	*DFP, Floropryl*
ecothiopate iodide	*Phospholine iodide*
edrophonium chloride	*Tensilon*
erythromycin	*Erythrocin, Erythroped, Ilotycin*
erythromycin estolate	*Ilosone*
ethacrynic acid	*Edecril, Edecrin, Endecril, Hydromedin, Lyovac*
ethambutol	*Myambutol*
ethinyloestradiol lynoestrenol	} *Minilyn*
ethinyloestradiol medroxyprogesterone	} *Provost*
ethinyloestradiol megestrol	} *Planovin, Volidan 21*
ethinyloestradiol norethisterone	} *Anovlar, Gynovlar 21, Minovlar, Norlestrin 21, Orlest 28*

OFFICIAL NAME	PROPRIETARY NAME	OFFICIAL NAME	PROPRIETARY NAME
ethionamide	Aetina, Trecator, Trescatyl	isoniazid	INH, Mybasan, Neumandin, Nicetal, Nydrazid, Pycazide, Rimifon, Tubomel, Vazadrine
ethionamide isoniazid	Trescazide		
ethopropazine	Lysivane	isoniazid ethionamide	Trescazide
ethyl biscoumacetate	Pelentan, Tromexan		
ethyloestrenol	Orabolin	isoprenaline	Aerotrol, Aleudrin, Isolevin, Isupren, Neodrenal, Neo-Epinine, Norisodrine
fludrocortisone	Alflorone, Florinef, Fludrocortone	isoprenaline (inhalation)	Iso-Autohaler, Isomist, Isovon, Medihaler-Iso, Medihaler-Iso-Forte, Meterdos-Iso, Meterdos-Iso-Forte, Prenomiser, Prenomiser-Forte
flufenamic acid	Arlef		
flumethasone	Locorten		
fluocinolone	Synalar, Synandone		
fluocortolone	Ultralanum	isoprenaline phenylephrine (inhalation)	Duo-Autohaler, Medihaler-Duo
5-fluorouracil	Fluracil, Fluril, 5-FU		
fluopromazine	Siquil, Vespral, Vesprin		
fluoxymesterone	Halotensin, Ultandren		
fluphenazine	Pacinol, Siqualon, Vespazine	kanamycin	Kamycin, Kannasyn, Kantrex, Resisto-mycin
fluprednisolone	Alphadrol		
frusemide	Lasilix, Lasix	laevomepromazine	Nazinan
furazolidone	Furoxone, Giardil, Medaron, Neftin, Nifulidone	lignocaine	Xylocaine, Xyloproct, Xylotox
		lincomycin	Frademicina, Lincocin, Mycivin
furosemide	see frusemide	lynoestrenol	Orgametril
		lynoestrenol ethinyloestradiol	Minilyn
gallamine	Flaxedil		
gamma benzene hexachloride	Gammexane, ItCH, Lindane, Lorex-ane, Viton	lynoestrenol mestranol	Lyndiol
		mebanazine	Actomol
gentamicin	Cidomycin, Garamycin, Gentricin	mecamylamine	Inversine, Mekamine, Mevasine, Pleg-angrin
glutethimide	Doriden, Elrodorm		
griseofulvin	Fulcin, Grisovin	medroxyprogesterone	Provera
guanethidine	Guethine Ismelin, Isobarin,	medroxyprogesterone ethinyloestradiol	Provost
haloperidol	Haldol, Serenace	mefenamic acid	Coslan, Parke-med, Ponstan, Ponstel
halothane	Fluothane	megestrol ethinyloestradiol	Planovin, Volidan 21
hexadimethrine bromide	Polybrene		
hexamethonium bromide	Vegolysen, Vegolystin	melphalan	Alkeran
		menadiol sodium diphosphate	Synkavit
hexamethonium chloride	Bistrium chloride, Hexameton chloride	menadoxime	Kapilon soluble
		mepacrine	Atebrin, Atebrine, Palacrin
hexamethonium iodide	Hexathide	mephenesin	Atensin, Avosyl, Lissephen, Myanesin, Tolseram
hexamethonium tartrate	Vegolysen T	mephenytoin	Insulton, Mesantoin, Phenantoin
hydracetin	Pyrodin	meprobamate	Anastress, Andaxin, Artolon, Equanil, Harmonin, Mepavlon, Miltown
hydrallazine	Apresoline, Hipoftalin, Hydrallazine, Hypothalin		
		mercaptomerin	Thiomerin
hydrochlorothiazide	Dichlotride, Direma, Esidrex, Hydro-diuril, Hydrosaluric, Salupres	mercaptopurine	Leukerin, Mercaleukin, Puri-Nethol
		mercuramide theophylline	Neptal, Unephral
hydrocortisone	Corlan, Cortril, Ef-Cortelan, Hydro-Adreson, Hydrocortistab, Hydro Cor-tisyl, Hydrocortone, Solu-Cortef		
		merphalan	Sarcoclorin
		mersalyl	Mersalyl
hydroflumethiazide	Bristab, Di-Ademil, Hydrenox, Hy-dril, Hydrol, Naclex, Rontyl	mestanolone	Androstalone
		mestranol lynoestrenol	Lyndiol
hydroxychloroquine	Ercoquin, Plaquenil, Quensyl		
hydroxyurea	Hydrea	mestranol norethindrone norethisterone	Norinyl-1, Orthonovin 1/50, Ovulen 50, see norethisterone
ibufenac	Dytransin		
iminopromazine	Lispamol	mestranol norethynodrel	Enavid E
imipramine	Berkomine, Deprinol, Dyna-Zina, Tofranil		
		metaraminol	Aramine
indomethacin	Amuno, Inacid, Indocid, Indomed, Mezolin	methacholine	Amechol
		methandienone	Dianabol
iproniazid	Marsilid	methandriol	see methylandrostenediol
isocarboxazid	Marplan	methenolone	Primobolan, Primobolan-Depot

OFFICIAL NAME	PROPRIETARY NAME	OFFICIAL NAME	PROPRIETARY NAME
methicillin	*Celbenin, Staphcillin*	pempidine	*Perolysen, Tenormal*
methimazole	*Favistan, Mercazole, Thycapsol*	*d*-penicillamine	*Cuprimine, Distamine, Metalcaptase*
methopromazine	*Mopazine*	pentamethonium	*Antilusin, Penthonium*
methotrexate	*Amethopterin, Methotrexate*	pentazocine	*Fortral*
methotrimeprazine	*Levoprome, Neuractil, Nirvan, Nozinan, Veractil*	pentolinium	*Ansolysen, Pentilium*
		perphenazine	*Fentazin, Trilafon*
methoxsalen	*Meladinin, Meloxine, Methoxa-Dome Oxsoralen*	phenactropinium	*Trophenium*
methylandrostenediol	*Androdiol, Crestabolic, Diolandrone, Masidol, Neosteron, Stenediol*	phenazone	*Anodynine, Parodyne, Sedatine*
		phenbenicillin	*Penspek*
methyldopa	*Aldomet*	phenelzine	*Nardil*
methylphenidate	*Ritalin*	phenindione	*Bindan, Danilone, Dindeval, Dindevan, Hedulin, Indon*
methylprednisolone	*Medrol, Medrone, Metastab*		
methyltestosterone	*Androteston, Dumogran, Metandren, Pantestin oral, Perandren, Virormone-Oral*	pheniprazine	*Catron, Catroniazid, Cavodil*
		phenobarbitone	*Gardenal, Luminal*
		phenoxybenzamine	*Dibenyline, Dibenzyline*
methyprylone	*Dimerin, Noctan, Noludar*	phenoxymethyl-penicillin	*Apsin, VK Distaquaine V, Eskacillin V, Icipen V, Penavlon V, Penicals, Penicillin V, Stabilin VK, V-Cil-K*
methysergide	*Deseril, Desernil, Sansert*		
		phenoxypropazine	*Drazine*
nalidixic acid	*Negram, Nogram, Wintomylon*	phentolamine	*Rogitine*
nalorphine	*Lehidrome, Lethidrone, Nalline*	phenylbutazone	*Alindor, Antadol, Butadion, Buta-zolidin, Buzon, Reudrox*
nandrolone	*Deca-Durabolin, Durabolin, Nortesto-sterone*		
		phenylephrine	*Neophryn, Neosynephrine*
neoarsphenamine	*Novarsenobillon*	phenytoin	*Alepsin, Dilantin, Epanutin, Eptoin*
neomycin	*Mycifradin, Myciguent, Mycostatin Neomin, Nivemycin*	phthalylsulphathiazole	*Sulfacetil, Thalazole*
		phytomenadione	*Konakion, Mephyton*
neostigmine	*Eustigmin, Proserine, Prostigmin*	polymyxin	*Aerosporin*
nialamide	*Niamid*	potassium menaphtho-sulphate	*Vikastab*
nicotinyl alcohol	*Roniacol, Ronicol*	prednisolone	*Codelcortone, Delta-Cortef, Delta-cortril, Deltastab, Di-Adreson-F, Pre-cortisyl, Prednelan, Predsol, Ultra-corten-H*
nicoumalone	*Sinthrome, Sintrom*		
nitrazepam	*Mogadon*		
nitrofurantoin	*Berkfurin, Furadantin, Furan, N-Fur*		
nitrofurazone	*Chemofuran, Furacin, Nitrofural*		
noradrenaline	*Levophed*	prednisone	*DeCortisyl, Delta-Cortelan, Delta-cortone, Di-Adreson, Ultracortenol*
norepinephrine	*see noradrenaline*		
norethandrolone	*Nilevar*	primidone	*Lepsiral, Mylepsin, Mysoline*
norethisterone	*Norlutin A, Primodos, Primolut N*	probenecid	*Benemid*
norethisterone ethinyloestradiol	*Anovlar, Gynovlar 21, Minovlar, Norlestrin 21, Orlest 28*	procainamide	*Novocamid, Procamide, Procardyl, Pronestyl*
norethisterone mestranol	*Norinyl-1, Orthonovin 1/50, Ovulen 50*	prochlorperazine	*Comazine, Compazine, Stemetil, Te-mentil*
norethynodrel mestranol	*Enavid E*	promazine	*Prazine, Sparine, Starazine, Talofen*
		promethazine	*Phenergan*
novobiocin	*Albamycin, Biotexin, Cathomycin, Streptonivicin*	propicillin	*Ultrapen*
		propranolol	*Inderal*
nystatin	*Nystan*	propylthiouracil	*Propacil, Propycil, Prothyran*
nystatin demethylchlortetra-cycline	*Lederstatin*	prothionamide	*Trevintix*
		pyrazinamide	*Zinamide*
		pyridostigmine	*Mestinon*
orciprenaline	*Alupent*	quinethazone	*Aquamox*
oxymesterone	*Oranabol*	quinidine bisulphate	*Kinidin*
oxymetholone	*Adroyd, Anapolon*	quinidine poly-galacturonate	*Cardioquin*
oxyphenbutazone	*Crovaril, Flogoril, Frabel, Tandearil, Tanderil*		
		quinidine sulphate	*Auriquin*
oxytetracycline	*Imperacin, Terramycin*		
		reserpine	*Alserin, Eskaserp, Sandril, Serpasil*
pamaquin	*Aminoquin, Plasmochin, Plasmoquine*	rifampicin	*Rifadin, Rimactane*
paramethadione	*Paradione*		
paramethasone	*Haldrate, Metilar*	salbutamol	*Ventolin*
pargyline	*Eutonyl*	sodium aurothio-malate	*Myocristin*
paromomycin	*Humatin, Pargonyl*		
pecazine	*Nothiazide, Pacatal, Paxital*	solapsone	*Sulphetrone*

OFFICIAL NAME	PROPRIETARY NAME	OFFICIAL NAME	PROPRIETARY NAME
spironolactone	Aldactone-A	tetracycline	Achromycin, Ambramycin, Steclin, Tetracyn, Thiozone
stanolone	Anabolex, Anaprotin		
stanozolol	Stanozol, Stromba, Tevabolin, Winstrol	tetracycline nystatin amphotericin B	} Mysteclin
stibophen	Fouadin, Fuadin, Neoantimosan, Pyrostib, Sodium antimosan	theophylline mercuramide	} Neptal, Unephral
streptoduocin	Dimycin, Mixtamycin	thiacetazone	Aktiran, Contebam, Seroden, Thioparamizone
streptomycin	Strepolin, Streptolin, Streptaquaine, Streptomycin		
succinylsulphathiazole	Kaoxidin, Sulfasuxidine, Thiacyl	thiambutosine	Ciba 1906
sulphadiazine	Debenal, Diazyl, Eskadiazine, Pyrimal	thiomersal	Thiomerosal, Thiomersalate
		thiopropazate	Dartal, Dartalan
sulphadimethoxine	Madribon	thioridazine	Malloral, Melleretten, Melleril
sulphadimidine	Paramez, S-Mez, Sulmet, Sulphix, Vertolan	thiotepa	Tespamin, Thiotepa, Tifosyl
		thiouracil	Deracil
sulphafurazole	Gantrisin	232-thorium dioxide	Collothor, Diagnothorine, Thoriophanin, Thorotrast, Tordiol, Toriofanina
sulphaguanidine	Resulfon, Ruocid		
sulphamerazine	Debenal M, Mesulfa, Pyrimal M, Veta-Merazine		
		tolbutamide	Artosin, Diabetamid, Diabuton, Orinase, Rastinon
sulphamethizole	Urolucosil		
sulphamethoxazole	Gantanol	tranylcypromine	Parnate
sulphamethoxazole trimethoprim	} Bactrim, Septrin	triacetyloleandomycin	Evramycin
		triamcinolone	Adcortyl, Adcortyl A, Aristocort Ledercort
sulphamethoxydiazine	Bayrena, Durenate, Kiron, Sulla, Ultrax		
sulphamethoxypyridazine	Davosin, Kynex, Lederkyn, Midicel, Opinsul	triamterene	Dytac
		trichlormethiazide	Esmarin, Eurinol, Fluitran, Flutra, Metahydrin, Salurin, Triclordiuride, Trichlormethiazide
sulphaphenazole	Orisulf		
sulphaproxyline	Dosulfin		
sulphapyridine	Dagenan, Eubasin, M & B 693, Pyriamid, Sulfidine	trifluoperazine	Stelazine
		trimetaphan	Arfonad
sulphasalazine	Salazopyrin	trimethoprim sulphamethoxazole	} Bactrim, Septrin
sulphasomidine	Elkosin		
sulphasomizole	Bidizole	trioxsalen	Trisoralen
sulphathiazole	Cibazol, Eleudron, Sulfamul, Sulzol, Thiazamide	triparanol	MER-29
		tripelennamine	Azaron, Dehistin, PBZ, Pyribenzamine, Tonaril, Vetibenzamina
sulphinpyrazone	Anturan, Enturen		
sulphomyxin	Thiosporin	troxidone	Epidione, Petidon, Ptimal, Tridione, Trimedal, Trimethadione
suxamethonium bromide	Brevidil M		
suxamethonium chloride	Anectine, Scoline	vinblastine	Velban, Velbe
		vincristine	Oncovin
suxethonium	Brevidil E	viomycin	Viocin, Vionactane
testosterone propionate	Neo-Hombreol, Pantestin, Virormone	warfarin	Marevan, Prothromadin, Tintorane
		zoxazolamine	Flexin

INDEX

Drug-induced disease, (contd.)
  genetic factors, (contd.)
    abnormalities of pseudocholineste-
      rase, 3
    antimalarials, 3
    glucose-6-phosphate dehydrogenase
      deficiency, 3
    isoniazid inactivation, 3
    suxamethonium, 3
  incidence, 1, 2
Drug interaction 9–18
  acceleration of metabolism, 9, 10
  antagonism, 9
    competitive, 9
    physiological, 9
  displacement from plasma or tissue
    protein, 9, 11, 12
  electrolyte imbalance, 9
  examples of known drug interactions,
    13–18
  metabolizing enzymes, 9, 10
  modification of absorption, 9
  modification of excretion, 9
  potentiation, 9, 10
  retardation of metabolism, 9, 10, 11
  summation, 9
  synergism, 9
Drug-metabolizing enzymes, 9, 10
  drugs influencing,
    anticoagulants, 10
    barbiturates, 10
    chloramphenicol, 10
    chlorcyclizine, 10
    dicoumarol, 10
    ethionine, 9
    glutethimide, 10
    hydrocortisone, 10
    imipramine, 9
    insecticides, 10
    iproniazid, 10
    morphine, 10
    nialamide, 10
    nikethamide, 9
    oestradiol, 10
    oxyphenbutazone, 10
    p-aminosalicylic acid, 10
    pentazocine, 10
    pentobarbitone, 9, 10
    pethidine, 10
    pheniprazine, 10
    phenylbutazone, 9, 10
    progesterone, 10
    SKF-525A, 10
    testosterone, 10
    triparanol, 10
    zoxazolamine, 9
Drug reactions, epidemiology, 1–7, 12, 13
  factors influencing,
    abnormal renal function, 12, 13
    age, 13
    clinical and personal variables, 12
    disease, 13
      gastro-intestinal, 13
      liver, 13
      renal, 13
    illness and infection, 12
    number of drugs administered, 13
    previous drug reactions, 13
Dyflos,
  cataract formation, 155
  treatment of esotropia, 155
Dyskinesia,
  drug-induced, 143, 144
Dystonia musculorum, 144

ECG,
  drugs inducing change,
    amitriptyline, 51
    digitalis, 48, 49
    emetine, 50, 51
    frusemide, 51, 52
    guanethidine, 51
    imipramine, 51
    quinidine, 48, 49, 50
    quinine, 49, 50
    thioridazine, 51
Ecothiopate,
  pseudocholinesterases, 140
Eczema, 24
  neomycin-induced, 26
Edrophonium, 12
  colistin neuromuscular block, 137,
    138
  suxamethonium neuromuscular block,
    3, 138, 139, 140
  viomycin neuromuscular block, 137
    138
Electro-oculogram,
  chloroquine retinopathy, 155
Emetine,
  amoebiasis, 50, 142
  cardiotoxicity, 50, 51, 142
  2-dehydroemetine, 51, 142
  myopathy, 142
  toxicity, 50, 51, 142
Encephalomyocarditis virus,
  ACTH, 166
  corticosteroids, 166
Encephalopathy,
  isoniazid, 145
Endocardial fibrosis,
  methysergide, 53, 54
Endocarditis, 36
Enema rash, 21
Entamoeba histolytica,
  corticosteroids, 166
Ephedrine,
  interaction with MAOI's, 17
  tolerance in asthma, 4
Epianhydrotetracycline, 126
Epidermophyton floccosum,
  topical corticosteroids, 167
Epinephrine, see Adrenaline
Ergot alkaloids,
  interaction with sympathomimetic
    amines, 18
Ergotamine, 130
Erythema multiforme, 21, 27
  bromides, 22
  chloral hydrate, 22
Erythema nodosum,
  drugs inducing,
    corticosteroids (withdrawal), 22
    oral contraceptives, 22
    penicillin, 22
    salicylates, 22
    sulphonamides, 22
    sulphonylureas (oral hypoglycae-
      mics), 22
    thiouracil, 22
Erythroid hypoplasia, 38
Erythromycin, 85, 137
  asthma, 65
  neophrotoxicity, 118
Erythromycin propionyl ester,
  intrahepatic cholestasis, 85
  jaundice, 85
Erythropoietic protoporphyria, 93
Esotropia, 155

Ethacrynic acid,
  diabetogenic action, 96, 98
  diuresis, 161, 162
  gastro-intestinal haemorrhage, 75
  hypercalcinuria, 106
  hyperglycaemia, 96, 98
  ototoxicity, 159, 161, 162
Ethacrynic acid plus aminoglycoside
    antibiotics, 162
  impaired renal function, 3, 161, 162
Ethambutol, 43, 80
Ethinyloestradiol, 59, 61
Ethinyloestradio plus medroxyproge-
    sterone,
  plasma triglyceride levels, 100–1
Ethionamide,
  acne, 22
  asthma, 65
  gynaecomastia, 115
  hair loss, 23
  intrahepatic cholestasis, 85
  jaundice, 85
  mammotropic action, 114, 115
Ethisterone, 113
Ethopropazine,
  interaction with MAOI's, 11
Ethylestrenol, see Ethyloestrenol
Ethyloestrenol, 113
Exfoliative dermatitis,
  drugs inducing,
    anticonvulsants, 22
    arsenicals, 22
    barbiturates, 22
    chloroquine, 22
    gold salts, 22
    griseofulvin, 22
    immunosuppressive agents, 22
    mercurial diuretics (organomer-
      curials), 22
    penicillins, 22
    phenothiazines, 22
    salicylates, 22
    sulphonamides, 22
    thiouracil, 22
Exophthalmos,
  corticosteroids, 154
  corticotrophin, 154
  Cushing's disease, 154
Extraocular muscle palsy,
  drugs inducing,
    chloroquine, 154
    hydroxychloroquine, 154
    phenothiazines, 151
Extrapyramidal reactions,
  acathisia, 143, 144
  akinesia, 143, 144
  drugs inducing,
    phenothiazines, 143, 144
      acetopromazine, 143
      chlorpromazine, 143
      fluphenazine, 143
      methotrimeprazine, 143
      pecazine, 143
      perphenazine, 143
      prochlorperazine, 143
      promazine, 143
      thiopropazate, 143
      thioridazine, 143
      trifluoperazine, 143
    rauwolfia alkaloids, 144
      deserpidine, 144
      reserpine, 144
  dyskinesia, 143, 144
  oculogyric crisis, 144